D0731229

Prevention
Diabetes Diet Cookbook

Prevention.
Diabetes Diet Cookbook
DISCOVER THE NEW FIBER-FULL EATING PLAN FOR WEIGHT LOSS

By the Editors of America's Leading Healthy Lifestyle Magazine
with Ann Fittante, MS, RD

RODALE

Direct edition was published as *Prevention's Diabetes Diet Cookbook* in 2007. Trade edition published in 2008.
© 2008 by Rodale Inc.

Rodale books may be purchased for business or promotional use or for special sales.
For information, please write to:
Special Markets Department, Rodale Inc., 733 Third Avenue, New York, NY 10017

Prevention is a registered trademark of Rodale Inc.
Some recipes have previously appeared in *Prevention* magazine.
Printed in the United States of America
Rodale Inc. makes every effort to use acid-free ∞, recycled paper ♲.

Interior photo credits appear on page 360.
Front cover photos © Pornchai Mittongtare (top left, bottom right);
© Alexandra Rowley (bottom left); © Jennifer Levy (top right)
Back cover photos © Elizabeth Watt (left);
© Mitch Mandel/Rodale Images (center); © Brian Hagiwara (right)
Cover design by Christina Gaugler
Interior design by Carol Angstadt

Library of Congress Cataloging-in-Publication Data

[Prevention's diabetes diet cookbook.] Diabetes diet cookbook : discover the new fiber-full eating plan for weight loss / from the editors of America's leading healthy lifestyle magazine ; with Ann Fittante.
　　　p.　　cm.
Includes index.
"Direct edition was published as Prevention's Diabetes Diet Cookbook in 2007."
ISBN-13 978–1–59486–671–5 paperback
ISBN-10 1–59486–671–6 paperback
1. Diabetes—Diet therapy—Recipes.　2. Reducing diets—Recipes.　3. High-fiber diet—Recipes.
4. Weight loss. I. Fittante, Ann. II. Prevention (Emmaus, Pa.)
RC662.P72　2008
641.5'6314—dc22　　　　　　　　　　　　　　　　　　　　　　　　　　　　　　2008030169

Distributed to the trade by Macmillan

2　4　6　8　10　9　7　5　3　1　paperback

We inspire and enable people to improve their lives and the world around them

For more of our products visit **rodalestore.com** or call 800-848-4735

CONTENTS

INTRODUCTION

If you or someone you cook for has recently been diagnosed with diabetes, you may feel very confused. You're not the only one. According to recent statistics, the number of Americans diagnosed with diabetes has risen to 17.9 million in 2008, reaching epidemic status in the minds of many health professionals. Worse, at least 57 million people over the age of 20 have prediabetes, a condition that puts them at risk for developing diabetes later in life. While it's urgent that we educate ourselves on how to prevent and hopefully reverse the damaging effects of this disease, the good news is that what you eat can have a tremendous impact on the way diabetes affects your life.

Consider this book your personal—extremely doable—road map to achieving greater vitality and overall health. Unlike many diets, this cookbook emphasizes making a gradual transition to foods you can enjoy forever. If you have type 2 diabetes, you'll learn to manage your blood glucose levels by losing excess weight, eating delicious and satisfying whole foods, becoming more physically active, and working with your doctor to find the treatment plan that's best for you. If you're at risk for or have prediabetes, you'll find a wealth of small but powerful steps you can take *right now* to help prevent the disease.

Our *Diabetes Diet Cookbook* provides you with the information, strategies, and above all the recipes, cooking, and lifestyle tips you need to protect yourself and your loved ones against this growing threat. You'll learn

- Smart strategies to *adapt* not *abandon* your favorite foods

- Positive lifestyle adjustments that will keep your energy levels soaring

- How to make intelligent choices so that no foods are off-limits

- Dozens of ways to decrease stress, a major factor in the acceleration of diabetes

- How to eradicate hunger from your vocabulary

- Why pricey "diabetic" foods are not beneficial and may even be harmful

Prevention is with you every step of the way to help you control your diabetes and enjoy a long, healthy, active life.

Z. Vaccariello

Liz Vaccariello

Editor-in-Chief, *Prevention*

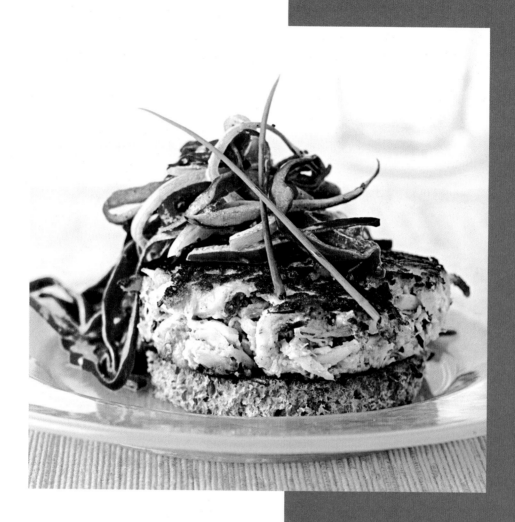

CHAPTER 1

THE FIBER-FULL DIET PLAN

Congratulations! The fact that you're reading this book means that you care deeply about your health and are taking steps to improve it. Yes, improve it—even if you've been diagnosed with type 2 diabetes or prediabetes.

Like most people, you probably weren't planning a life with diabetes or prediabetes. No, you most likely had other things on your mind—things like caring for a family and home, paying the bills, volunteering in your community, coaching a youth sports team perhaps. However you fill your days, diabetes was probably not on the agenda.

In fact, odds are you were consumed with taking care of everyone and everything except yourself. That is the first thing that is going to change in your life. Caring for yourself will be the first item on your "to do" list from this day forward. When you are well, everything else will fall into place.

DIABETES DEFINED

If left unchecked, diabetes wreaks harm that can progress stealthily, becoming noticeable only once the damage reaches advanced stages. So if you have been newly diagnosed with diabetes, have prediabetes, or are planning and cooking meals for someone with either of these challenges, understanding the disease is critical.

Broadly defined, diabetes is a metabolic disorder that disrupts the way our bodies use the energy from food. During digestion, most of what we eat, particularly carbohydrate, is broken down into glucose, the form of sugar in the blood that provides energy. To reach all of the cells in our bodies, glucose hitches a ride in the bloodstream. But to actually get into the cells to feed them, glucose requires a hormone called insulin that is produced by the pancreas, a small gland situated just behind the stomach.

When a healthy person eats, the pancreas produces just the right amount of insulin to move glucose from the blood into the cells. In people with diabetic conditions, however, either the pancreas produces little or no insulin or the cells don't respond appropriately to the insulin that is produced. As a result, glucose backs up in the blood, overflows into the urine, and passes out of the body without even nourishing it. It's like trying to fuel your car with the gas cap locked.

Under the broad category of diabetes, however, there are some specific forms the disease can take.

- **Type 1 diabetes.** Also referred to as juvenile diabetes, type 1 diabetes is an autoimmune disease that causes the body to attack and destroy the cells in the pancreas that produce insulin. A person with type 1 diabetes must take insulin to survive.

- **Gestational diabetes.** As the name implies, this type of diabetes develops in women during pregnancy but often disappears after the birth of the baby. However, women who've experienced gestational diabetes carry a 20 to 50 percent chance of developing type 2 within a decade.

- **Type 2 diabetes.** By far the most widespread form of the disease, about 90 to 95 percent of people with diabetes have type 2. Risk factors include older age, obesity, family history, previous gestational diabetes, physical inactivity, and certain ethnicities. About 80 percent of people with type 2 are overweight. Unlike type 1, type 2 develops gradually. At first, the body has trouble using its insulin effectively, a condition called insulin resistance. After several years, insulin production decreases, glucose builds up in the blood, and the body can't make efficient use of its main source of fuel.

- **Prediabetes.** Also referred to as metabolic syndrome, prediabetes is a condition in which blood glucose levels are higher than normal but not high enough to classify as diabetes. This condition is identified by impaired fasting glucose (IFG)/impaired glucose tolerance (IGT) depending on the test used to diagnose it. People with prediabetes are at higher risk to develop type 2 diabetes, heart disease, and stroke.

Despite the sobering reality of diabetes, there is some very hopeful news for most people. If you have prediabetes, you have the power to prevent or delay the onset of type 2 diabetes. If you have type 2 diabetes, you have the power to manage, or even lower, your blood glucose levels.

Studies have clearly shown that even modest weight loss can help you lower your risk of developing diabetes. One major study of more than 3,000 people with prediabetes found that diet and exercise resulting in a 5 to 7 percent weight loss—that's only 7 to 10 pounds for a woman who weighs 150 pounds—lowered the incidence of type 2 diabetes by nearly 60 percent.

Two easy tools that can help determine your weight loss goals are the Body Mass Index (BMI) Table on page 358 and taking a waistline measurement. The BMI is a measure of your weight relative to your height. You can determine your waist circumference by placing a measuring tape snugly around your waist. It is a good indicator of your abdominal fat, which is another predictor of your risk for developing heart disease and other diseases. This risk increases with a waist measurement of more than 35 inches in women and 40 inches in men.

But before revealing our plan to help you achieve your weight loss goals, let's look into what many others (with interests other than your well-being) would have you believe you should be eating.

The naked truth about the "diabetic diet"

In the Hans Christian Andersen fairy tale "The Emperor's New Clothes," it's a child whose purity of perception exposes the falsity of grown-ups' group thinking, what we call conventional wisdom.

In the tale, con men posing as tailors convince the vain emperor that the "suit" they fabricated for him is exquisitely rendered in the finest silks and brocades. But, when the monarch flaunts his attire in procession, the child shouts the obvious, "But he has nothing on!" Everyone in the crowd is shocked into seeing the true situation. The moral? Just because everyone thinks something is true doesn't make it true.

In our society, the idea of a "diabetic diet" that requires a severly limited range of specialized foods is, much like the emperor's suit—it just doesn't exist.

"A big part of our mission is to teach patients with diabetes, as well as the general public, about healthy eating," explains Ann Fittante, MS, RD, a registered dietitian and certified diabetes educator at the Joslin Diabetes Center education affiliate at Swedish Medical Center in Seattle. "Healthy eating is eating balanced meals that are high in fiber, contain lean protein and healthy fats, and contain minimally processed ingredients. In my opinion, it is exactly the way all of us should be eating whether we have diabetes or not."

Another common misunderstanding is that people with diabetes must avoid sugar. That's just false. Small amounts of sugar worked into a balanced meal plan are acceptable. The fact is, nobody should consume tremendous amounts of sugar. It's a nutritionally empty food. If eaten in excess and teamed with saturated fat and refined white flour as it often is, it can add up to a lot of extra calories that spike glucose levels.

So, this train of logic eventually leads to the question, what *should* you be eating? The answer is so simple that a child in a fable could figure it out: Eat real foods.

A NEW APPROACH TO DIABETES AND DIET

The Joslin Diabetes Center, with divisions dedicated to both research and treatment, has a reputation for being at the forefront of the latest scientific developments in diabetes care. In line with this, Joslin has recently revised its dietary guidelines to increase the recommended dietary fiber intake for overweight and obese adults with type 2 diabetes, prediabetes, or high risk for developing type 2 diabetes. Joslin now recommends a goal of up to 50 grams of fiber daily (in proportion with the recommended daily calorie intake), more than tripling the amount that the average American consumes.

The research behind this recommendation is compelling. For example, one study conducted at the University of Texas Southwestern Medical Center at Dallas Southwestern Medical School concluded that by significantly increasing their intake of dietary fiber derived solely from natural foods (not fiber supplements), obese type 2 diabetes patients reduced their blood glucose levels as much as would be expected with some diabetes medications.

Along the same lines, a research review headed by James W. Anderson, MD, of the department of internal medicine at the University of Kentucky in Lexington analyzed data published over the last 25 years by nine international diabetes associations. In addition, because of the link between chronic heart disease and diabetes, the recommendations of the American Heart Association and the National Cholesterol Education Panel were also considered. Based on the available data, Dr. Anderson's team concluded that people with diabetes can enjoy long-term benefits to their health with a diet that assumes 55 percent of calories from carbohydrates; a desirable range of 55 to 65 percent of calories from carbohydrates was identified as being even more practical.

Daily doses of delicious

To translate these guidelines into delicious daily meals (see Chapter 5 for Menu Plans), we consulted dietitian Ann Fittante. With her expertise, we've created the Fiber-FULL Plan for lasting weight loss and lowered blood glucose levels. As the name indicates, fiber provides the foundation upon which the F-U-L-L program pillars stand.

- Fill Up on Whole Foods
- Unleash Nutrients
- Loosen Up/Get Moving
- Let Yourself Go/Stress Less

Throughout this book, we'll explain why fiber is so important to our health, as well as dozens of easy ways to enjoy more of it. One immediate benefit you'll likely notice is that eating fiber-rich foods tends to leave you feeling full longer and free of the cravings that refined carbohydrates can trigger. That's because your body has to work harder and longer to convert high-fiber carbs into blood glucose, resulting in a longer, steadier fuel source.

Another benefit to the Fiber-FULL diet is that when your meals revolve around fiber-rich foods, you automatically eat more nutritiously. Many important nutrients, including trace elements that many Americans are sorely lacking, are embedded in fiber-rich foods. Some of these nutrients are especially important for people with diabetes, since the disease increases one's risk for so many other conditions. For example, getting enough potassium, magnesium, and calcium every day has been shown to decrease blood pressure, a major risk factor for cardiovascular disease that often accompanies diabetes. Look for the Unleash Nutrients tips throughout the book to learn more about what you'll gain by eating foods that are best for your body.

Once you start following the meal plans in this book, you're also likely to notice a newfound spring in your step. Increased energy and stamina are natural by-products of a healthier diet. The most important thing to remember when such feelings strike is to take advantage of them. Keep moving! Exercise is proven to reduce blood glucose levels, and when combined with a carb-controlled, high-fiber diet, losing pounds and keeping them off is guaranteed. Look for the Loosen Up/Get Moving tips throughout this book to inspire you to get going!

With a healthful diet and exercise as part of your everyday lifestyle, you also find a natural vent for the potentially damaging stress that contributes to elevated blood glucose. This is especially important since people with diabetes are four times more likely to develop depression even prior to their diabetes diagnosis. If you want to seek out other ways to calm your mind and spirit, look for the Let Yourself Go/Stress Less tips for precious insights into the mind-body connection for maximum health.

How the Fiber-FULL Diet Plan works

The Fiber-FULL meal plan is structured in two easy-to-follow phases. Meals in the initial 2 weeks of the plan are slightly lower in (fiber) carbohydrate so your body can adjust to digesting these nutrient-rich whole foods.

Phase 1

- Meal plans are between 1,400 and 1,600 calories, approximately 40 percent carbohydrate (not less than 130 grams of carbohydrate total/day), 20 to 30 percent lean protein, and 30 to 35 percent predominantly healthy fats. Each plan includes three meals (breakfast, lunch, dinner) and three snacks.
- Goal for fiber: a minimum of 20 grams/day

Phase 2

- Meal plans are between 1,400 and 1,600 calories, approximately 45 to 60 percent carbohydrate, 15 to 25 percent protein, and 25 to 35 percent predominantly healthy fats, and include three meals (breakfast, lunch, dinner) and three snacks.
- Goal for fiber: a minimum of 30 grams/day

In addition to being fiber-rich, the meals in the menus in this book are designed to help you better control your sodium intake, which can help lower blood pressure. People with diabetes can lower their risk of heart disease and stroke by up to 50 percent by keeping their blood pressure under control; the risk of microvascular complications (eye, kidney, and nerve diseases) lowers as well, by approximately 33 percent. In general, for every 10 mm Hg reduction in systolic blood pressure, the risk for any complication related to diabetes is reduced by 12 percent.

For meal plans and sample menus, turn to Chapter 5.

Why whole foods?

In 2003, Belinda Hovde-Klingman of Seattle was diagnosed with type 2 diabetes. Since then, she has dropped 45 pounds, reduced her blood glucose levels, and gained energy and alertness. That Belinda feels better now than she ever has in her adult life may sound paradoxical (read Belinda's "I'm Beating Diabetes" story on page 8), but it's not. In fact, many people who've heeded the wake-up call of a type 2 diagnosis have dramatically changed their way of eating and living, and subsequently their overall health, for the better.

Throughout the upcoming chapters, we'll share stories about people like Belinda who have declared their independence from processed refined food products that may have contributed to the development of the disease. For example, public enemy number one on Belinda's hit list is high-fructose corn syrup, a cheap refined sweetener that's dumped into everything from canned soup to "healthy" low-calorie dinners. "As soon as I stopped eating those foods, I felt more alert," says Belinda, who now bases her meals and snacks on vegetables, beans, seafood, lean meats, whole grains, fruits, and other whole foods.

What are whole foods anyway?

Whole foods are foods in their natural state, or nearly so, as they were cultivated, caught, picked, or otherwise harvested. Strawberries plucked from the bush are an example of a whole food. In addition to carbohydrate, fiber, and vitamin C, the berries contain trace minerals such as magnesium, potassium, and phosphorus that are hard to come by in refined foods. In contrast, a shelf-stable strawberry fruit roll-up, flagged on the box as a "fruit-flavored snack," has very little to do with strawberries, real or otherwise. The ingredients are: pears from concentrate, corn syrup, dried corn syrup, sugar, partially hydrogenated cottonseed oil, citric acid, sodium citrate, pectin, distilled monoglycerides, malic acid, vitamin C (ascorbic acid), acetylated mono and diglycerides, natural flavor, and color (Red 40, Yellow 5 & 6, Blue 1, Red 3).

Another compelling health reason to select whole foods is to avoid dangerously high amounts of sodium that can elevate blood pressure. Manufacturers add sodium to virtually all processed foods as a preservative and flavoring. The plan recipes start with naturally flavorful ingredients seasoned to perfection with sodium-free seasonings and small amounts of table salt. (See Chapter 3 for more information on cooking.)

Contrary to what food processors and product advertising would like us to believe, whole foods are incredibly simple to shop for and eat. You don't have to spend time poring over nutritional labels and ingredients lists worrying that you're buying the "right" foods for your health. You certainly don't need a label to figure out that a juicy orange, a succulent salmon fillet, or a crisp stalk of broccoli is good for your body and health. You don't need to "do" anything to make a vine-ripened garden tomato taste fabulous.

Even with food products that require minimal processing and packaging for mass distribution, opting for the choice that's closest to the food's original state makes the selection process quicker and easier. Look for five or fewer ingredients on the product

(continued on page 10)

NOW YOU KNOW

What's the Real Cost?

If you look at the valuable role whole foods play in preventing and managing diabetes, they are dirt cheap. An apple costs about 40 cents. A ¼ cup of dried beans costs 10 cents. A slice of stone-ground whole wheat bread costs 15 cents. Compare that paltry expenditure with total health care and related costs for the treatment of diabetes. Drugs, medical treatment, and disability costs run about $132 billion each year in the United States. That's a lot of apples, beans, and whole grain bread.

I'M BEATING DIABETES

BELINDA HOVDE-KLINGMAN

When she delivered a healthy 6 pound, 1 ounce baby girl in November 2002, Belinda Hovde-Klingman's life was about to change dramatically—even more so than the average new mother's.

"I was diagnosed with gestational diabetes when I was 4 months pregnant," recalls the 40-year-old Seattle resident. "I dramatically changed my diet and lost 10 pounds during the pregnancy because I was so concerned about the situation. Then, immediately after Heidi Rose was born, I was diagnosed with type 2 diabetes."

Belinda, who had struggled with carb cravings since childhood, had kept her weight to 130 pounds during college, but in the 12 years after graduation, she reached an all-time high of 220 pounds on her 5-foot-4½-inch frame.

The demands of her job as a water quality inspector for the Washington state Department of Ecology, sometimes working up to 70 hours a week, combined with the stress of trying to conceive a child (she unknowingly suffered from polycystic ovary syndrome, or PCOS), left her little time or energy for self-care.

"I was in a real rut," Belinda says. "But after Heidi was born healthy, everything realigned. All my focus shifted so that I wanted to make sure I was going to be healthy enough to take care of her. I have the constant reinforcement to feed her healthy food so she doesn't develop diabetes."

After dietary counseling at the Joslin Diabetes Center in Seattle, Belinda dramatically increased both the amount and the variety of fruits and vegetables she eats, particularly broccoli, cauliflower, and spinach and other dark green leafy vegetables. She also incorporates more lean protein, beans, and whole grains into her diet.

"I love cooking. I've gotten into a healthy cooking habit. I'm looking for healthier recipes all the time," says Belinda. "Also, I'm much more aware of portion sizes now, especially with carbs, and of eating meals more slowly."

She credits much of her newfound energy to eating whole foods. "I've tried to eliminate 95 percent of high-fructose corn syrup and sugar substitutes like sucralose from my diet. They made me feel bad. As soon as I stopped eating those foods, I felt more alert and balanced throughout the day."

A typical breakfast is a piece of fresh fruit, two eggs, 1 percent organic milk, and whole grain toast. For midmorning and midafternoon snacks, she carries sustaining foods with her such as raw nuts, sunflower seeds, whole grain granola bars, or a packaged cheese stick.

Lunch could be a peanut butter and jelly sandwich on whole grain bread, with raw fruit, broccoli, or cauliflower. "When I eat whole grain breads, they don't create the bread cravings I used to have," Belinda says.

Dinner might be tilapia with salsa or a stir-fry of vegetables with beef or poultry. She's even dabbled with ostrich and beefalo.

Dining isn't all that's different these days. Belinda has also started practicing relaxation techniques and exercising regularly, such as walking and swimming, with her husband and daughter. "I've made a whole lifestyle change."

Today, at 175 pounds, Belinda notes that her diabetes is under control. Because she gained weight in increments over a number of years, she's realistic about losing it gradually. She's set on reaching her target weight of 140 pounds by increasing her exercise and strength training to build more fat-burning muscle.

"Once you add up a bunch of small changes, you can see how much you can accomplish," Belinda says. "I feel better and I'm losing weight—slowly, but losing. Both of those are two big positive changes I'm making in my life. That's what keeps me going."

label, making sure the first ingredient is what you're seeking: "100 percent stone-ground whole wheat flour" in a loaf of whole wheat bread, "pumpkin" in a can of cooked pumpkin, "peanuts" in all-natural peanut butter, "steel-cut oats" in hot cereal. For a more detailed discussion of ingredients and how to use them, turn to page 38. Not only are commercially marketed "diabetic foods" unnecessary and frequently costly, they sometimes contain very unhealthy ingredients.

"Whole foods are always the healthiest choice since they are minimally processed and contain important nutrients. People tend to be more satisfied and have fewer cravings when eating whole foods over processed ones," says Fittante. "For instance, a so-called health bar is an example of an edible product fabricated in the laboratory—fortified with fiber, vitamins, and minerals—that still may contain unhealthy saturated fat such as palm oil. For the same number of calories, between 150 and 200, we're all better off eating a medium piece of fruit and a small handful of nuts that contain predominantly healthy monounsaturated fat."

Fiber is the foundation

The Fiber-FULL Diet Plan is so simple to follow because in choosing foods that naturally contain dietary fiber—plant foods such as whole grains, dry beans, vegetables, fruits, and nuts—most of our other nutrients will fall into place. That's because these

---

FILL UP ON WHOLE FOODS

What Does Fiber Do?

Fiber is part of all plant foods we eat. It's a carbohydrate that passes through our bodies undigested. But the benefits of fiber to our health are many and continually unfolding. Dietary fiber generally is characterized as "soluble" (dissolves in water; examples are beans, oats, strawberries, apples) and "insoluble" (doesn't dissolve in water; examples are whole wheat bread, brown rice, and carrots). Some fiber foods contain higher amounts of each type, but in fact, most plant foods contain a combination of both. Fiber has been credited with a myriad of health boosters, from ushering "bad" LDL cholesterol out of the body to improving long-term glucose control in individuals with type 2 diabetes. The American Dietetic Association recommends a diet high in fiber-rich plant foods for the treatment of obesity, cardiovascular disease, and type 2 diabetes. This type of diet is lower in calories, is often lower in fat (particularly saturated fat), is larger in volume, and is richer in micronutrients, all of which have beneficial health effects.

foods haven't been stripped of vital nutrients by the refining process.

Getting the most for your money is a time-honored American tradition. You wouldn't consider buying a new dining table if the legs were visibly splintered and glued back together. You'd laugh if someone tried to sell you a suit with crudely mended rips in the fabric. Yet every day, millions of us hand over our hard-earned money for products with ingredients that have first been stripped of fiber and essential nutrients and then "fortified" to make them seem more nutritious than they are. Added to these processed products are plenty of high-fructose corn syrup and salt—cheap additives that act as preservatives, bulking agents, and fat substitutes, among other functions. We're not actively choosing these additives, but we're passively getting plenty of them if most of what we eat is comprised of processed products. It's as if that damaged dining table also harbors termites at no extra charge!

So if you're interested in reaping the nutritional values whole foods have to offer, read on. Chapter 2 shows you how to tailor the Fiber-FULL Diet Plan to meet your specific needs.

CHAPTER 2

THE FOODS AND LIFE YOU LOVE— ONLY BETTER!

For most people, living with diabetes means improving their relationship with food. And *that* is a complicated task. No other disease has such an intimate connection to food as does diabetes. At the same time, food is much more than fuel for your body. It's tied up with memories of people and places. Good foods and good times naturally go hand in hand.

Pumpkin pie buried under a blizzard of whipped cream takes you back to Grandma's at Thanksgiving. A cheeseburger sizzling from the grill conjures up Dad's grin as he slides it onto your plate. Chocolate chip cookies make you feel as good as Mom did after you got that C in geometry.

Fast-forward to present life in a world hooked on speed. Sometimes, it seems impossible to put on the brakes, even when it comes to food. With the boss who wants that report now, the child who's late for the soccer game, the laundry that's piling up, convenience foods may seem like the smartest, quickest option. Unfortunately, some of the food products that are the fastest to eat are also the fastest to harm us.

In this chapter, we'll explore the range of challenges inherent in making lasting dietary change, and we'll supply realistic strategies to *adapt* instead of *abandon* the

(continued on page 16)

I'M BEATING DIABETES

KATHY ROOT

Fifty-one-year-old Kathy Root's hazel eyes shine with vitality. Perhaps that's because, as she puts it, she now has the "vision" for the vibrant life she was always meant to lead.

In March 2000, Kathy's eyes were clouded by self-doubt and sickness. That was the year the St. Peters, Missouri, resident was diagnosed with type 2 diabetes. She wasn't surprised. At 5 feet 7¾ inches, Kathy weighed 288 pounds. "Both my parents and three of my grandparents had diabetes. My brother has been insulin dependent since his early thirties. My blood sugar had been rising for a couple of years before the diagnosis," Kathy recalls.

Years of on-again, off-again dieting only left her heavier and more discouraged after each failed attempt to lose weight. When her children, David, Michael, Joseph, and Clarissa, were little, Kathy loved cooking for them, but, as she now understands, it was the wrong kinds of food.

"We ate lots of pasta, cereal, tons of sugary stuff, plenty of fried food, chips, cookies—it was high calorie and empty carbs. Then we'd drink skim milk and diet pop," Kathy says. "I think I ate constantly. Food was my drug of choice for loneliness, boredom, hurt, stress, anger, you name it. I used food as my primary coping mechanism."

After her diabetes diagnosis, her physician prescribed two different oral diabetes medications, plus blood pressure and arthritis medications. Still her blood glucose levels hovered around 150.

Kathy came to understand that she needed to break her emotional connection to food yet find a healthful way to nourish her true hunger. "No one can live on salad, celery sticks, and cottage cheese for long. I need to eat real, whole foods and be able to eat when I'm hungry. I don't *do* hungry! No one can keep that up for long."

In April 2004, Kathy joined Weight Watchers and lost weight steadily throughout the spring and summer. When the TurnAround Program Core Plan was introduced in August, Kathy switched to it. It really appealed to her because it's centered on wholesome, nutritious foods (beans, vegetables, fruits, fat-free dairy, whole grains, lean meats, seafood) without the need for tracking or counting that's part of other Weight Watchers programs.

By mid-2005, Kathy had lost 100 pounds, and she's now down to 164 pounds. Her doctor has taken her off all diabetic and blood pressure medications. Her blood glucose levels are between 65 and 70, and her A1C (the regular blood test that evaluates the stability of glucose levels) is steady around 5. Her husband Donald, who also has diabetes, has benefited, too. While enjoying Kathy's delicious and nourishing dishes, such as bean tacos, pasta fagioli, and cassoulet, he's shed 50 pounds and no longer requires insulin. He currently requires a very small dose of one oral medication.

"I have become very picky about foods I'm willing to make a part of me," says Kathy. "Food has to *earn* the right to get inside of me, and only quality food passes the test."

Physical activity is also now the agenda. "Before I lost the weight, I would get out of breath taking laundry upstairs. Now I jog or ride my bike for hours. I'm healthier and stronger than I have been for years. I exercise 5 or 6 days a week now, and I always take the stairs. When I'm bored, I take a walk—get out of the house and grab life by the tail!"

Now that she is educated, she's on a mission to enlighten others. She shares her progress with the National Weight Control Registry (NWCR)—a research tool that tracks more than 5,000 individuals who have lost significant amounts of weight and kept it off for long periods of time. (For more information about NWCR, visit www.nwcr.ws). And she has a new job working for Weight Watchers.

"People tell me all the time 'I could lose weight if I had your willpower.' But it's not willpower at all. It's vision," Kathy says. "I hope I can show others who are overweight and have diabetes the vision of how they can transform their bodies, their health, and their lives. I got my life back, and I'm 51! It's not too late. It is possible to improve your health."

dishes you love or have gotten into the habit of eating. Favorite dishes and good health can sit down at the same table. You won't have to give up the foods you love altogether—*once you know how to make the right choices*. We'll also look at physical activity and stress reduction, two other ways to significantly improve the quality of the life you live.

TALK TO YOURSELF

What do a plumber unclogging a drain, a student writing a term paper, and a surgeon poised to operate have in common? Before they lift a finger, they each need to do their research in order to do a good job. Information is power, and you are singularly powerful in your ability to research the way you eat and the way you live. Here's a six-step plan to finding the answers that will work for you.

1. Start a food and activity journal. First, chronicle what and when you eat, plus when and how you are physically active. Keep honest records for a week. When jelly doughnuts, french fries, sodas, and evenings on the couch stare back at you in cold print, they actually become easier to confront.

2. Look for small habits to break. Review your food and activity journal and make a list of food and fitness goals that are small changes you can easily make to your existing habits. Remember, you have to achieve only a 5 to 7 percent weight loss to reap significant health benefits. And, according to David M. Nathan, MD, director of the Massachusetts General Hospital Diabetes Center and author of *Beating Diabetes*, eating fewer calories and increasing exercise can lower blood sugar levels *before* even a pound of weight is lost.

3. Personalize your plan. Analyze your notes to develop specific strategies that address your individual challenges. (If it helps, pretend you're doing this for a friend or someone you love.) Do you snack constantly? Are your portions larger than they need to be? Do you eat late at night? Do you skip breakfast because you have "no time"? A big part of setting your strategies is learning as much as you can about healthy eating (the overriding goal), preferably from a registered dietitian or a certified diabetes educator. If that isn't an option, log onto the Internet at home or at your public library.

4. Think ahead and troubleshoot early. As the Boy Scouts always say, "Be prepared." Consider how you will deal with common eating situations. For example, sometimes you might be forced to grab a fast-food meal. So, research ahead of time (go online or ask for nutrition information at the fast-food restaurant) about the healthiest and most satisfying options. How can you deal with poor food options at work parties and holiday meals? Having a plan puts you in control of situations instead of letting situations control you.

5. Remember to crawl before you walk. To ingrain healthier habits *that last a lifetime*, you have to crawl before you walk and walk before you run (with exercise, sometimes literally!). If your current vegetable palate is off-white, is it realistic and attainable to set a goal to "eat five orange, red, or deep green vegetables each day"? A more reasonable idea might be to introduce one serving a day of a vegetable you've never eaten before to find ones you really like (see Chapter 8 for delicious recipes to get you started). "Get more exercise" is a commendable but vague ideal. "Walk 5 miles a day" is specific, but is it attainable? "Walk 30 minutes every day" is more attainable, but what happens on days when you have to work late or it's sleeting? "Walk 30 minutes, 5 days each week, indoors on a treadmill if necessary" is specific, attainable, and forgiving. In short, a great goal!

6. Reward yourself for good habits. Recognize the good changes that you make with small rewards along the way. An effective reward is desirable, timely, and contingent on meeting your goal. Choose tangible items such as a new garment, CD, or spa massage. Or make the treat intangible—a mental health day from work or a hike in the woods. Numerous small rewards will keep your motivation high.

STEERING YOUR NEW COURSE

In diabetes control, it's far better to adjust your course gradually than to jump ship altogether and try to swim for shore. Of course, sometimes it also helps to lighten the load by throwing unwanted cargo overboard. Do you really L-O-V-E sweet rolls, or do you just eat them out of habit because they're always in the office break room? Would some peanut butter spread on a few whole grain crackers (conveniently tucked into your briefcase by you!) satisfy you even more?

Once again, use some honest self-reflection to help determine what foods give you real pleasure and which aren't worth the baggage they carry. It's worth the time and effort to figure out how to tweak your favorites to your best advantage.

Is pasta your passion?

If so, cut your typical serving amount in half and opt for whole wheat pasta—instead of white—to increase the fiber intake. You can make it half whole wheat and half white pasta to start. Remember that all carbohydrates will raise blood glucose levels if eaten in too large of quantities. One cup of cooked whole wheat pasta combined with 1½ cups of cooked red, dark green, or orange vegetables and 3 ounces of lean protein will fill you up, will nourish you with vitamins and minerals, and won't significantly raise your blood glucose. Try other cooked whole grains (see page 32)—barley, buckwheat, or quinoa—with your favorite tomato sauce. You may discover it's really the sauce that you love most after all.

Do sweet pastries push your pleasure buttons?

Replace nutritionally empty pastries with the natural flavors that inspire them. Opt for nutrient-dense, fiber-filled, and naturally sweet dried dates, apricots, plums, or raisins. Just keep track of carb choices because these foods are relatively high in carbohydrates. If it's the creamy texture you crave, dip the fruit (or stuff pockets in the fruits) with reduced-fat cream cheese or homemade yogurt cheese flavored with orange or lemon extract.

LOOSEN UP/GET MOVING

Shaping the Shape You're In!

Shaping is a behavioral technique in which you select a series of short-term goals that get closer and closer to the ultimate goal. If you currently eat one serving of whole grain a day, you can make a goal to eat two servings daily and then later three servings daily. It is based on the concept that "nothing succeeds like success." Shaping uses two important behavioral principles: Consecutive goals that advance you gradually are the best way to reach a distant point; and consecutive rewards keep you excited about reaching that point.

Are you a fried-food fanatic?

Kick the fast-food french fry habit with homemade oven veggie fries. The reduction in fat can be phenomenal—you'll eat less than 2 grams of fat per 3½-ounce serving compared to 15 grams of fat (one quarter of the daily allowance on an 1,800-calorie eating plan) for a comparable fast-food portion! Cut kohlrabi, rutabaga, sweet potatoes, russet potatoes, or another starchy vegetable (unpeeled for extra fiber and nutrients) into thick sticks. Pat dry and place on a large baking sheet. Coat lightly with extra virgin olive oil from a spray bottle. Toss and spread into a single layer. Bake in a preheated 375°F oven, turning occasionally for 40 minutes or until browned and crispy.

Is "chocoholic" your middle name?

You've no doubt read about scientific studies showing the heart-healthy effects—such as lower oxidation levels of bad LDL cholesterol, higher blood antioxidant levels, and higher levels of good HDL cholesterol—derived from the antioxidants contained in unsweetened cocoa powder and plain solid dark chocolate. One brand in particular, Dove Dark, made by Mars, contains Cocoapro cocoa, a proprietary, specially processed cocoa that contains superhigh levels of flavanols. Just remember that 1 ounce of dark chocolate can contain up to 11 grams of fat, so it must be factored wisely into your total eating plan. In Chapter 10, you'll find a variety of delectable desserts that will fit into your meal plans and satisfy your darkest desires.

Are you sinking in soda?

It's now common knowledge (or should be) that soft drinks are a major source of empty calories in our diets, the equivalent of liquid candy. Drinking just one 12-ounce soda (150 calories) most days can add approximately 10 pounds to our weight each year. But instead of simply replacing your sugary drinks with diet cola, think about other beverage choices first. That's because there's some evidence that artificial sweeteners may actually make us fatter.

In a study conducted at the University of Texas Health Science Center School of Medicine, San Antonio, the consumption of diet soft drinks in study subjects over a 7- to 8-year period was associated with increased incidence of overweight and obesity.

Experts think that artificial sweeteners may hinder our bodies' natural ability to count calories based on a food's sweetness. Drinking a diet soda instead of a sweetened soda eliminates calories, but the body may be tricked into thinking other sweet foods are also calorie free.

Try unsweetened brewed regular or herbal iced tea, sparkling water with a wedge of lemon or lime, fat-free milk, or just good old H_2O.

A BAKER'S DOZEN INDULGENCES

The challenge of adapting the way you eat—especially at the beginning—can feel daunting. For times like these, Ann Fittante, MS, RD, a registered dietitian and certified diabetes educator at the Joslin Diabetes Center education affiliate at Swedish Medical Center in Seattle, gives the green light to "indulgences" that are okay to eat once in a while (two or three times a month). Eating the amounts listed should not increase blood glucose levels significantly or ruin your weight loss efforts. Each "indulgence" is approximately 30 grams of carbohydrate and 250 calories or fewer.

½ cup regular ice cream (not gourmet or premium types,
which are much higher in fat)

1 ounce milk, semisweet, or bittersweet chocolate

1 ounce snack chips

½ bag microwave popcorn

2 or 3 small cookies

¼ cup chocolate chips

8 chocolate kisses

3 cups kettle corn

1 small serving french fries

1 doughnut

1 small flavored latte, mocha, or frappuccino coffee drink

2 small "Halloween"-size candy bars

1 small cannoli

Is junk food jinxing your health?

Junk food, in the form of fast food and highly processed packaged products, is a recent fixation. Within the last 50 years, it has made rapid inroads into our collective tastebuds, but a bit of reeducation may help weaken its grip.

"It can be difficult at first for someone conditioned to the taste of highly processed foods to appreciate the subtlety of natural whole foods," says Chris Fenn, PhD, a nutrition author and motivational speaker based in Aberdeen, Scotland.

According to Fenn, the process of eating—how we decide what to eat, how much to put on a plate, and when to stop eating—is complex. In large part, it's all in our heads because the brain is constantly receiving signals from the eyes, mouth, nose, and stomach that influence appetite. Another factor at play is the junk food itself, since food manufacturers add artificial colors to make their products eye-catching. In the mouth, the combination of added flavorings, fat, and/or sugar blasts our taste buds with a hit of intense flavors. This is the "hook." Our palate gets a jolt, but our appetite will not be satiated. This keeps us coming back for more of the same.

Even if we're "hooked" on phony flavors that don't follow up with honest appetite satisfaction, Fenn assures us that it *is* possible to reeducate our taste buds.

"The trick is to stimulate the thousands of taste and aroma detectors, called chemoreceptors, that reside on our tongue and in our nose. Our sense of smell accounts for around 50 percent of the initial satisfaction from eating. When we eat, these chemoreceptors are stimulated and send pleasure signals to the brain. The more chemoreceptors stimulated, the greater the satisfaction," Fenn says.

"Whole foods naturally stimulate a greater number of chemoreceptors because they require more chewing. When we thoroughly chew food and allow it to linger in our mouths, we can actually savor the flavor. We've gotten out of this habit because highly processed foods can practically be swallowed with little or no actual chewing. It's almost as if they're predigested at the factory. Compare the amount of chewing required between a hunk of crusty whole grain bread studded with seeds and nuts and a slice of puffy white bread."

Every time we choose to eat a whole food instead of a processed one, we reward our senses with genuine satisfaction.

SMART STEPS (SKIPS AND JUMPS, TOO!)

With newfound energy from eating nutrient-rich whole foods, you'll likely have some extra energy to burn—and the sooner you light your fire, the better.

"No other intervention will do more to burn fat and improve your health than physical activity," explains exercise physiologist Richard Weil, MEd, CDE, director of the New York Obesity Research Center weight loss program at St. Luke's–Roosevelt Hospital Center. "Remember that you don't have to do Herculean amounts of activity. If performed regularly and at a moderate intensity, any type of physical activity, such as walking, biking, swimming, or dancing, will help you burn fat, achieve good health, improve your diabetes control, and perhaps most important of all, improve the quality of your life."

If the word *exercise* sounds too daunting, call it something else that makes it sound more fun—activity, movement, or grown-up play time! Weil, who serves on the board of the Diabetes Exercise and Sports Association, encourages this kind of thinking outside the gymnasium box. "Walking, biking, dancing, weight lifting, swimming, climbing stairs, hiking, gardening, housework, and many other activities of daily living such as walking your dog, washing your car by hand, and mowing your lawn with a push mower will all do the trick," he says. "In most studies of physical activity, even modest amounts of activity help the body reduce fat, if not all over the body, then certainly in the abdomen and deeper in the visceral fat where it counts most for good health.

"In one study of 24 people with type 2 diabetes who exercised for 45 minutes three times per week for 8 weeks, visceral fat and subcutaneous abdominal fat—the fat just below the skin—was reduced significantly," Weil says. "Moreover, insulin resistance improved by 46 percent. Most interesting was that the subjects lost significant amounts

FOCUS ON WHAT YOU CAN EAT

Ann Fittante, MS, RD, a registered dietitian and certified diabetes educator at the Joslin Diabetes Center education affiliate at Swedish Medical Center in Seattle, likes to keep it real when dispensing healthy eating advice to her patients. One of her teaching techniques involves a show-and-tell basket filled with the promise of good food for better health.

"One of my strategies for helping people improve their diets is to focus on which foods they should be eating instead of not eating. It's not very helpful to be told to avoid sweets, soda, and chips. What's more important is to suggest which foods to include so that people can improve their health, feel satisfied, and lose weight," explains Fittante.

"In my basket of healthy foods are food labels that include nuts, popcorn that is made with healthy fat, whole grain tortilla chips, whole grain crisp breads and crackers, yogurts that do not have artificial sweeteners and have 30 grams (or fewer) of carbohydrates, oatmeal, hummus, whole wheat pasta, a package of edamame, whole grain bread, and healthier potato chips (only two ingredients—potatoes and peanut oil). I also show food models of serving portions: 1½ cups of veggies and two fruits, which should be eaten daily; 1 cup of legumes; 1 ounce of nuts, which should be eaten weekly; 1 tablespoon of peanut butter; a 3-ounce portion of protein (3 to 6 ounces for lunch and dinner is a good goal for most people); and 1 cup of milk."

of abdominal fat and improved their insulin sensitivity even though they lost very little body weight."

To help set your "smart steps" in motion, look for our Loosen Up/Get Moving tips throughout this book.

DON'T WORRY, BE HEALTHY

For most of us, stress is an unavoidable by-product of life, just part of the price we pay. But for people with type 2 diabetes, research shows that stress can accelerate the disease's progress.

"Patients with type 2 diabetes might be at increased health risk from the effects of stress," says Richard S. Surwit, PhD, vice chairman of the department of psychiatry and behavioral sciences at Duke University Medical Center in Durham, North Carolina, and author of *The Mind-Body Diabetes Revolution.* "Experiencing stress is associated with the release of hormones that lead to energy mobilization—known as the 'fight or flight' response. Key to this energy mobilization is the transport of glucose into the bloodstream, resulting in elevated glucose levels, which is a health threat for people with diabetes."

But according to the results of a yearlong research study led by Surwit, patients with type 2 diabetes who incorporate simple, cost-effective stress management techniques into their routine care can significantly reduce their average blood glucose levels.

"The stress management techniques—such as progressive muscle relaxation and breathing exercises—when added to standard care, helped reduce glucose levels," says Surwit. "The amount of glucose level reduction is nearly as large as you would expect to see from some diabetes-control drugs."

"Managing stress can significantly improve a patient's control of their diabetes," says Surwit. "These techniques are simple, quick to learn, and have been shown to work for multiple conditions, including coronary syndromes. There are many self-help books and other commercially available materials about stress management from which patients can learn these techniques."

Be on the lookout throughout the book for Let Yourself Go/Stress Less tips that can enable you to "don't worry, be healthy!"

GO—SLOW—WHOA FOODS

Post this chart on your refrigerator or take it along when you shop for food. Refer to your personalized meal plan or consult the Meal Plans in Chapter 5, to see how these choices fit in with your daily nutrient needs.

GO Foods—Eat almost anytime. Nutrient-dense foods that are the highest in quality and the least processed. Low in fat, sugar, sodium, and calories. In the plant groups, they are highest in fiber.

SLOW Foods—Eat sometimes, at most several times a week. These foods are more processed and may be high in fat, added sugar, sodium, and calories.

WHOA Foods—Eat only once in a while or for special treats, about three times a month. These are low-nutrient foods that may be highly processed and may contain unnecessary additives. Highest in fat, sugar, and sodium. In the plant food groups, they are lowest in fiber.

VEGETABLES	
GO	Fresh, plain frozen, or low-sodium canned vegetables with no added fat and sauces; homemade oven-baked "french fries"
SLOW	All vegetables cooked with moderate amounts of healthy unsaturated fats (such as olive and canola oils) and low-fat tomato sauces
WHOA	French fried potatoes, hash browns, or other fried potatoes; other deep-fried vegetables; frozen vegetables in cheese or other high-fat sauces
FRUITS	
GO	All fresh, frozen, dried, and canned (in juice) fruits
SLOW	Fruits canned in light syrup
WHOA	Fruits canned in heavy syrup
BREADS AND CEREALS	
GO	Whole grain types of the following: breads, pitas, crackers, tortillas, pasta, brown rice, waffles; steel-cut oats and other hot breakfast cereals; cooked bulgur, barley, and quinoa; homemade low-fat whole grain muffins; homemade whole grain French toast and pancakes
SLOW	Refined-flour products or other refined grains: bread, white rice, pasta, French toast, biscuits, and pancakes
WHOA	High-fat, refined-flour products: commercially prepared croissants, muffins, doughnuts, sweet rolls, and crackers made with trans fats; sweetened breakfast cereals
MILK AND DAIRY PRODUCTS	
GO	Fat-free or 1% milk; fat-free or low-fat plain yogurt; part skim, reduced-fat, and fat-free cheese; 1% or fat-free cottage cheese

SLOW	2% milk; cream cheese, goat, and feta cheese; small amounts of regular full-fat cheese such as American, Cheddar, Swiss, Monterey Jack, Colby, Parmesan (no more than 2 to 3 ounces per week)
WHOA	Whole milk; whole-milk yogurt; processed cheese spread

BEANS, SOY, FISH, POULTRY, MEATS, EGGS, AND NUTS

GO	All dried beans or canned beans, split peas, lentils, hummus; tofu; tuna canned in water; baked, broiled, steamed, or grilled fish and shellfish; chicken and turkey without skin; fat-trimmed beef and pork; extralean ground beef; eggs (limit four egg yolks per week); Canadian bacon; all-natural peanut butter; 1 ounce nuts (three or four times per week)
SLOW	Frozen veggie burgers; lean ground beef, broiled hamburgers; ham; chicken and turkey with skin; low-fat hot dogs; tuna canned in oil
WHOA	Fried fish and shellfish; fried chicken, chicken nuggets; untrimmed beef and pork; regular ground beef; fried hamburgers; ribs; bacon; hot dogs, delicatessen meats, pepperoni, sausage

SWEETS AND SNACKS

GO	Popcorn made with healthy fats, whole grain tortilla chips, baked chips, whole grain crackers and crispbreads, homemade muffins or quick breads made with healthy fats and whole grain flour; homemade desserts with quality ingredients; dark chocolate; ice milk bars and low-fat ice cream; boxed gingersnaps, animal crackers, graham crackers (Though some of these "GO" choices are lower in fat and calories, all sweets and snacks need to be limited in order not to exceed one's daily calorie requirements.)
SLOW	Frozen fruit juice bars; low-fat frozen yogurt or sorbet; packaged fig bars, pretzels, low-fat microwave popcorn
WHOA	Commercial cookies and cakes; pies; cheesecake; ice cream; candy; chips; microwave popcorn

FAT

GO	Olive, canola, and other unsaturated vegetable oils; unsaturated oil-based salad dressing, mayonnaise, and low-fat mayonnaise; low-fat sour cream; 1 ounce nuts (three or four times per week); pesto; ⅛ avocado, Better Butter (page 323)
SLOW	Tartar sauce; sour cream; olives; trans-fat free spread; butter
WHOA	Margarine, solid vegetable shortening, lard; salt pork; gravy; regular creamy salad dressing; cheese sauce; cream sauce; cream cheese dips

BEVERAGES

GO	Water, fat-free milk, 1% milk, club soda or seltzer water, mineral water, unsweetened iced tea with lemon, herbal tea
SLOW	2% milk, wine, beer, hard liquor, sports drinks
WHOA	Whole milk; regular and diet soda; sweetened iced teas and lemonade; fruit drinks and fruit juice, diet iced teas, and diet lemonade

Source: Adapted from the National Heart, Lung, and Blood Institute (NHLBI). Published by the US Department of Health and Human Services; Public Health Service; National Institutes of Health; and the National Heart, Lung, and Blood Institute, Bethesda, MD.

CHAPTER 3

COOKING REAL FOODS IN THE REAL WORLD

By her mid-sixties, Nancy Boughn had struggled with type 2 diabetes for nearly a decade. Despite adhering to the typically prescribed eating plan and intense drug therapy, by early 2004 her A1C number (the regular blood test that evaluates the stability of glucose levels) had reached a high of 8.3 and her weight had soared to 196 pounds.

Today, Nancy weighs 147 pounds, she has an A1C of 6.4, and she is glad to report that she is free of medications and happier than she has been in years. It may sound as if Nancy experienced a miracle, but this dramatic transformation actually came about through much humbler means. As a subject in a diabetes and diet study, Nancy simply switched to eating plant foods—legumes (beans, peas, and lentils), whole grains, vegetables, and fruits. (For Nancy's complete story, turn to "I'm Beating Diabetes" on page 36.)

In Chapter 2, we took the food industry to task for what they're doing wrong (marketing too many processed food products). This time, we're going to praise them for what they're doing right. In response to increasing consumer demand, there are many more choices of convenience whole foods available today. So if your reason for not eating more whole foods has been something like "they take too much time and effort to prepare," that excuse is evaporating fast.

"B" HEALTHIER RIGHT AWAY WITH SUPER SWAPS

If you want to jump-start the health benefits of whole foods, start by adding some "B" foods to your diet right now (think "B" for "better" nutrition).

"B" is for beans, plus lentils and dried split peas. At least three or four times a week, replace a typical meat or poultry main dish with a bean dish.

"B" is for bulgur—cracked partially cooked wheat seeds—plus other whole foods such as 100 percent whole wheat bread and whole wheat couscous. Cook bulgur or couscous as a breakfast cereal or as a side dish instead of white rice, or cool and toss it into a hearty salad (tabbouleh is the classic whole wheat salad). Replace white bread with 100 percent whole wheat.

"B" is for broccoli and its cruciferous vegetable cousins: Brussels sprouts, cabbage, cauliflower, collard greens, kale, kohlrabi, mustard greens, rutabaga, turnips, bok choy, Chinese cabbage, arugula, and radishes. Try raw broccoli stems as a delicious snack. Add several servings of stir-fried or steamed broccoli, several times a week, to luncheon salads or as a side dish at supper.

"B" is for berries such as strawberries, blueberries, blackberries, and raspberries that offer needed nutrients and fiber in a low-carbohydrate package. Plus, they are convenient because they're readily available frozen loose-pack with nothing added. Eat some berries several times a week stirred into fat-free plain yogurt or breakfast oats. For a wonderful snack, simply partially thaw ½ cup of berries and toss in a bowl with 1 teaspoon of sugar, honey, or maple syrup.

A BUYER'S GUIDE TO WHOLE FOODS

When you start your journey down the whole foods path, it may be helpful to play a game of make-believe. Pretend that you've never been to the supermarket before. In truth, some departments may be uncharted territory (quick, name the aisle where the dried beans are stocked!). Of course, you may also find some whole foods in your usual stomping ground. Perhaps you frequently pick up processed frozen "diet" meals, so instead stop and take a closer look to find frozen whole foods. Pick a day when you can spare some time for research. The investment will pay off handsomely. Consider it an educational field trip for your health. But before you head out the door, read on to see what exactly you should be looking for.

Choose *prepped* instead of *processed*

If you think whole foods require more time and energy in the kitchen, think again. The key is to choose ingredients that are *partially prepared* (eliminating a good portion of the usual work and cooking time in the kitchen) but not *processed* (food products based upon refined grains, to which salt, high-fructose corn syrup, saturated fat, artificial colorings, and flavorings are added). Feel free to load up on the following:

- Prechopped onions, broccoli, bell peppers, minced garlic in oil, and pre-washed bagged salad greens, just a few of the prepped foods in the produce department

- Instant boxed whole grains such as brown rice, barley, and whole wheat couscous (partially cooked with no salt or other additives)

- Individual Quick Frozen (IQF) strawberries, blueberries, raspberries, peaches, and other fruits (nothing added) for convenience when local fresh fruit is out of season

- IQF broccoli, baby peas, corn, and other vegetables (nothing added) for convenience when fresh might not be readily available

- Pretrimmed and cut-up fish, poultry, beef, pork, and turkey (select types without any added fats or seasonings)

- Canned black, cannellini, great Northern, kidney, lima, pink, navy, and other beans. Some health food stores carry sodium-free canned varieties.

- Canned reduced-sodium or sodium-free diced tomatoes

- Canned fat-free reduced-sodium chicken broth and vegetable broth (home-made or available in natural food stores) instead of high-sodium canned broth or bouillon cubes

Primed for produce

While it's fun to take an outing to a local farmers' market during the growing season, many supermarkets now feature regionally grown produce, so it's a good idea to educate yourself about what fruits and vegetables grow in your area at what time of the year.

The benefits to buying seasonally harvested vegetables and fruits grown closer to home are threefold. First, the produce will be fresher because it didn't have to travel thousands of miles to get to your plate. Second, the fruits and vegetables are likely to be more flavorful varieties that are cultivated for maximum taste instead of shipping attributes. Third, they are more likely to be a good value. At a farm market in August or

FIBER-FULL FOODS

Stock your pantry with foods that provide valuable dietary fiber as well as essential nutrients.

- ½ cup all-bran dry cereal—14 grams
- ½ cup cooked navy beans— 9.5 grams
- ½ cup baked beans, canned— 9 grams
- ½ cup cooked lentils—7.8 grams
- ½ cup cooked black beans— 7.5 grams
- 1 cup raisin bran cereal—7 grams
- ½ cup cooked lima beans— 6.7 grams
- ½ cup cooked kidney beans— 6.5 grams
- ½ cup cooked chickpeas— 6.2 grams
- ½ cup homemade bean with ham soup—5.6 grams
- ½ cup fresh or frozen red raspberries—5.5 grams
- 1 medium homemade bran muffin— 5 grams
- ½ cup edamame—5 grams
- ½ Asian pear—5 grams
- ½ cup cooked artichokes— 4.5 grams

- ½ cup frozen peas—4.4 grams
- 1 cup oatmeal—4 grams
- ½ cup frozen mixed vegetables— 4 grams
- ½ cup raw blackberries— 3.8 grams
- ¼ cup dates—3.6 grams
- ½ cup canned pumpkin— 3.5 grams
- ½ cup cooked whole wheat spaghetti—3.4 grams
- 24 almonds (1 ounce)—3.3 grams
- 1 apple with skin—3.3 grams
- ½ cup cooked barley—3 grams
- ¼ cup dried plums—3 grams
- 1 slice (34 grams) sprouted wheat bread—3 grams
- 1 cup broccoli—2.4 grams
- 1 red sweet pepper—2.4 grams
- 1 nectarine—2.3 grams
- 28 peanuts (1 ounce)—2.3 grams
- 1 slice whole grain bread—2 grams
- 15 walnut halves (1 ounce)—2 grams

September, you can buy an entire bag of red or yellow bell peppers for less than a single supermarket pepper would cost in January.

If you're the resourceful type, you can freeze fruits and vegetables to enjoy when the season is done. Simply wash and pat dry whole tomatoes, raspberries, blueberries, and so forth in a single layer on a large tray or baking sheet with sides. Place, uncovered, in the freezer for about 24 hours or until frozen solid. Pack the frozen foods into resealable plastic freezer bags. Because they're not frozen in a clump, you can take out just the amount you want and put the rest back in the freezer. Come January, stir some frozen blueberries into your steaming oatmeal for a mighty sweet treat.

Many people are confused about just how to choose the best-tasting vegetables and fruits, but it's actually no more complicated than selecting a bouquet of flowers. Rely on your senses of sight, smell, and touch. Is the head of cauliflower creamy white with no brown patches? Does the blossom end (a soft indented round green patch where the fruit was attached to the vine) of a cantaloupe smell like a sweet melon or like nothing? Do the green beans feel crisp in your fingers or limp and mushy? Which of these previous foods would you prefer to eat?

Storing produce properly can also contribute greatly to the final flavor on your palate. For example, many fruits that are still hard to the touch when purchased—bananas, peaches, nectarines, mangoes, and pears—will actually ripen further if stored at room temperature in a large brown paper bag. When the fruits become fragrant and slightly soft to the touch, either eat or refrigerate them.

KISS UNWANTED ADDITIVES GOOD-BYE!

The KISS principle—Keep it simple, stupid—is handy in evaluating packaged food products. Compare two seemingly similar boxed foods: instant brown rice and a seasoned rice mix.

The instant brown rice contains one ingredient—precooked parboiled brown rice—and no sodium. The seasoned rice mix has 10 lines of ingredients that include corn syrup and a whopping 660 milligrams of sodium, which is 28 percent of the daily value for sodium in a single serving. The better choice is to season the instant brown rice with sodium-free seasoning blend to taste.

Goodness grains

Even as recently as a few years ago, if you wanted to buy steel-cut oats, unhulled barley, and toasted buckwheat groats (kasha), you had to make a special trip to the natural foods store. That situation has changed dramatically with the advent of whole foods sold in regular supermarkets, not to mention entire supermarket chains devoted to whole foods. Many even carry whole grains in bulk, which is often a better value than boxed grains.

Look for a store that does a brisk business in whole grains so that the inventory turns over quickly. Whole grains contain more natural, nutritious oil than refined grain, so they are more perishable. When you get them home, store the grains in an airtight container in a cool dark spot, the refrigerator, or the freezer.

As with any new food, it's a good idea to introduce different grains gradually into your diet. Wheat, probably the most familiar grain for most people, is an easy place to start. See page 28 for great ways to add more whole wheat to your diet right away. Other whole grains can be used in stuffings, soups, casseroles, salads, pilafs, and nontraditional risottos. Consider the following:

- **Barley**—Hulled (whole grain) is the most nutritious. Pearl barley is polished to remove the outer bran layer. Quick-cooking barley is sold in boxes.

- **Buckwheat**—Available as buckwheat groats or more intensely flavored toasted buckwheat groats, called kasha.

STAMP OF APPROVAL

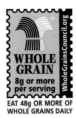 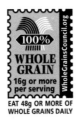

It's getting easier to identify whole grain foods in the market. The Whole Grains Council, a not-for-profit association affiliated with the Oldways Preservation Trust in Boston, is undertaking a consumer education campaign to increase consumption of whole grains to provide better nutrition. Just look for the Whole Grain Stamps on food packages. One stamp indicates an 8-gram half serving, the other a 16-gram whole serving, making it simpler to achieve the recommended goal of 48 grams of whole grains daily.

Eating three whole grain food products labeled "100% Whole Grain" does the trick—or six products bearing *any* Whole Grain Stamp.

"Refined" Redefined

A Harvard study found that an eating plan high in whole grains reduced the risk of diabetes by 38 percent, but a high intake of refined grains was associated with a 31 percent increase in the likelihood of diabetes.

- **Millet**—Hulled. If you feed the birds in your backyard, you're familiar with millet. This seed is easily digested because it is alkaline, whereas most other grains are acidic.

- **Oats**—Whole groats, steel-cut, and old-fashioned are the types you should buy. Quick cooking oats, while convenient, have a different texture.

- **Quinoa**—(pronounced *keen-wa*). This is a high-protein grain originating in South America. When cooked, its light texture belies its high protein content. Be sure to rinse well under cold water before cooking to remove a bitter-tasting substance called saponin that coats the seeds.

- **Rice**—Opt for brown rice in long and medium grain or in more exotic incarnations such as basmati, with its enticing aroma and flavor. Convenient instant brown rice is sold in boxes, and cooked brown rice is available frozen.

- **Teff**—These seeds of a North African grass resemble millet but are tinier. High-protein teff contains all eight essential amino acids.

- **Triticale**—Berries that offer a full-bodied texture and light rye flavor. They can be sprouted for a nice addition to salads.

- **Wild rice**—This is actually a native long-grain marsh grass that enjoys a gourmet reputation for its nutty flavor and toothsome texture.

Protein possibilities

Perhaps because the United States is the richest country in the world, we've always been a bit obsessed about making red meat (the most expensive source of protein to produce) our primary source of protein. Yet meat, along with our other primary "proteins"—poultry, seafood, eggs, and cheese—is not comprised solely of protein. In fact, very few foods are. Meat, poultry, seafood, eggs, and cheese also all contain fats, both saturated and unsaturated, in varying amounts.

Dried beans, lentils, and some grains contain good amounts of protein and virtually no fat of any kind, but they are often categorized as carbohydrates because that is their predominant nutrient. If feeling hungry on a weight-loss program is a challenge for you, the solution may be to eat more dried beans and lentils. Other recommended sources of lean protein are fish, skinless poultry, tofu, and fat-free or low-fat dairy. Higher-fat cuts of beef, pork, lamb, as well as high-fat dairy products should be eaten only occasionally, if at all. Consult the "Go—Slow—Whoa Foods" chart on page 24 for the healthiest options.

Finding fats

Our approach to dietary fat is simple: Eat moderate amounts of the healthiest types, aiming for at least two-thirds of your daily intake to come from healthy sources. Healthful fat, derived from plants and cold-water fish, is essential to our health. It supplies our bodies with essential fatty acids and aids the absorption of certain vitamins and carotenoids.

Choose monounsaturated oils such as olive oil, peanut oil, and canola oil, or polyunsaturated oils such as safflower or sunflower, as the healthiest choices. A daily weight-loss plan of about 1,600 calories affords about 30 percent of total calories to come from fat. Keeping in mind the ideal two-thirds ratio, that equals 320 calories, or 3 tablespoons, of healthy oils added to foods for cooking and flavoring. (Of course, this amount would be less if you get some oil from other natural sources of monounsaturated fats such as peanuts or almonds.)

The remaining recommended 10 percent of fat can be less healthful saturated fat, for instance, butter if you like the flavor. In a daily weight-loss plan of about 1,600 calories, that equals 160 calories, or roughly 1½ tablespoons of butter added to foods for cooking and flavoring. (Of course, this amount would be less on a daily basis if you get some saturated fat from other natural sources such as beef or poultry.)

"It seems to me that most people are confused, and rightly so, by all the messages to 'avoid trans fat.' In fact, if you eat mostly whole foods, trans fat becomes a nonissue. Trans fats, which occur in hydrogenated vegetable shortening, are found in processed food products—crackers, frozen diet dinners, chips, snacks, bottled salad dressings, preseasoned rice and grain mixes, and so on," explains Ann Fittante, MS, RD, a registered dietitian and certified diabetes educator at the Joslin Diabetes Center education affiliate at Swedish Medical Center in Seattle.

"As for trans-fat free spreads, I personally don't recommend them to my patients because they often contain palm oil, which is a saturated fat. Plus, many brands are loaded with artificial colors and other unnecessary additives. I suggest they avoid any spreads that contain more than three ingredients. The ingredients in butter are simple: cream and natural flavorings!

"Some of the trans-fat free spreads promote their healthy ratio of omega-3 to omega-6 fatty acids, but really none of us should be eating so much margarine spread that it plays a significant role in our fatty acid intake. I prefer to advise patients to take in fatty acids in the form of salmon, ground flaxseed, walnuts, and other whole foods. The fact is many foods are good sources of fatty acids—scallops, halibut, sardines, soy, flaxseed oil—and it all adds up," Fittante says.

The editors of *Prevention,* however, support the use of trans-free margarine as a cholesterol-free alternative to butter, so the recipes in this collection are written to provide readers with many options.

EQUIP YOURSELF

A few well-chosen pieces of the right kitchen tools will make preparing whole foods a snap.

- **Kitchen scale.** Even an inexpensive model can enable you to accurately gauge portions.

- **Kitchen scissors.** Very handy for cutting a range of ingredients, from raw poultry to fresh herbs.

(continued on page 38)

I'M BEATING DIABETES

NANCY BOUGHN

Soft-spoken grandmother Nancy Boughn, 66, may not look the part, but she's a real fighter. As someone who has struggled with the symptoms of type 2 diabetes since 1996, Nancy is proactive when it comes to self-care.

"I had worked hard to control my diabetes with the American Diabetes Association diet, but my A1C number had risen to 8.3," recalls the Herndon, Virginia, resident, who was also requiring intensified drug therapy. "I had two friends who went on kidney dialysis and lost their eyesight as a result of type 2 diabetes. Just about that time I read the ad in the *Washington Post* about a diabetes diet study. I thought it was time for me to take another step in the right direction of making sure this did not happen to me. I was personally motivated to be healthy."

"The study" for which Boughn volunteered was a randomized controlled dietary trial conducted by doctors and dietitians with the Physicians Committee for Responsible Medicine (PCRM), George Washington University, and the University of Toronto.

"I was assigned the vegan diet. That means absolutely no animal products. We eat four categories of food—fruits, vegetables, whole grains, and beans, peas, and lentils are where our protein comes from," Boughn explains. The vegan diet represents a major departure from current diabetes diets in that it places no limits on calories, carbohydrates, or portions of the foods that are approved in the diet. (Because vegan means no dairy, no seafood, no poultry or eggs, and no meat, saturated fat and cholesterol are virtually eliminated.) The researchers believe that if the participants eat the right foods, the amounts they eat will naturally fall in line.

"Almost immediately upon starting this diet, I noticed that I felt better generally. I could tell that my blood glucose numbers were dropping because I checked them frequently. Within 5 months, my A1C dropped from 8.3 to 6.4. I also lost all my joint pain. I consider that an extra added bonus. After 18 months in the study, I lost 48 pounds."

Boughn, who lives alone and has a demanding job schedule working sometimes 10-hour days as an executive assistant, finds that sticking to vegetable foods is easy for her. "People say to me, 'I don't know how you can do that,' but just by a little planning ahead, even when I'm traveling, it's very simple to do it.

"When I was following the ADA diet, I typically had oatmeal with milk and coffee with cream in the morning. I had fruit for a snack, and lunch was 3 ounces of fish or chicken, whole wheat bread, and veggies. Dinner was again 3 ounces of fish or chicken, salad with no dressing, and veggies. I ate dairy products, meat, and fish," Boughn says.

"The difference now that I eat vegan is that I don't weigh or measure portions. I don't worry about eating before I go to bed if I'm hungry. I do get about 40 grams of fiber a day. My diet consists of 75 percent complex carbohydrates (I use the glycemic index as a guide to food choices), 15 percent protein from beans, peas, or lentils, and 10 percent fat. I use a nonfat vanilla soymilk in my coffee. I try not to eat too many processed foods. I make my own soup in the winter. I buy a share in an organic farm during the summer and fall for fresh vegetables. I eat more fruit on the vegan diet. Fruit is my snack when I'm stressed.

"The study is over and we've had the final results. Everything about my numbers looks great across the board," Boughn says, beaming with victory. "It's definitely something that I'll continue to do."

- **Slow cooker.** Not essential, but useful for stews and cooking dried beans.
- **Food processor.** A kitchen workhorse for grinding, pureeing, and combining ingredients.
- **Cookware.** Have a few nonstick saucepans and skillets (great for sticky foods like eggs, beans, and oatmeal) and baking pans (silicone is the next-generation nonstick) but also at least one regular heavy skillet for browning foods to develop flavor. Browning a mix of chopped carrots, onion, and celery (and sometimes bell pepper) is a classic cooking technique that builds layers of flavor in many dishes. Stainless clad with an aluminum core, cast iron, or enameled cast iron are good options.
- **Silicone kitchen brush.** Won't melt under high heat. Very handy for spreading small amounts of oil in a skillet.
- **Spray bottle or two for oil.** Real oils such as olive and canola taste better on food than aerosol sprays. With a spray bottle, you can apply very small amounts for greatest effect.
- **Plastic freezer containers and resealable freezer bags.** Cook once and store leftovers for healthy "convenience" meals and snacks.
- **Digital instant-reading thermometer.** Foolproof method to check doneness of lean meats so they don't dry out. Also an accurate gauge for testing the temperature of yeast water for pizza dough.
- **Salad spinner.** A plastic colander set inside a large bowl to spin-dry lettuce leaves and other greens.
- **Microplane grater.** Based on a carpentry tool with razor-sharp teeth, this tool makes quick work of grating cheeses, citrus peels, fresh ginger, chocolate, garlic, and more.

ABOUT INGREDIENTS

For best results, we recommend you consult the following information about the ingredients called for in the recipes before you start cooking.

Beans

Dried and cooked (preferred for lower sodium) or canned beans, rinsed and drained. Some markets carry no-sodium-added canned beans. These make it really easy to prepare wonderful dishes anytime. When you find a brand you like, stock up.

Broth

Low-sodium canned chicken broth. Low-sodium packaged vegetable broth is sold in some supermarkets and natural foods stores. If using regular canned vegetable broth, use only half the amount called for and use water for the remaining measure.

Citrus juice

Always use fresh squeezed orange, lemon, and lime juice for finest flavor. Frozen 100 percent pure lemon juice (not sweetened lemonade concentrate) is an acceptable substitute for lemon or lime juice.

Dairy

Milk. Fat-free offers the best nutrition profile for the least fat. Sometimes higher-fat milks are used in smaller amounts in recipes where results would be unacceptable without them.

Dry fat-free milk is called for in some recipes as an ingredient to boost protein and calcium.

Cheese. A variety of fat-free, low-fat, and full-fat milk products are used depending upon the requirements of the individual recipe. Full-fat cheeses are very flavorful and melt beautifully but are used as a condiment because of their high saturated fat content. The fat content is indicated in recipes.

Yogurt is almost exclusively fat-free plain. It has the best nutritional profile and is the most versatile for cooking because you can control the added sweetener and flavorings.

Eggs

US Grade AA large eggs

Flours

Whole wheat pastry flour is sold in most supermarkets. It is softer than regular whole wheat and can replace all-purpose flour in most recipes. Store in a cool cupboard, refrigerator, or freezer.

COOKING FOR ONE OR TWO?

If you have only yourself (or maybe one other) to feed, consider yourself lucky! You can prepare what you want to eat, in the way you want it, when you want to eat it.

First of all, plenty of the foods recommended in the Fiber-FULL Diet Plan require no cooking and are portable to boot. Apples, oranges, pears, and other fresh fruits; dried plums, dried apricots, raisins; almonds, walnuts, pistachios, and other raw nuts are all 100 percent edible as is. Pack these foods for yourself in resealable plastic bags for convenient snacks.

Now for the cooking part. Some recipes in this book are designed for one serving or two servings. With recipes where it would be silly or impractical to create one serving, like the Cinnamon Buckwheat Pancakes with Honeyed Strawberries (page 99), we share tips for freezing the extras to create your own healthful convenience breakfast foods to have on hand. We also offer recipes that are delicious enough for entertaining, like the Monterey Strata (page 112) for brunch.

And so it goes through the recipe chapters. You'll find menu items such as sandwiches and wraps made in one- or two-serving amounts, and again, you can freeze individual portions.

SMART SHOPPING STRATEGIES

Seek out supermarkets that sell produce stacked loose in bins so you can buy only the number of pieces you need. Ditto for seafood, poultry, and meat. If you shop at a store with a service counter, you can buy only the amount you need. If your only choice is to shop at

Whole wheat flour or white whole wheat flour (100 percent whole wheat from a special strain of "white" wheat)

Ginger, fresh

Scrub the fresh ginger, dry it, and peel if desired. Store in a plastic resealable freezer bag. To use, grate just the amount needed and return the rest to the freezer.

Grains, whole

Consult page 32.

a store that prepacks foods, ring the bell and politely ask the service person to take out just the amount you need.

A store that sells grains in bulk allows you to select smaller amounts. If you can only purchase whole grains and whole grain flours in packages, just store the amount you're not using right away in the freezer to keep the nutrients in the oil-rich germ fresher longer.

Food manufacturers are catching on to the demand for whole grains in smaller portions. For instance, individual portions of cooked brown rice are now sold in shelf-stable cups. Keep a few of these on hand in the pantry for quick side dishes.

CELEBRATE YOURSELF

The final component of eating for one or two is to nourish your spirit along with your body. Sit down and savor the food you have taken the time and effort to prepare. Experts advise that slow, mindful eating that engages all of the senses allows our brains time to register that we are getting the nutrition we need.

If morning is your most relaxed time, sit down at the table and thoroughly engage in your first meal of the day (with no toxic TV news on the side).

The midday meal, especially for those who work outside the home, is often the most difficult to eat at a civilized pace. But make the effort, even if it's just for 15 solid minutes, to extricate yourself from your work environment. You'll be renewed in body and spirit when you return to work.

Oils and fats for cooking

For cooking, choose monounsaturated olive oil, canola oil, or peanut oil, or unsaturated safflower oil, corn oil, or sunflower oil. For salad dressings and some cooked dishes, extra virgin olive oil gives the most flavor. Some recipes call for Better Butter (see page 323), a healthier blend of 60 percent canola oil and 40 percent butter, when the flavor of butter is desired in a recipe.

Sweeteners

Sugar (granulated, brown, and confectioners'), honey, pure maple syrup. Because sugar substitutes can mislead us into thinking that desserts made with them are "free" foods, the Fiber-FULL plan instead uses moderate amounts of real sugar combined with whole grains and other whole ingredients to create desserts that truly satisfy with one serving.

Vegetables

Prechopped and minced fresh vegetables save time in many recipes. Frozen and canned vegetables are also called for in some recipes.

ABOUT COOKING TIMES, SERVING SIZES, AND THE NUTRITIONAL DATA

To help you schedule your time in the kitchen, each recipe includes preparation time and cooking time, plus any standing or cooling time required.

SUGAR VS. ARTIFICIAL SWEETENER

Ann Fittante, MS, RD, a registered dietitian and certified diabetes educator at the Joslin Diabetes Center education affiliate at Swedish Medical Center in Seattle, believes Mary Poppins may have been on to something when she warbled "just a spoonful of sugar helps the medicine go down."

"I'm not an advocate of artificial sweeteners. This is my own personal philosophy, as they have been approved by the American Diabetes Association and the American Dietetic Association," Fittante says. "My concern is that many people assume sugar-free food products are better, healthier for them. Most of these products still have a fair amount of bad fat and the same carbohydrate and calorie content as the regular item. For example, low-fat ice cream versus sugar free; sugar-free cookies versus regular cookies. I think it's fine to have regular sugar in moderation. Sweets are empty calories and should be limited for everyone, whether they have diabetes or not. One teaspoon of sugar, honey, jam, jelly, or maple syrup is 4 grams carbohydrate. This amount will not raise blood glucose levels. My general rule of thumb is not to worry about 1 to 2 teaspoons of sugar at one time. If having 1 tablespoon of sugar (15 grams carbohydrate), then count it as one carbohydrate choice in the total amount of carbohydrate in the meal or snack. Limiting cookies, ice cream, and other desserts to 30 grams carbohydrate and 200 calories per serving keeps blood glucose levels from spiking and keeps calories within an acceptable range. Go for quality, not quantity!"

Nutritional information is included for one serving of a recipe. Depending upon your personal calorie needs, you may require more or fewer than one serving of a particular dish.

The nutritional numbers for each recipe look like this:

Per serving: 000 calories, 00 g carbohydrate, 00 g protein, 00 g fat, 00 g saturated fat, 000 mg cholesterol, 00 mg sodium, 00 g fiber

Carbohydrate Choices: 0

Dietary Exchanges: 0 starch, 0 fruit, 0 milk, 0 vegetable, 0 meat, 0 fat

Carbohydrate Choices are the current, flexible system for managing carbohydrate intake. Because carbohydrate has the biggest effect on blood glucose, clinicians believe that if individuals are allocated a number of grams of carbohydrate to eat at each meal, they can choose which carbohydrate they want to eat and still keep their blood glucose under control. One Carbohydrate Choice = 15 grams carbohydrate.

The Dietary Exchange meal planning system is an older program that divides all food into six categories—starch, fruit, milk, vegetable, meat, and fat groups. A defined serving or "exchange" of each food item in one of these categories has the same calories, grams of fat, protein, and starch in it as every other food item in that category. So, under the "fruit choices" in the exchange system, for example, ½ cup of applesauce and a small banana each equal one "fruit exchange" that has 60 calories, 15 grams of starch, and no protein or fat. Individuals can use food lists to figure out how to "spend" those exchanges at each meal.

CHAPTER 4

ASK THE DIABETES EDUCATOR

For people living with type 2 diabetes, dozens of questions can arise. With insights on some of the most common questions her clients face, Ann Fittante, MS, RD, a registered dietitian and certified diabetes educator at the Joslin Diabetes Center education affiliate at Swedish Medical Center in Seattle, offers answers. Of course, before undertaking any weight-loss program or change in your eating plan, talk with your personal physician, dietitian, or certified diabetes educator to make sure it's the right decision for you.

1. *How can I tell if a specific food raises my blood glucose?*

   The best way to determine the effects of food on blood glucose levels is to monitor your glucose before the meal and then either 1, 2, or 3 hours after the meal. I prefer using the 2-hour test.

   Blood glucose targets for most people with diabetes are:

   - 90–130 mg/dl before meals
   - Less than 180 mg/dl 1 hour after meals
   - Less than 160 mg/dl 2 hours after meals
   - Less than 140 mg/dl 3 hours after meals

For example, if your glucose level before eating chicken, 1 cup of rice, and 1 cup of broccoli is 120 mg/dl and 2 hours later it is 150 mg/dl, you know the portion sizes in that meal (more specifically the carbohydrate amounts) are appropriate for you. If, however, before a meal of pasta, bread, and chocolate cake your glucose level is 120 mg/dl and 2 hours later it is 250 mg/dl, you know the carbohydrate amounts of that meal are too high for you.

2. *I always thought that regular sugar was forbidden for those with diabetes, but lately I've been seeing recipes that call for sugar. Is it okay to eat sugar?*

Yes, it's okay to eat sugar. Sugar is a carbohydrate and does not raise glucose levels more than other sources of carbohydrate. Because foods that contain quite a bit of sugar and fat (like desserts) are sources of empty calories, it is best to limit the amount. One teaspoon of sugar, honey, jam, or jelly has 4 grams of carbohydrate, which will not raise glucose levels very much. I recommend limiting sugar to 1 to 2 teaspoons at one time and limiting desserts to 30 grams or fewer of carbohydrate. If you are going to eat a high-carbohydrate dessert like cake or pie, combining it with a lower-carbohydrate meal like fish and nonstarchy vegetables will keep glucose levels in a better range than if you ate it with a higher-carbohydrate meal such as pasta.

3. *Should I stick to the same foods every day?*

Eating a variety of foods ensures a healthier diet. But I know many people with diabetes tend to stick to the same foods since they can better predict how these foods will affect their glucose levels. Learning the carbohydrate amounts in new foods can help you decide the right portion sizes so that your glucose level stays on target. Eating seasonally is a good strategy for increasing variety. Fruits and vegetables taste much better and cost less when they are newly harvested. Another strategy is to eat foods by the color of a rainbow. Choose red foods (red apples, red peppers), orange (carrots, winter squash), yellow (banana, yellow peppers), green (kiwifruit, spinach), blue (blueberries), and violet (eggplant, concord grapes). Aim for variety if possible since you get different nutrients from different foods. Your diet is likely to be healthier.

4. *Is broccoli some kind of magic food for diabetes? My blood glucose always tests normal after I eat it, no matter what other "bad" foods I have with the meal.*

I think broccoli is a magic food because it is packed with nutrients and fiber! I have not heard specifically that eating it seems to cause blood glucose levels to be lower, however. Most nonstarchy vegetables are very low in carbohydrate and have minimal impact on blood glucose levels. It may be that when you eat the "bad" food with broccoli, the entire meal is not very high in carbohydrate, and it is for that reason your blood glucose level is lower.

5. *I heard alcohol lowers blood glucose levels. Is this true?*

It is true that alcohol can lower blood glucose levels in some people with diabetes. This is especially true if you are on a medication like insulin or some pills for diabetes that can cause low blood glucose. To prevent low blood glucose if you drink, it is best to include a carbohydrate snack like whole grain crackers or popcorn or have it with a meal. Mixed drinks can increase blood glucose levels because the "mixer" is usually high in carbohydrates (sugar). Beer, wine, and hard liquor have minimal impact on blood glucose levels if consumed in small amounts. General recommendations for alcohol are to limit to one drink per day for women and two drinks per day for men. Remember, alcohol contributes excess calories and can make weight loss more difficult. One drink is approximately 80 to 150 calories.

6. *Dried cereal seems to raise my blood glucose significantly. Why is that?*

Many dried cereals are very high in carbohydrate even though they may be high in beneficial fiber and have little or no sugar. The combination of a medium to large bowl (one to three servings) of cereal, fruit, and milk increases the carbohydrate content of the meal significantly. To see the effects of dried cereal on your blood glucose levels, test glucose levels before and 2 hours after eating. Remember the 2-hour blood glucose goal is 160 mg/dl or less. Hot cereals are less processed and tend not to raise glucose levels as much as dried cereals.

7. *I heard fruit raises blood glucose levels. Is this true?*

Fruit is a carbohydrate and if eaten in large quantities can increase blood glucose levels. Fruit is high in fiber and important nutrients, as well as relatively low in calories, so fruit should be eaten daily. A medium piece of fruit (like an apple, an orange, or 1 cup of grapes) is approximately 30 grams of carbohydrate and should not increase glucose levels too much. My general recommendation is to include one to three pieces of fruit per day, eating one piece at one time (spacing it out over the course of several meals). If fruit seems to be increasing your blood glucose level, include it with some protein or fat (cottage cheese or nuts), which may slow the absorption and prevent the glucose from increasing too much.

8. *Will eating too much protein put a strain on my kidneys?*

If you already have kidney disease, eating too much protein may put more of a strain on your kidneys. For this reason, high-protein diets are discouraged. Limiting animal protein to 6 ounces per day is a good place to start if you already have kidney disease. Ask your physician or dietitian for more specific recommendations. If you do not have kidney disease, eating more protein should not negatively affect your kidneys; however, a more balanced meal plan approach (eating carbohydrate, protein, and healthy fat with meals) is still recommended for best nutrition.

9. *Can I eat salt? Does it raise my blood glucose levels?*

Salt, or sodium chloride, does not raise blood glucose levels. If you have high blood pressure, kidney disease, or congestive heart failure, limiting sodium in your diet is very important. Too much sodium can also cause fluid retention. *Prevention* recommends limiting sodium to 2,300 milligrams per day for optimal health. If you have high blood pressure, kidney disease, or congestive heart failure, limiting sodium further to 1,500 to 2,000 milligrams per day may be beneficial. Avoiding processed food products that typically contain high amounts of sodium can eliminate a great deal of sodium from your diet.

10. *My trainer wants me to eat a snack before exercise. What should I be eating?*

If the reason your trainer wants you to snack before exercise is to prevent low blood glucose, first consider if you are at risk for low blood glucose (hypoglycemia). People who are not on medication for diabetes are not at risk for hypoglycemia. Some medications for diabetes also do not cause hypoglycemia, and therefore having a snack may not be necessary. Consuming snacks may add extra calories that are unnecessary, especially if weight loss is your goal. However, if it's been several hours since your last meal, having a snack before exercise may provide extra fuel and maximize your workout. I suggest 15 to 30 grams of carbohydrate and fewer than 200 calories (i.e., fruit and six nuts; ½ serving crackers and 1 teaspoon peanut butter; or 1 cup of plain, low-fat yogurt with ½ cup berries).

11. *How do protein and fat affect blood glucose levels?*

Protein and fat have minimal effects on blood glucose levels. They both slow absorption of carbohydrate. As the carbohydrate, such as bread, in a meal is digested and transformed into blood glucose, the protein and fat, such as turkey and mayonnaise, in the meal slow the absorption of the glucose and prevent spikes in blood glucose levels. In some situations, very high fat meals can slow down the absorption process too much, keeping blood glucose levels higher than desired for a longer period of time. Generally, the highest blood glucose level is approximately 1 hour after eating, and by 2 hours it should come back down (remember the target is less than 160 mg/dl). A very fatty meal of fish and chips may cause blood glucose levels to stay higher for 3 to 5 hours after eating because the fat in the meal slows absorption and keeps the glucose levels higher for a longer period of time. In situations like this, decreasing the fat in the meal will not only decrease extra calories but will help bring your glucose levels back to target sooner. Fried fish and a salad or baked fish with fries would be a better balance. Baked fish with salad and a small baked potato is the best choice.

12. *When my blood glucose level drops too low, what should I be eating to bring it back up?*

Symptoms of hypoglycemia (low blood glucose) include feeling shaky, sweaty, and dizzy, and being irritable, light-headed, or very hungry. This can happen if blood glucose levels drop below 80 mg/dl. To bring blood glucose levels back up to normal as quickly as possible, have 15 grams of carbohydrate, like ½ cup juice, 1 tablespoon of honey, a small fruit, 2 tablespoons of raisins, or 3 glucose tablets. Wait 15 minutes and retest. If blood glucose levels are not above 80 mg/dl, have another 15 grams of carbohydrate. Once blood glucose levels are above 80 mg/dl, you can eat a meal or have another carbohydrate/protein snack (such as toast with peanut butter) to sustain you until your next meal. Avoid carbohydrates that have added fat, like chocolate, granola bars, or cookies, to treat hypoglycemia. These foods do not work quickly enough to bring your glucose levels back to normal.

13. *What is a hemoglobin A1C test, and when should I have it done?*

Glycohemoglobin, or hemoglobin A1C or A1C, is a blood test that measures your long-term blood glucose control. The test is an average of what your blood glucose level has been for the last 3 months. The A1C target for most people with diabetes is less than 7.0 percent (normal range is between 4.2 and 6.3 percent, so some physicians are recommending less than 6.5 percent). People with diabetes should have an A1C test every 3 to 4 months.

14. *I've heard that diabetes is hereditary, and I'm worried my kids will develop the disease. How can I make sure they don't?*

Type 2 diabetes is hereditary and in the last several years becoming more prevalent in overweight children. Type 2 diabetes can be prevented or at least delayed until older age by maintaining a healthy weight, staying active, and eating healthfully. Eating right and being active is important for the entire family. Modeling these behaviors for your children helps them establish healthy lifestyle habits that they can maintain for life. Encourage the family to eat fruits and veggies daily; milk, yogurt, and cheese for calcium; lean meats; healthy fats; and snacks like popcorn, nuts, and peanut butter crackers. Limit the amount of soda, fast food, and unhealthy store-bought cookies and cake, chips, and doughnuts your family consumes.

15. *I had a cold last week and my blood glucose levels went up to 200 mg/dl and I was barely eating anything. Is this normal?*

Yes, it's very normal for blood glucose levels to increase when you are sick. Being sick is a stressor to the body. When you are sick, you should continue monitoring your glucose levels. You may need to increase the frequency of testing to two to four times per day if your numbers are high. It's important to continue taking your diabetes medications when you are sick even if you are not eating very much. If blood glucose levels are 300 mg/dl or higher, you need to call your doctor.

16. *Can a person with diabetes ever get off diabetes medications?*

Yes, it is possible for some people with type 2 diabetes to either need less diabetes medication or get off it altogether with lifestyle changes. Typically those people who no longer need their diabetes medications are those who lose weight if they are overweight and those who improve their fitness by exercising regularly. Although some people strive to get off their diabetes medicines, it is not a sign of failure if that does not happen. Sometimes the body doesn't cooperate, and the amount of insulin your pancreas makes decreases and medications are necessary. It is important to remember that good blood glucose control is the goal whether it is controlled by diet, exercise, medication, or a combination of the three.

17. *Are there vitamin/mineral supplements I should be taking?*

My overall recommendation is to try to obtain the nutrients you need through a balanced eating plan. However, taking a multivitamin for added insurance of obtaining necessary nutrients is a good idea. If you are not getting three servings of a high-calcium food (milk, yogurt, cheese, dried fish, sardines, fortified soymilk), consider taking a calcium supplement with vitamin D in addition to the multivitamin. (The goal is 1,000 to 1,200 milligrams of calcium per day and 400 to 600 IU of vitamin D.) Deficiencies in minerals such as chromium, magnesium, and potassium may cause higher blood glucose levels in some people with diabetes. These nutrients can be obtained through both diet and the multivitamin supplement. Additional supplementation should not be necessary. There has been interest in antioxidant supplementation in people with diabetes. Currently the recommendation is to obtain antioxidants through diet (fruits, veggies, whole grains).

18. *My dietitian gave me a meal plan with recommended percentages of carbohydrate, protein, and fat, but I don't know how to translate those into actual meals. Any advice?*

If you are unclear how to incorporate your dietitian's advice, I suggest calling him or her for clarification. Having a sample meal plan based on the recommendations will give you a better idea of how to translate the guidelines into actual meals. Using a healthy plate method is another meal plan approach. With the plate method, fill half of your plate with vegetables, one-quarter of your plate with carbohydrate (rice, bread, pasta, fruit, milk), and one-quarter of your plate with protein and fat (meat, chicken, fish). If you don't eat vegetables for breakfast, fill one-third of your plate with protein, one-third with carbohydrate, and one-third with healthy fat. This guideline proportions the amount of carbohydrate, protein, and fat that is appropriate for most people with diabetes.

19. *At the pharmacy, I noticed special "diabetic foods" like energy bars and shakes that promise to help control my blood glucose levels. Do I need to buy these kinds of products to be healthy?*

No, you do not need to buy specialty foods marketed to people with diabetes. Many times the carbohydrate content is slightly lower but not significantly lower than the traditional food. A "diabetes" bar might have 25 grams of carbohydrate compared to a regular granola bar with 30 grams of carbohydrate. Calories are the same. Fat content is the same, and in some cases the saturated fat (bad fat) is higher in the "diabetic" product. I've noticed that the specialty foods are more expensive and don't always taste as good. Check the ingredient list as well. Many times specialty foods have many more ingredients. They have been heavily fortified with vitamins and minerals. I believe the key to healthy eating is choosing foods that are less processed, and that means choosing foods with the fewest ingredients possible.

CHAPTER 5

THE FIBER-FULL DIET PLAN

MENUS FOR LOSING WEIGHT AND CONTROLLING BLOOD GLUCOSE

We hope by now you're convinced that with positive lifestyle adjustments—eating whole foods, exercising, and stressing less—you can beat the advance of diabetes if you are already diagnosed and even prevent the onset of the disease if you have prediabetes.

If your first goal is weight loss, our plan can help you to safely lose up to 2 pounds a week by eating six satisfying meals and snacks each day. This will not only keep your hunger in check but will balance your blood glucose levels. The meal plans are based on a new approach to the treatment of diabetes through diet. The latest scientific studies are proving that an eating plan based upon whole, fiber-rich foods can not only control but in many cases reduce blood glucose levels. That means you can say good-bye to high-priced, highly processed "diabetic" foods, artificial sweeteners, and any other food product that doesn't give you maximum nutritional bang for your buck. Say hello to whole foods bursting with flavor, mouth appeal, and the fiber to keep you feeling full for longer periods of time.

If you have diabetes or prediabetes, we know that your motivation for losing weight goes far beyond cosmetic reasons. You want to be the healthiest you can—lowering

NUTRITIOUS MEAL PLANNING TIPS AND SUGGESTIONS

- Take advantage of washed and precut bagged vegetables whenever possible. They make very convenient snacks and reduce meal preparation time considerably.

- Plain low-fat yogurt is the healthiest choice and is used almost exclusively in the meal plans. If you prefer, add 1 teaspoon of sweetener (sugar, honey, jam, maple syrup). If choosing commercially sweetened yogurts, select those that are fruit juice sweetened and contain 30 grams of carbohydrate or less per serving, with no artificial colors or flavorings. (See "Brand Names of Recommended Whole Foods" on page 356.) Limit your intake of commercially sweetened and artificially sweetened yogurts.

- One percent milk is included as a beverage in many of the menus. If you prefer, you can replace the 1 percent milk with fat-free milk to save an extra 2 grams of fat per 8-ounce serving.

- Homemade salad dressing in the menus is a combination of ½ tablespoon olive oil, preferably extra virgin for the most flavor, and ½ tablespoon wine vinegar or lemon juice. A batch of Better Butter (see page 323), a combination of 60 percent canola oil and 40 percent butter, can be kept on hand in the refrigerator or freezer.

- Hot cereals like steel-cut oatmeal, rolled oatmeal, and oat bran are foods that are very high in soluble fiber and should be included regularly in your diet. These cereals are included twice a week for breakfast.

body weight, blood glucose, and blood pressure—to dramatically cut your risk of developing heart disease, stroke, nerve damage, and other life-threatening complications.

For a full explanation of the Fiber-FULL Diet Meal Plan and Menus for Losing Weight and Controlling Blood Glucose, refer to Chapter 1. But if you want to get started right away, simply follow our easy two-phase weight-loss menu program followed by maintenance guidelines.

Phase 1 gradually introduces your system to the fiber-rich whole foods that will literally transform your health. You can follow it for the full 2 weeks or move directly into Phase 2 whenever you feel ready.

In Phase 2, you'll continue your steady weight loss while increasing your intake of fiber-rich whole foods, balanced by lean protein and healthy fats to maximize your

- Remember to select 100 percent whole grain baked goods so you derive the maximum nutrients and fiber.

- Alcohol is extra calories. One drink (4 ounces of wine, 12 ounces of beer, 1 ounce of hard liquor) is approximately 80 to 150 calories. The American Diabetes Association recommends that women with diabetes limit alcohol to one drink daily and men limit to two drinks daily. Mixed drinks are generally high in carbohydrate and can increase glucose levels. An occasional glass of wine has been included in the meal plans. If you prefer not to drink alcohol, you may substitute another "treat" (½ ounce chocolate, ½ cup low-fat ice cream or pudding, or two small cookies) if desired.

- Plain tea and coffee, decaffeinated or regular, are "free" beverages that can be included with any meal or snack.

- Sweets and desserts can be high in carbohydrate and raise glucose levels considerably. For better blood glucose control, choose to have dessert with a low-carbohydrate meal. For example, cake following a chicken breast and broccoli will not raise glucose levels as much as having cake with a pasta meal.

health benefits. You should follow the meal plans in Phase 2 until you achieve your healthy body weight.

Remember to monitor your glucose levels closely during both phases of the plan. As an individual, your body's reaction to various foods can be different from others. So, make adjustments to the menus accordingly.

KNOWING THE NUMBERS

While it's ideal to follow the menus in this book exactly as written, in the real world things are rarely so easy. So with that in mind, here's a quick overview of the numbers you'll need to know in order to tailor meals as necessary. In general, the meal plans in the Fiber-FULL Diet Plan provide between 1,400 and 1,600 calories per day, which is a suitable range to help most people achieve a healthy rate of weight loss of 1 to 2 pounds per week. However, if your calorie needs differ, make sure to stay above the following ranges as you reach your goals:

Men: No lower than 1,500 calories per day

Women: No lower than 1,200 calories per day

If you need fewer calories than the meal plans provide:

- Substitute 1 cup of raw vegetables for one snack and
- Eliminate 1 ounce of protein and one fat serving per day

If you need more calories than the meal plans provide:

- Increase the number of snacks to four a day (instead of three)
- Increase protein by 1 ounce, and
- Increase fat by one serving

Foods to add and enjoy every day:

- Minimum 1½ cups dark green, orange, or red vegetables, raw or cooked
- One to three fruits (one serving should equal 30 grams of carbohydrate or 2 carbohydrate choices)
- One to three servings of low-fat dairy

Foods to add to your diet two to four times per week:

- ½ to 1 cup legumes (beans)
- ½ to 1 cup oatmeal or oat bran hot cereal
- 2 to 4 tablespoons unsalted or raw nuts, and
- A good source of omega-3 fats (salmon, sardines, or mackerel; ground flaxseed or flaxseed oil; walnuts; soy; or canola oil)

Keep in mind that fruit is an excellent choice to include in a healthy diet, but because it is also moderately high in carbohydrate, enjoy only one serving at one time and space your servings evenly throughout the day. Regarding snacks and desserts, the general guidelines for weight loss and blood glucose control are to limit portions to 30 grams of carbohydrate and 200 calories or fewer per serving.

PHASE 1

If you're unaccustomed to eating fiber-rich foods regularly, make sure to start the Fiber-FULL Diet Plan with Phase 1. If your blood glucose numbers remain steady or drop, you can move into the higher-fiber, higher-carbohydrate Phase 2. If on Phase 2 you find your glucose readings rising, simply move back into the lower carbohydrate of Phase 1. You'll still lose weight at a healthy rate. Continue with the menus on whichever phase works best for you until you reach your ideal weight. Then consult the section on maintenance.

- Meal plans are between 1,400 and 1,600 calories, 40 percent carbohydrate (not less than 130 grams of carbohydrate total per day), 20 to 30 percent protein, and 30 to 35 percent predominantly healthy fat. They include three meals (breakfast, lunch, and dinner) and three snacks.

- Goal for fiber: a minimum of 20 grams per day

Week 1

RECIPES FOR WEEK 1

Seasonal Fruit Salad (page 92)

Almond and Mixed Berry Muffins with Flaxseed (page 102)

Cheese and Pepper Frittata (page 106)

Mediterranean Veggie Burger (page 155)

Chicken-Cranberry Sandwich (page 158)

Peanut Butter and Raisin Porcupines (page 172)

Summer Tomato Soup with Fresh Dill (page 184)

Fresh Pea Soup with Mint (page 188)

Barley, Butternut, and Black Bean Salad (page 192)

Orange-Soy Salmon with Vegetables (page 238)

Roasted Flounder with Artichokes (page 256)

Lime-Marinated Chicken with Salsa (page 265)

Greek Meatballs (page 284)

Week 1 ▪ Sunday

BRUNCH

    1 serving Cheese and Pepper Frittata (page 106)

    1 slice whole grain toast with 1 teaspoon Better Butter (page 323)

    1 cup 1% milk

LUNCH

    ½ tuna sandwich on whole grain bread with lettuce and tomato (½ cup tuna, 1 teaspoon mayonnaise, 1 teaspoon chopped onion, and 1 teaspoon chopped celery)

    1 cup chopped tomato and cucumber salad with a splash of balsamic vinegar

    1 peach

SNACK

    1 small apple with 1 teaspoon cashew butter

    ½ cup raw sugar snap peas

DINNER

    1 serving Lime-Marinated Chicken with Salsa (page 265)

    1 medium whole wheat tortilla

    Tossed salad with 1 tablespoon Homemade Salad Dressing (page 54)

SNACK

    ½ cup low-fat ice cream

DAILY ANALYSIS		CARBOHYDRATE CHOICES	
	Calories: 1,499		10
	Carbohydrate: 151 grams		
	Protein: 100 grams		
	Fat: 55 grams	**DIETARY EXCHANGES**	Starch: 4
	Saturated Fat: 15 grams		Fruit: 2
	Cholesterol: 428 milligrams		Milk: 2
	Sodium: 1,787 milligrams		Vegetable: 6
	Fiber: 27 grams		Meat: 7
			Fat: 6

Week 1 ▪ Monday

BREAKFAST

½ cup cooked rolled oats with 1 tablespoon ground flaxseed

½ cup sliced peaches topped with ¼ cup low-fat cottage cheese

SNACK

2 pieces whole grain crispbread with 1 teaspoon almond butter

LUNCH

1 serving Fresh Pea Soup with Mint (page 188)

1 ounce Swiss cheese with ½ medium pear

SNACK

1½ servings Peanut Butter and Raisin Porcupines (page 172)

DINNER

1 serving Orange-Soy Salmon with Vegetables (page 238)

⅓ cup cooked brown rice

Mixed greens with 1 tablespoon Homemade Salad Dressing (page 54)

SNACK

½ serving whole grain crackers with 1 tablespoon cream cheese

DAILY ANALYSIS		CARBOHYDRATE CHOICES	
	Calories: 1,484		10
	Carbohydrate: 153 grams		
	Protein: 92 grams		
	Fat: 56 grams	**DIETARY EXCHANGES**	Starch: 7
	Saturated Fat: 14 grams		Fruit: 2
	Cholesterol: 140 milligrams		Milk: 0
	Sodium: 1,403 milligrams		Vegetable: 3
	Fiber: 31 grams		Meat: 9
			Fat: 5

Week 1 ▪ Tuesday

BREAKFAST

> 1 cup plain low-fat yogurt topped with ½ serving Seasonal Fruit Salad (page 92) and 2 tablespoons walnuts, toasted or raw

SNACK

> 2 pieces whole grain crispbread with ¼ cup low-fat cottage cheese and 1 sliced plum tomato

LUNCH

> 2 ounces grilled *or* baked chicken
>
> 1 serving Barley, Butternut, and Black Bean Salad (page 192)
>
> ½ cup steamed broccoli with 1 teaspoon lemon juice

SNACK

> ½ serving Seasonal Fruit Salad (page 92)

DINNER

> 3 ounces baked pork chop
>
> ½ cup unsweetened applesauce sprinkled with apple pie spice
>
> 1 cup green beans sautéed with 1 teaspoon olive oil and garlic
>
> Small spinach salad with 1 tablespoon Homemade Salad Dressing (page 54)

SNACK

> 1 ounce almonds, raw or toasted

Note: Save remaining ½ serving Seasonal Fruit Salad for afternoon snack; save ½ serving Barley, Butternut, and Black Bean Salad for Wednesday's afternoon snack.

DAILY ANALYSIS	Calories: 1,478	**CARBOHYDRATE CHOICES**	10
	Carbohydrate: 162 grams		
	Protein: 77 grams		
	Fat: 58 grams	**DIETARY EXCHANGES**	Starch: 4
	Saturated Fat: 11 grams		Fruit: 3
	Cholesterol: 110 milligrams		Milk: 1
	Sodium: 1,101 milligrams		Vegetable: 6
	Fiber: 30 grams		Meat: 6
			Fat: 6

Week 1 ■ Wednesday

BREAKFAST

1 slice whole grain toast

1 teaspoon Better Butter (page 323)

Scrambled eggs (beat 1 egg and 1 egg white; cook with 1 teaspoon olive oil)

1 cup 1% milk

SNACK

1 cup blueberries with a dollop of plain low-fat yogurt with ¼ teaspoon orange extract

LUNCH

½ turkey sandwich on whole grain bread with lettuce and tomato, 2 ounces turkey, and 1 teaspoon Dijon mustard

Side salad with 1 tablespoon Homemade Salad Dressing (page 54)

1 cup 1% milk

SNACK

½ serving Barley, Butternut, and Black Bean Salad (page 192)

DINNER

1 serving Summer Tomato Soup with Fresh Dill (page 184)

1 serving Mediterranean Veggie Burger (page 155)

1 medium corn on the cob with 1 teaspoon Better Butter (page 323)

SNACK

½ cup low-fat vanilla ice cream topped with 2 tablespoons chopped walnuts

DAILY ANALYSIS		CARBOHYDRATE CHOICES	
	Calories: 1,453		10
	Carbohydrate: 151 grams		
	Protein: 84 grams		
	Fat: 57 grams	DIETARY EXCHANGES	Starch: 6
	Saturated Fat: 16 grams		Fruit: 1
	Cholesterol: 292 milligrams		Milk: 2
	Sodium: 1,499 milligrams		Vegetable: 4
	Fiber: 23 grams		Meat: 5
			Fat: 7

Week 1 ▪ Thursday

BREAKFAST

15g carb ½ cup steel-cut oatmeal with 1 tablespoon ground flaxseed and 2 tablespoons walnuts, toasted or raw ~ *cooked*

SNACK

½ cup blackberries with a dollop of plain low-fat yogurt

LUNCH

1 large spinach salad with 2 ounces feta, goat, or blue cheese; 3 ounces grilled chicken; ¼ cup chickpeas; ¼ cup sliced grapes; and 1 tablespoon Homemade Salad Dressing (page 54)

2 pieces whole grain crispbread

SNACK

½ cup plain low-fat yogurt with ½ cup mandarin oranges (add ½ teaspoon almond extract if desired)

DINNER

1 serving Greek Meatballs (page 284)

1 cup steamed carrots

SNACK

3 cups popcorn with 1 tablespoon grated Parmesan cheese

DAILY ANALYSIS	Calories: 1,599	**CARBOHYDRATE CHOICES**	11
	Carbohydrate: 170 grams		
	Protein: 97 grams		
	Fat: 59 grams	**DIETARY EXCHANGES**	Starch: 6
	Saturated Fat: 17 grams		Fruit: 3
	Cholesterol: 178 milligrams		Milk: 1
	Sodium: 1,738 milligrams		Vegetable: 5
	Fiber: 37 grams		Meat: 9
			Fat: 4

Week 1 ■ Friday

BREAKFAST

Breakfast Smoothie with 1 cup 1% milk, 1 cup frozen strawberries, 2 tablespoons fat-free dry milk powder, 1 tablespoon ground flaxseed, and ice cubes

SNACK

1 piece whole grain crispbread

1 ounce string cheese

LUNCH

1 cup lentil soup

½ serving whole grain crackers with 2 ounces sliced turkey

½ cucumber sliced and sprinkled with ground black pepper

SNACK

1 ounce unsalted peanuts

DINNER

1 serving Roasted Flounder with Artichokes (page 256)

Small baked potato topped with 2 tablespoons sour cream and chives

Tossed salad with 1 tablespoon Homemade Salad Dressing (page 54)

4 ounces wine

SNACK

1 cup melon with a dollop of plain low-fat yogurt

DAILY ANALYSIS		CARBOHYDRATE CHOICES	
	Calories: 1,400		10
	Carbohydrate: 148 grams		
	Protein: 85 grams		
	Fat: 52 grams	**DIETARY EXCHANGES**	Starch: 6
	Saturated Fat: 14 grams		Fruit: 2
	Cholesterol: 117 milligrams		Milk: 1
	Sodium: 1,820 milligrams		Vegetable: 4
	Fiber: 27 grams		Meat: 7
			Fat: 5

Week 1 ▪ Saturday

BREAKFAST

    1 Almond and Mixed Berry Muffin with Flaxseed (page 102)

    Herbal tea or coffee

SNACK

    ½ cup sugar snap peas

LUNCH

    1 Chicken-Cranberry Sandwich (page 158)

    1 cup raw green, yellow, and red bell pepper strips

SNACK

    1 kiwifruit

    1 ounce unsalted peanuts

DINNER

    3 ounces baked chicken

    ⅔ cup whole wheat pasta mixed with 1 cup total of sautéed chard, mushrooms, garlic, and onion; ¼ cup marinara sauce; 2 tablespoons grated Parmesan cheese

SNACK

    ½ cup low-fat ice cream topped with 1 teaspoon cocoa powder and 2 tablespoons chopped walnuts

Note: Save 1 Almond and Mixed Berry Muffin with Flaxseed for Monday's breakfast.

DAILY ANALYSIS		CARBOHYDRATE CHOICES	
	Calories: 1,487		10
	Carbohydrate: 156 grams		
	Protein: 92 grams		
	Fat: 55 grams	**DIETARY EXCHANGES**	Starch: 6
	Saturated Fat: 16 grams		Fruit: 2
	Cholesterol: 219 milligrams		Milk: 1
	Sodium: 1,357 milligrams		Vegetable: 3
	Fiber: 32 grams		Meat: 8
			Fat: 6

Week 2

RECIPES FOR WEEK 2

Week 2 ▪ Sunday

BREAKFAST

Veggie omelet with 1 egg and 1 egg white, ½ cup sautéed mixed veggies, and 1 ounce feta cheese

1 slice whole grain toast with 1 teaspoon Better Butter (page 323)

½ grapefruit, sprinkled with 1 teaspoon brown sugar and a pinch of apple pie spice; broiled, if desired

SNACK

1 cup plain low-fat yogurt with ⅛ teaspoon cinnamon and a dash of maple extract (optional)

LUNCH

1 serving (¼ cup) Edamame Hummus (page 116) in 1 small whole wheat pita (filled with chopped lettuce, ½ tomato)

½ cup raw broccoli or cauliflower

SNACK

2 pieces whole grain crispbread with 1 teaspoon cashew butter

DINNER

1 serving Roasted Catfish with Cumin Sweet Potatoes (page 254)

1 large spinach and mushroom salad with chopped onion and ¼ avocado and 1 tablespoon Homemade Salad Dressing (page 54)

SNACK

1 plum and ¼ cup low-fat cottage cheese

Note: Save one serving of Edamame Hummus for Monday's snack.

DAILY ANALYSIS	Calories: 1,570	**CARBOHYDRATE CHOICES**	11
	Carbohydrate: 170 grams		
	Protein: 83 grams		
	Fat: 62 grams	**DIETARY EXCHANGES**	Starch: 5
	Saturated Fat: 16 grams		Fruit: 2
	Cholesterol: 303 milligrams		Milk: 1
	Sodium: 1,583 milligrams		Vegetable: 9
	Fiber: 32 grams		Meat: 8
			Fat: 6

Week 2 ▪ Monday

BREAKFAST

1 Almond and Mixed Berry Muffin with Flaxseed (page 102)

Herbal tea or coffee

SNACK

1 tangerine

6 cashews

LUNCH

1 serving Sloppy Tom Sandwich (page 160)

Salad with mixed greens, celery, and shredded carrots with 1 tablespoon Homemade Salad Dressing (page 54)

SNACK

1 serving Edamame Hummus (page 116)

1 cup raw veggies (baby carrots, green beans, broccoli) to dip in hummus

DINNER

1 serving Dijon Pepper Steak (page 288)

1 cup kale *or* collards sautéed in 3 tablespoons broth and garlic

1 serving Clementine Latte Cotta with Blueberry Sauce (page 332)

SNACK

3 cups popcorn with 1 tablespoon grated Parmesan cheese

DAILY ANALYSIS		CARBOHYDRATE CHOICES	
	Calories: 1,563		10
	Carbohydrate: 152 grams		
	Protein: 97 grams		
	Fat: 63 grams	**DIETARY EXCHANGES**	Starch: 5
	Saturated Fat: 14 grams		Fruit: 2
	Cholesterol: 201 milligrams		Milk: 1
	Sodium: 1,732 milligrams		Vegetable: 6
	Fiber: 25 grams		Meat: 10
			Fat: 4

Week 2 ■ Tuesday

BREAKFAST

1 frozen whole grain waffle with 1 teaspoon Better Butter (page 323), sprinkled with 1 teaspoon confectioners' sugar *or* spread with 1 teaspoon jam

1 cup 1% milk

SNACK

1 small orange

1 ounce string cheese

LUNCH

1 serving Chinese Chicken Salad with Toasted Almonds (page 203)

1 piece whole grain crispbread

SNACK

Fruit smoothie with 1 cup 1% milk, ½ banana, 1 tablespoon ground flaxseed, and ice cubes

DINNER

3 ounces grilled chicken

2 servings Cauliflower, Green Bean, and Tomato Gratin (page 215)

½ cup steamed carrots tossed with chopped fresh mint or parsley

SNACK

½ cup pudding made with 1% milk

DAILY ANALYSIS		**CARBOHYDRATE CHOICES**	10
	Calories: 1,472		
	Carbohydrate: 154 grams		
	Protein: 97 grams		
	Fat: 52 grams	**DIETARY EXCHANGES**	Starch: 3
	Saturated Fat: 15 grams		Fruit: 2
	Cholesterol: 174 milligrams		Milk: 3
	Sodium: 1,267 milligrams		Vegetable: 7
	Fiber: 28 grams		Meat: 7
			Fat: 5

Week 2 ▪ Wednesday

BREAKFAST

½ cup hot oat bran cereal with 1 tablespoon ground flaxseed

1 ounce string cheese — *cooked*

SNACK

1 piece whole grain crispbread topped with ⅛ avocado, 1 slice tomato, and 1 slice onion with fresh basil leaves

LUNCH

1 cup tomato soup made with water

½ serving whole grain crackers

½ cup tuna fish salad with ½ cup tuna, 1 teaspoon mayonnaise, 1 teaspoon chopped onion, and 1 teaspoon celery

½ cup radishes

SNACK

¼ cup grapes, frozen if desired

½ cup low-fat cottage cheese *or* 1 ounce string cheese

DINNER

1 serving Better-for-You Burritos (page 167)

Mixed greens with mushrooms and cauliflower with 1 tablespoon slivered almonds and 1 tablespoon Homemade Salad Dressing (page 54)

SNACK

2 ribs celery with 1 tablespoon peanut butter

DAILY ANALYSIS		CARBOHYDRATE CHOICES	
	Calories: 1,418		9
	Carbohydrate: 145 grams		
	Protein: 97 grams		
	Fat: 50 grams	**DIETARY EXCHANGES**	Starch: 6
	Saturated Fat: 10 grams		Fruit: 1
	Cholesterol: 85 milligrams		Milk: 0
	Sodium: 2,132 milligrams		Vegetable: 6
	Fiber: 33 grams		Meat: 8
			Fat: 6

Week 2 ■ Thursday

BREAKFAST

Raspberry Yogurt Parfait (page 92)

6 almonds, raw or toasted, sprinkled on top

SNACK

½ whole wheat English muffin with 1 teaspoon Better Butter (page 323)

¼ cup low-fat cottage cheese

LUNCH

1 open-faced egg salad sandwich on 1 slice whole grain bread (2 hard-cooked eggs, use one yolk, 2 teaspoons chopped onion, 2 teaspoons chopped celery, and 1 teaspoon mayonnaise)

1 cup chopped tomato and cucumber salad with lemon juice and 1 teaspoon chopped fresh basil

1 ounce dark chocolate

SNACK

¼ cup cut-up mango

4 walnut halves, toasted if desired

DINNER

1 serving Salmon with White Bean and Citrus Salad (page 245)

Spinach salad with 1 tablespoon Homemade Salad Dressing (page 54)

SNACK

3 cups popcorn with 1 tablespoon grated Parmesan cheese

DAILY ANALYSIS	Calories: 1,386	**CARBOHYDRATE CHOICES**	9
	Carbohydrate: 142 grams		
	Protein: 83 grams		
	Fat: 54 grams	**DIETARY EXCHANGES**	Starch: 5
	Saturated Fat: 16 grams		Fruit: 2
	Cholesterol: 308 milligrams		Milk: 1
	Sodium: 1,784 milligrams		Vegetable: 5
	Fiber: 26 grams		Meat: 7
			Fat: 6

Week 2 ■ Friday

BREAKFAST

1 slice whole grain toast *or* ½ whole wheat English muffin with 1 teaspoon almond butter

1 cup 1% milk

SNACK

1 ounce cashews

LUNCH

1 large salad with mixed greens; chopped peppers and broccoli florets; 1 ounce feta, goat, or blue cheese; 3 ounces cut-up chicken; ¼ sliced avocado; and 1 tablespoon Homemade Salad Dressing (page 54)

2 pieces whole grain crispbread

SNACK

½ cup plain low-fat yogurt with ½ cup crushed pineapple

DINNER

1 serving Five-Spice Pork Medallions (page 296)

½ cup mashed sweet potato

½ cup steamed green beans with lemon juice

4 ounces wine

SNACK

1 cup watermelon

DAILY ANALYSIS			
Calories: 1,436		**CARBOHYDRATE CHOICES**	10
Carbohydrate: 152 grams			
Protein: 90 grams			
Fat: 52 grams		**DIETARY EXCHANGES**	Starch: 4
Saturated Fat: 15 grams			Fruit: 2
Cholesterol: 189 milligrams			Milk: 2
Sodium: 1,390 milligrams			Vegetable: 6
Fiber: 23 grams			Meat: 8
			Fat: 5

Week 2 ■ Saturday

BREAKFAST

Breakfast Burrito with 1 whole wheat tortilla; ¼ cup black beans; ½ ounce shredded extra sharp Cheddar cheese; 1 egg and 1 egg white, scrambled; and 2 tablespoons Salsa Fresca (page 119)

SNACK

1 cup raw veggies dipped in 1 tablespoon Homemade Salad Dressing (page 54)

LUNCH

1 serving Herb and Mesclun Salad with Grilled Shrimp (page 200)

1 nectarine

1 cup 1% milk

SNACK

2 graham cracker squares with 2 teaspoons cream cheese or peanut butter

DINNER

1 serving Sage Turkey Cutlets with Squash (page 282)

½ cup steamed asparagus with lemon juice and red-pepper flakes

SNACK

1 serving Chocolate Strawberries (page 330)

DAILY ANALYSIS		CARBOHYDRATE CHOICES	10
	Calories: 1,435		
	Carbohydrate: 149 grams		
	Protein: 95 grams		
	Fat: 51 grams	DIETARY EXCHANGES	Starch: 5
	Saturated Fat: 15 grams		Fruit: 2
	Cholesterol: 502 milligrams		Milk: 1
	Sodium: 1,680 milligrams		Vegetable: 6
	Fiber: 32 grams		Meat: 9
			Fat: 4

PHASE 2

- Meal plans are between 1,400 and 1,600 calories, 45 to 60 percent carbohydrate, 15 to 25 percent protein, and 25 to 35 percent fat and include three meals (breakfast, lunch, and dinner) and three snacks.
- Fiber: minimum 30 grams per day

Week 3

RECIPES FOR WEEK 3

Mixed Berry Muesli (page 94)

Strawberry-Banana Topped French Toast (page 98)

Bacon, Spinach, and Tomato Scrambled Eggs (page 108)

Golden Pepper Dip (page 126)

Blue Cheese–Walnut Spread on Asian Pear Slices (page 129)

Double-Cheese Double-Stuffed Pizza Pockets (page 150)

Salad Pita (page 164)

Chocolate-Dipped Almond Apricot Pouches (page 171)

Candied Spiced Nuts (page 173)

Autumn Harvest Minestrone (page 178)

Hearty Chickpea Soup (page 180)

Farmers' Market Pasta Salad (page 187)

Wheat Berry Salad with Red Pepper, Eggplant, and Zucchini (page 196)

Warm Quinoa Salad (page 198)

Stir-Fried Curly Kale (page 225)

Poached Halibut in Vegetable Broth (page 244)

Tangerine-Sesame Noodles with Seared Scallops (page 257)

Kidney Beans and Beef Chili (page 285)

Steak Burgers (page 290)

Magic Lasagna (page 302)

Chocolate Almond Biscotti (page 350)

Week 3 ■ Sunday

BREAKFAST

1 serving Strawberry-Banana Topped French Toast (page 98)

1 cup herbal tea or coffee

SNACK

½ cup steamed edamame (unshelled)

LUNCH

1 serving Double-Cheese Double-Stuffed Pizza Pockets (page 150)

Tossed salad with a splash of balsamic vinegar

SNACK

1 Chocolate Almond Biscotti (page 350)

1 cup 1% milk

DINNER

3 ounces grilled salmon with lemon and garlic

1 serving Wheat Berry Salad with Red Pepper, Eggplant, and Zucchini (page 196)

½ cup grilled asparagus

SNACK

½ cup plain low-fat yogurt mixed with 1 chopped date

Note: Save 2 Chocolate Almond Biscotti for Monday and 2 for Tuesday.

DAILY ANALYSIS		CARBOHYDRATE CHOICES	13
	Calories: 1,627		
	Carbohydrate: 195 grams		
	Protein: 88 grams	**DIETARY EXCHANGES**	Starch: 9
	Fat: 55 grams		Fruit: 1
	Saturated Fat: 14 grams		Milk: 1
	Cholesterol: 246 milligrams		Vegetable: 6
	Sodium: 1,251 milligrams		Meat: 6
	Fiber: 30 grams		Fat: 6

Week 3 ▪ Monday

BREAKFAST

½ serving Mixed Berry Muesli (page 94)

1 cup herbal tea or coffee

SNACK

½ serving whole grain crackers

½ tablespoon almond butter

LUNCH

1 cup low-sodium vegetable soup

1 chicken salad sandwich with 2 slices 100 percent whole wheat bread, 2 ounces chicken, 1 teaspoon mayonnaise, 1 tablespoon chopped celery, spinach leaves, and sliced tomato

SNACK

2 Chocolate Almond Biscotti (page 350)

DINNER

1 serving Tangerine-Sesame Noodles with Seared Scallops (page 257)

½ cup steamed broccoli drizzled with balsamic vinegar and red-pepper flakes

SNACK

1 small baked apple with 1 teaspoon brown sugar and a sprinkling of cinnamon

DAILY ANALYSIS		CARBOHYDRATE CHOICES	
	Calories: 1,641		15
	Carbohydrate: 229 grams		
	Protein: 71 grams		
	Fat: 49 grams (27%)	**DIETARY EXCHANGES**	Starch: 12
	Saturated Fat: 7 grams (4%)		Fruit: 1
	Cholesterol: 107 milligrams		Milk: 0
	Sodium: 2,159 milligrams		Vegetable: 6
	Fiber: 34 grams		Meat: 5
			Fat: 4

Week 3 ▪ Tuesday

BREAKFAST

1 egg sandwich on a whole wheat English muffin with ½ ounce Cheddar cheese, ½ ounce Canadian bacon, and 1 poached egg

SNACK

1 small orange

LUNCH

1 serving Hearty Chickpea Soup (page 180)

2 pieces whole grain crispbread spread with 2 teaspoons cream cheese

½ cup sliced yellow or red peppers and scallions

1 cup soymilk (or 1% milk)

SNACK

½ cup unsweetened applesauce mixed with several dashes cinnamon

1 Chocolate Almond Biscotti (page 350)

DINNER

1 serving Steak Burgers (page 290)

Oven fries (1 medium potato, sliced lengthwise, drizzled with 1 teaspoon olive oil, sprinkled with pepper, and baked in 375°F oven until crisp)

½ cup homemade or delicatessen coleslaw

SNACK

1 Chocolate Almond Biscotti (page 350)

DAILY ANALYSIS	Calories: 1,576	**CARBOHYDRATE CHOICES**	13
	Carbohydrate: 198 grams		
	Protein: 79 grams		
	Fat: 52 grams	**DIETARY EXCHANGES**	Starch: 9
	Saturated Fat: 15 grams		Fruit: 2
	Cholesterol: 353 milligrams		Milk: 1
	Sodium: 2,399 milligrams		Vegetable: 3
	Fiber: 33 grams		Meat: 6
			Fat: 5

Week 3 ■ Wednesday

BREAKFAST

½ cup steel-cut oatmeal with 1 tablespoon ground flaxseed, ½ cup plain low-fat yogurt, and 1 teaspoon raspberry jam or all-fruit spread. Top with 1 slice kiwifruit.

SNACK

1 serving Chocolate-Dipped Almond Apricot Pouches (page 171)

LUNCH

1 serving Salad Pita (page 164)

½ ounce almonds, raw or toasted

SNACK

1 cup raw veggies with 1 serving Golden Pepper Dip (page 126)

DINNER

3 ounces grilled chicken

1 serving Warm Quinoa Salad (page 198)

1 serving Stir-Fried Curly Kale (page 225)

SNACK

Soymilk smoothie with 1 cup soymilk, ½ peach, and ice cubes

DAILY ANALYSIS		CARBOHYDRATE CHOICES	
	Calories: 1,620		14
	Carbohydrate: 214 grams		
	Protein: 83 grams		
	Fat: 48 grams	**DIETARY EXCHANGES**	Starch: 8
	Saturated Fat: 9 grams		Fruit: 2
	Cholesterol: 90 milligrams		Milk: 2
	Sodium: 1,263 milligrams		Vegetable: 6
	Fiber: 40 grams		Meat: 5
			Fat: 5

Week 3 ▪ Thursday

BREAKFAST

2 slices whole grain toast with 1 teaspoon Better Butter (page 323) and 1 teaspoon jam *or* all-fruit spread

SNACK

1 cup plain low-fat yogurt with 4 chopped dried apricots

LUNCH

1 serving Farmers' Market Pasta Salad (page 187)

1 cup strawberries

SNACK

1 serving Candied Spiced Nuts (page 173)

DINNER

1 serving Kidney Beans and Beef Chili (page 285)

1 small whole grain roll with 1 teaspoon Better Butter (page 323)

Chiffonade-cut savoy cabbage with 1 tablespoon Homemade Salad Dressing (page 54)

SNACK

1 cup honeydew melon topped with 1 tablespoon plain low-fat yogurt

DAILY ANALYSIS		CARBOHYDRATE CHOICES	
	Calories: 1,447		12
	Carbohydrate: 183 grams		
	Protein: 64 grams		
	Fat: 51 grams	DIETARY EXCHANGES	Starch: 6
	Saturated Fat: 12 grams		Fruit: 3
	Cholesterol: 64 milligrams		Milk: 1
	Sodium: 1,486 milligrams		Vegetable: 6
	Fiber: 30 grams		Meat: 3
			Fat: 7

Week 3 ▪ Friday

BREAKFAST

½ cup hot oat bran cereal with 2 tablespoons raisins and 1 tablespoon ground flaxseed

SNACK

½ cup baby carrots dipped in 2 tablespoons hummus

LUNCH

Chop-chop salad with chopped lettuce, spinach, and veggies; 1 ounce turkey; 1 ounce ham; and ¼ avocado with 1 tablespoon Homemade Salad Dressing (page 54)

2 pieces whole grain crispbread

½ cup grapes, frozen if desired

SNACK

1 ounce whole grain tortilla chips with ¼ cup salsa

DINNER

1 serving Poached Halibut in Vegetable Broth (page 244)

1 small baked sweet potato with 1 teaspoon Better Butter (page 323)

4 ounces wine

SNACK

1 cup homemade hot chocolate. Mix 1 cup 1% milk or soymilk, 2 teaspoons unsweetened cocoa powder, 2 teaspoons sugar, and a splash of vanilla extract. Heat in microwave for 1–2 minutes.

DAILY ANALYSIS	**CARBOHYDRATE CHOICES**	
Calories: 1,431	11	
Carbohydrate: 175 grams		
Protein: 59 grams		
Fat: 55 grams	**DIETARY EXCHANGES**	Starch: 6
Saturated Fat: 10 grams		Fruit: 2
Cholesterol: 94 milligrams		Milk: 1
Sodium: 1,815 milligrams		Vegetable: 6
Fiber: 32 grams		Meat: 5
		Fat: 6

Week 3 ▪ Saturday

BRUNCH

    1 serving Bacon, Spinach, and Tomato Scrambled Eggs (page 108)

    ½ whole grain English muffin with 1 teaspoon Better Butter (page 323)

    ½ grapefruit

LUNCH

    2 servings Autumn Harvest Minestrone (page 178)

    Mixed greens with 1 tablespoon Homemade Salad Dressing (page 54)

SNACK

    1 serving Blue Cheese–Walnut Spread on Asian Pear Slices (page 129)

DINNER

    1 serving Magic Lasagna (page 302)

    1 cup stir-fried cauliflower with 1 teaspoon olive oil, a splash of balsamic vinegar, and red-pepper flakes, if desired

SNACK

    ½ cup tapioca pudding made with 1% milk, drizzled with 1 teaspoon maple syrup

Note: Save 1 serving Autumn Harvest Minestrone for Sunday's dinner.

DAILY ANALYSIS		CARBOHYDRATE CHOICES	
	Calories: 1,591		12
	Carbohydrate: 187 grams		
	Protein: 69 grams		
	Fat: 63 grams	**DIETARY EXCHANGES**	Starch: 7
	Saturated Fat: 18 grams		Fruit: 2
	Cholesterol: 371 milligrams		Milk: 1
	Sodium: 2,357 milligrams		Vegetable: 6
	Fiber: 33 grams		Meat: 7
			Fat: 5

Week 4

RECIPES FOR WEEK 4

Green Tea, Blueberry, and Banana Smoothies (page 95)

Baked Rice and Raisin Pudding (page 96)

Salsa Fresca (page 119)

Creamy Chipotle Spread on Cucumber Slices (page 128)

Turkey Couscous Roll-Ups (page 138)

Roasted Vegetable Sandwich (page 162)

Autumn Harvest Minestrone (page 178)

Garden Vegetable Soup with Grilled Chicken (page 183)

Cajun Blackened Zucchini (page 218)

Roasted Root Vegetables (page 231)

Wild Pacific Salmon with Creamy Avocado Sauce (page 240)

Mediterranean Cod (page 250)

Chinese Beef and Rice (page 292)

Cinnamon-Rubbed Pork Loin with Roasted Apples and Onions (page 294)

Broccoli and Tofu Stir-Fry with Toasted Almonds (page 301)

Provençal Lentil Ragout (page 313)

Red, White, and Blue Cheesecake (page 334)

Dark Chocolate Mint Cookie Bars (page 352)

Week 4 ▪ Sunday

BREAKFAST

1 serving Baked Rice and Raisin Pudding (page 96)

1 cup blackberries topped with 1 tablespoon plain low-fat yogurt and 1 teaspoon maple syrup

SNACK

¼ cup mandarin oranges mixed with ¼ cup low-fat cottage cheese

LUNCH

1 serving Roasted Vegetable Sandwich (page 162)

SNACK

Peanut butter and banana (slice small banana lengthwise, spread ½ tablespoon peanut butter, top with other half of banana, freeze if desired)

DINNER

1 serving Autumn Harvest Minestrone (page 178)

1 serving Mediterranean Cod (page 250)

½ cup steamed Brussels sprouts

1 serving Red, White, and Blue Cheesecake (page 334)

SNACK

1 cup 1% milk

Note: Save 2 servings Baked Rice and Raisin Pudding for Monday's breakfast.

DAILY ANALYSIS		CARBOHYDRATE CHOICES	
	Calories: 1,595		14
	Carbohydrate: 209 grams		
	Protein: 102 grams		
	Fat: 39 grams	**DIETARY EXCHANGES**	Starch: 7
	Saturated Fat: 14 grams		Fruit: 3
	Cholesterol: 253 milligrams		Milk: 2
	Sodium: 2,049 milligrams		Vegetable: 6
	Fiber: 32 grams		Meat: 5
			Fat: 5

Week 4 ▪ Monday

BREAKFAST

2 servings Baked Rice and Raisin Pudding (page 96)

SNACK

3 cups popcorn, with salt-free Cajun or other favorite seasoning

LUNCH

Ham and cheese sandwich with 2 ounces ham, 1 ounce cheese, 1 teaspoon mustard or mayonnaise, lettuce and tomato, and whole grain bread

1 cup raw sugar snap peas, yellow peppers, and cherry tomatoes

1 small apple

SNACK

1 cup plain low-fat yogurt topped with ¼ cup fruit cocktail

DINNER

1 serving Broccoli and Tofu Stir-Fry with Toasted Almonds (page 301)

Mixed green salad with 1 tablespoon Homemade Salad Dressing (page 54)

1 cup 1% milk

SNACK

1 cup blackberries topped with 1 tablespoon plain low-fat yogurt and 1 teaspoon brown sugar

DAILY ANALYSIS		
Calories: 1,548	**CARBOHYDRATE CHOICES**	14.5
Carbohydrate: 223 grams		
Protein: 83 grams		
Fat: 36 grams	**DIETARY EXCHANGES**	Starch: 6
Saturated Fat: 10 grams		Fruit: 3
Cholesterol: 118 milligrams		Milk: 4
Sodium: 2,027 milligrams		Vegetable: 5
Fiber: 30 grams		Meat: 5
		Fat: 3

Week 4 ▪ Tuesday

BREAKFAST

1 whole grain frozen waffle with 1 teaspoon Better Butter (page 323) and 1 teaspoon confectioners' sugar

1 cup 1% milk

SNACK

½ cup sliced mango

6 almonds

LUNCH

Spinach salad with 2 ounces sardines, ¼ cup red beans, sliced mushrooms, scallions, sliced red pepper, and 1 tablespoon Homemade Salad Dressing (page 54)

3 pieces whole grain crispbread

1 small pear

SNACK

½ turkey sandwich with 1 slice whole grain bread, 1 teaspoon mustard, 1 ounce turkey, lettuce, and tomato

DINNER

1 cup whole wheat pasta with ½ cup (1 ounce ground beef) meat sauce and 1 tablespoon grated Parmesan or Romano cheese

½ cup steamed asparagus

½ cup sliced navel oranges and red onions drizzled with 1 teaspoon extra virgin olive oil

SNACK

½ cup low-fat ice cream

DAILY ANALYSIS		CARBOHYDRATE CHOICES	13
	Calories: 1,461		
	Carbohydrate: 195 grams		
	Protein: 69 grams		
	Fat: 45 grams	DIETARY EXCHANGES	Starch: 7
	Saturated Fat: 11 grams		Fruit: 3
	Cholesterol: 153 milligrams		Milk: 2
	Sodium: 2,282 milligrams		Vegetable: 3
	Fiber: 35 grams		Meat: 3
			Fat: 5

Week 4 ■ Wednesday

BREAKFAST

½ serving (8 ounces) Green Tea, Blueberry, and Banana Smoothie (page 95)

1 hard-cooked egg

SNACK

1 cup plain low-fat yogurt sprinkled with 1 teaspoon brown sugar and a sprinkling of cinnamon

LUNCH

1 serving Turkey Couscous Roll-Ups (page 138)

1 cup raw veggies plain *or* dipped in ½ tablespoon Homemade Salad Dressing (page 54)

SNACK

½ serving (8 ounces) Green Tea, Blueberry, and Banana Smoothie

DINNER

2 servings Provençal Lentil Ragout (page 313)

Radicchio salad with 1 tablespoon Homemade Salad Dressing (page 54)

1 Dark Chocolate Mint Cookie Bar (page 352)

SNACK

1 cup cut-up fresh fruit topped with 1 tablespoon plain low-fat yogurt and 1 tablespoon chopped walnuts

Note: Save the other ½ serving (8 ounces) Green Tea, Blueberry, and Banana Smoothie for midafternoon snack.

DAILY ANALYSIS	
Calories: 1,640	
Carbohydrate: 242 grams	
Protein: 78 grams	
Fat: 40 grams	
Saturated Fat: 8 grams	
Cholesterol: 260 milligrams	
Sodium: 1,623 milligrams	
Fiber: 46 grams	

CARBOHYDRATE CHOICES	15.5

DIETARY EXCHANGES	
Starch: 7	
Fruit: 4	
Milk: 3	
Vegetable: 5	
Meat: 5	
Fat: 3	

Week 4 ▪ Thursday

BREAKFAST

½ cup steel-cut oats with 1 tablespoon ground flaxseed

1 slice whole grain toast with 1 teaspoon almond butter

SNACK

½ cup pineapple chunks

1 ounce string cheese

LUNCH

1 serving Garden Vegetable Soup with Grilled Chicken (page 183)

½ serving whole grain crackers

¾ cup radish and broccoli stems cut into coins

SNACK

2 servings Creamy Chipotle Spread on Cucumber Slices (page 128)

½ serving whole grain crackers

DINNER

1 serving Chinese Beef and Rice (page 292)

½ cup additional fried rice

1 cup steamed bok choy

SNACK

1 cup 1% milk

2 graham cracker squares

Note: Save 2 servings Creamy Chipotle Spread on Cucumber Slices for Friday morning snack.

DAILY ANALYSIS	CARBOHYDRATE CHOICES	
Calories: 1,539	12	
Carbohydrate: 190 grams		
Protein: 89 grams		
Fat: 47 grams	**DIETARY EXCHANGES**	Starch: 8
Saturated Fat: 12 grams		Fruit: 1
Cholesterol: 122 milligrams		Milk: 1
Sodium: 1,630 milligrams		Vegetable: 8
Fiber: 30 grams		Meat: 7
		Fat: 4

Week 4 ■ Friday

BREAKFAST

½ cup rolled oatmeal with 1 tablespoon ground flaxseed topped with ½ cup plain low-fat yogurt, 1 tablespoon dried cranberries, and 2 tablespoons slivered almonds

SNACK

2 servings Creamy Chipotle Spread on Cucumber Slices (page 128)

LUNCH

1 cup low-sodium black bean *or* split pea soup

½ turkey sandwich on whole grain bread with lettuce, 2 ounces turkey, 1 slice tomato, and 1 teaspoon mustard

SNACK

1 cup mixed berries topped with 1 tablespoon plain low-fat yogurt

DINNER

1 serving Wild Pacific Salmon with Creamy Avocado Sauce (page 240)

2 servings Cajun Blackened Zucchini (page 218)

2 servings Roasted Root Vegetables (page 231)

4 ounces wine

SNACK

½ cup low-fat ice cream

DAILY ANALYSIS		CARBOHYDRATE CHOICES	
Calories: 1,466		11	
Carbohydrate: 171 grams			
Protein: 92 grams			
Fat: 46 grams	**DIETARY EXCHANGES**	Starch: 7	
Saturated Fat: 7 grams		Fruit: 2	
Cholesterol: 134 milligrams		Milk: 1	
Sodium: 2,179 milligrams		Vegetable: 4	
Fiber: 31 grams		Meat: 8	
		Fat: 4	

Week 4 ■ Saturday

BRUNCH

1 poached egg

1 whole wheat English muffin *or* 2 slices whole grain toast

1 teaspoon Better Butter (page 323)

1 ounce Canadian bacon

LUNCH

Healthy nachos with 1 ounce whole grain tortilla chips; ½ cup pinto, black, or low-fat refried beans; ½ ounce shredded extra-sharp Cheddar cheese. Heat in oven or microwave. Top with 1 serving Salsa Fresca (page 119) and ⅛ avocado, sliced.

SNACK

1 tangerine

DINNER

1 serving Cinnamon-Rubbed Pork Loin with Roasted Apples and Onions (page 294)

½ cup cooked quinoa

Tossed salad with 1 tablespoon Homemade Salad Dressing (page 54)

SNACK

½ cup plain low-fat yogurt blended with ½ cup blackberries and ¼ teaspoon apple pie spice, frozen if desired

DAILY ANALYSIS		CARBOHYDRATE CHOICES	12
	Calories: 1,589		
	Carbohydrate: 182 grams		
	Protein: 87 grams		
	Fat: 57 grams	**DIETARY EXCHANGES**	Starch: 7
	Saturated Fat: 17 grams		Fruit: 2
	Cholesterol: 351 milligrams		Milk: 1
	Sodium: 1,389 milligrams		Vegetable: 6
	Fiber: 27 grams		Meat: 7
			Fat: 5

MAINTAINING YOUR IDEAL WEIGHT

Congratulations! You have reached your goal weight and plan to stay here for the rest of your life. Hopefully, you also have more energy and vitality than you've had in years. That's incentive enough to keep up your healthy ways.

Now that you've reached your weight goal, it's time to increase calories to maintain your weight. To get started, you can follow the Phase 2 menus, increasing the size or number of snacks or increasing portion sizes at meals. Since one of the goals is to maintain good blood glucose control, continue monitoring your glucose levels as you make dietary changes and adjust food choices and portion sizes as necessary.

To fully realize the benefits of fiber-rich whole foods, we suggest increasing high-fiber foods to reach a fiber goal of 50 grams per day. Some ways to increase your intake of high-fiber foods are:

- Add an extra serving or two of nuts, popcorn, whole grain crackers, or whole grain tortilla chips.
- Increase the portion size of whole grain pasta, brown rice, millet, barley, or quinoa to 1 to 1½ cups.
- Add fruit to hot cereal at breakfast.
- Add one serving of dried fruit to plain low-fat yogurt.
- Make fruit smoothies for snacks using berries, 1 cup low-fat milk, ground flaxseed, and ½ cup low-fat ice cream.
- Have a snack of natural peanut butter and whole grain crackers.
- Increase portion sizes of beans to 1 cup.

Increasing fiber foods will also increase the amount of carbohydrate in your diet. Remember to spread out carbohydrates throughout the day to keep blood glucose levels on target. Two to four servings of carbohydrate per meal for women and four to five servings per meal for men is reasonable. By testing your glucose levels, you can determine the appropriate amount of carbohydrate for you.

If you prefer not to increase carbohydrate in your meals, you can increase the amount of lean protein in a meal by 1 to 2 ounces or add an extra one to two servings of a healthy fat like ¼ avocado, 1 tablespoon salad dressing, or 1 tablespoon olive oil for stir-frying.

Soon it will become second nature to select just the perfect mix of whole foods that's right for your body.

CHAPTER 6

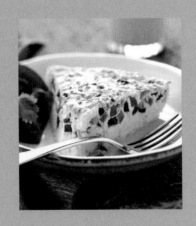

BREAKFASTS

SEASONAL FRUIT SALAD

The local fruits of summer will taste the best. Feel free to vary the selections in this recipe by replacing plums with peaches, blueberries with strawberries, or honeydew with cantaloupe.

Preparation time: 10 minutes

 1 medium plum, sliced
½ cup blueberries
½ medium nectarine, sliced
⅛ honeydew
⅛ teaspoon ground nutmeg
 2 tablespoons apricot nectar

In a small bowl, combine the plum, blueberries, and nectarine. Stir to mix. Sprinkle the fruit mixture over the honeydew. In a small bowl, whisk the nutmeg into the nectar. Drizzle over the fruit.

MAKES 1 SERVING

Per serving: 193 calories, 47 g carbohydrate, 3 g protein, 1 g fat, 0 g saturated fat, 0 mg cholesterol, 31 mg sodium, 5 g fiber

Carbohydrate Choices: 3

Dietary Exchanges: 3 fruit

RASPBERRY YOGURT PARFAIT

If you can spare some added calories, toss some chopped toasted walnuts atop this refreshing breakfast bowl.

Preparation time: 5 minutes

½ cup red raspberries, fresh or (thawed) frozen
 1 teaspoon lemon juice
 1 cup low-fat plain yogurt

In a small bowl, combine the raspberries and lemon juice. Toss. In a parfait dish, alternate layers of yogurt and raspberries.

MAKES 1 SERVING

Per serving: 190 calories, 29 g carbohydrate, 15 g protein, 3 g fat, 1.5 g saturated fat, 15 mg cholesterol, 190 mg sodium, 4 g fiber

Carbohydrate Choices: 2

Dietary Exchanges: ½ fruit, 2 milk

PEAR CRISP WITH CREAMY ORANGE SAUCE

If you like, you can bake this special fruit dish and prepare the sauce ahead of serving. Refrigerate separately for several days. Reheat individual servings of the crisp on a microwaveable plate and then top with the sauce.

Preparation time: 25 minutes ● **Baking time: 55 minutes**

FRUIT

- 1 tablespoon confectioners' sugar
- 2 teaspoons cornstarch
- 4 cups (about 2 pounds) peeled and sliced Anjou or Bartlett pears
- 2 teaspoons vanilla extract

TOPPING

- ½ cup old-fashioned oats
- 2 tablespoons slivered almonds
- ¼ teaspoon ground nutmeg
- 2 tablespoons cold Better Butter (page 323) or trans-fat free spread

SAUCE

- 1 cup fat-free plain yogurt
- 1 tablespoon maple syrup
- ¼ teaspoon orange extract

1. Preheat the oven to 350°F. Coat an 8" x 8" baking dish with vegetable oil spray. Set aside.

2. To prepare the fruit: In a bowl, combine the confectioners' sugar and cornstarch. Stir until well blended. Add the pears and vanilla. Toss to coat evenly. Transfer to the reserved dish. Set aside.

3. To prepare the topping: Wipe the bowl dry with a paper towel. Add the oats, almonds, and nutmeg. Toss with a fork to mix. With the fork, break the Better Butter or spread into small chunks. Add to the mixture. Use the fork to cut into smaller pieces that blend with the oats mixture. Sprinkle over the reserved fruit. Bake for about 55 minutes, or until bubbly.

4. To prepare the sauce: In a small bowl, combine the yogurt, syrup, and extract. Stir to mix. Serve the crisp warm or at room temperature, topped with the sauce.

MAKES 9 SERVINGS

Per serving: 124 calories, 23 g carbohydrate, 3 g protein, 3 g fat, 1 g saturated fat, 0 mg cholesterol, 37 mg sodium, 4 g fiber

Carbohydrate Choices: 1½

Dietary Exchanges: 1 fruit, ½ fat

NOTES: Select pears that are ripe but still somewhat firm to the touch for this crisp. They will soften during baking. For additional fiber and nutrients, scrub the pears but leave the peel on.

Apples, plums, nectarines, or peaches can replace the pears. The baking time may vary depending upon the type of fruit.

Grated orange peel can replace or be added to the orange extract in the sauce.

MIXED BERRY MUESLI

Did you know you don't always have to cook oatmeal? In this fast breakfast, all that's required is to mix the oats into yogurt, then combine with fruit and nuts.

Preparation time: 7 minutes

1 cup fat-free vanilla yogurt

2 tablespoons old-fashioned oats

2 tablespoons chopped walnuts

¼ cup blueberries, fresh or (thawed) frozen

¼ cup raspberries, fresh or (thawed) frozen

½ small cantaloupe, seeds removed

1. In a medium bowl, combine the yogurt and oats. Stir well to mix. Fold in the walnuts and then gently fold in the berries.

2. Cut the melon into 2 wedges. Scoop the yogurt mixture over each wedge.

MAKES 2 SERVINGS

Per serving: 226 calories, 38 g carbohydrate, 9 g protein, 6 g fat, 1 g saturated fat, 2 mg cholesterol, 96 mg sodium, 4 g fiber

Carbohydrate Choices: 2½

Dietary Exchanges: 2 starch, 1 fruit, 1 fat

ORANGE, DRIED PLUM, AND ALMOND COMPOTE

A mélange of juicy fresh fruit, sweet dried fruit, and protein-rich nuts is a healthy addition to the morning meal.

Preparation time: 4 minutes

1 navel orange

⅓ cup canned crushed pineapple with juice

6 dried plums, cut into slivers

¼ teaspoon almond extract

2 tablespoons slivered almonds

Peel the orange and separate into sections. Cut the sections into small pieces. Transfer to a bowl. Add the pineapple, plums, and extract. Sprinkle the almonds on each serving.

MAKES 3 SERVINGS

Per serving: 95 calories, 19 g carbohydrate, 2 g protein, 2 g fat, 0 g saturated fat, 0 mg cholesterol, 2 mg sodium, 3 g fiber

Carbohydrate Choices: 1

Dietary Exchanges: 1 fruit, ½ fat

GREEN TEA, BLUEBERRY, AND BANANA SMOOTHIES

This nutritious beverage is a healthful snack or breakfast on the go. Since it's easier to prepare 2 servings at one time, just store the extra serving in a closed glass jar in the refrigerator.

Preparation time: 5 minutes

3	tablespoons water
1	green tea bag
2	teaspoons honey
1½	cups frozen blueberries
½	medium banana
¾	cup calcium-fortified light vanilla soymilk

1. In a small glass measuring cup or bowl, microwave water on high until steaming hot. Add the tea bag and allow to brew for 3 minutes. Remove the tea bag. Stir the honey into the tea until it dissolves.

2. In a blender with ice-crushing ability, combine the berries, banana, and soymilk.

3. Add the tea to the blender. Blend ingredients on ice crush or the highest setting until smooth. (Some blenders may require additional water to process the mixture.) Pour the smoothie into tall glasses and serve.

MAKES 2 SERVINGS

Per serving: 150 calories, 35 g carbohydrate, 2 g protein, 2 g fat, 0 g saturated fat, 0 mg cholesterol, 37 mg sodium, 4 g fiber

Carbohydrate Choices: 2

Dietary Exchanges: ½ starch, 1½ fruit, ½ milk

NOTE: You can transport this smoothie to work with you to enjoy for a snack. If stored several hours in a thermos, shake vigorously before pouring. The smoothie will be tasty but thinner than when freshly made.

BAKED RICE AND RAISIN PUDDING

Make this on a weekend afternoon or some evening while you're doing other activities. It takes only a few minutes to assemble and then requires no attention as it bakes and cools. Enjoy it for breakfast or snacks all through the week.

Preparation time: 8 minutes ● **Baking time: 1 hour 15 minutes**

---

2   cans (12 ounces each) evaporated fat-free milk

3   tablespoons raisins

1   tablespoon ground flaxseed

½   teaspoon cinnamon

1   egg

2   teaspoons vanilla extract

½   cup regular brown rice

8   teaspoons brown sugar or honey

1. Preheat the oven to 325°F. Lightly coat an 8" × 8" baking dish with canola oil spray. Heat the milk in a small saucepan for about 3 minutes, or until hot but not boiling.

2. In a spice grinder or small food processor fitted with a metal blade, combine the raisins, flaxseed, and cinnamon. Process for about 2 minutes, or until the raisins are finely chopped. Place in the baking dish.

3. In a mixing bowl, beat the egg with a fork. Add about ½ cup of the milk, beating constantly, to warm the egg. Add the remaining milk and the vanilla. Stir to mix. Pour into the baking dish. Add the rice. Stir with a fork. Cover with aluminum foil.

4. Bake for 1 hour and 15 minutes. Turn off the heat. Let stand in the oven for 30 minutes. Serve right away or cool to room temperature before refrigerating. Serve cold or warm garnished with 1 teaspoon brown sugar or honey.

MAKES 8 SERVINGS

Per serving: 160 calories, 28 g carbohydrate, 7 g protein, 2 g fat, 0 g saturated fat, 25 mg cholesterol, 120 mg sodium, 1 g fiber

Carbohydrate Choices: 2

Dietary Exchanges: 1 starch, 1 milk

NOW YOU KNOW

When going for flaxseed, select the ground seeds, which make the nutrients more accessible. Keep a bag of nutritious ground flaxseed in your refrigerator. Adding just a tablespoon or two to baked goods or hot cereal will increase your intake of omega-3 fatty acids and fiber. Ground flaxseed is sold in natural food stores and many supermarkets.

ENGLISH MUFFINS TOASTED WITH CINNAMON CHEESE AND MAPLE APPLES

The elements are simple and few, but they combine to create a wonderful result in this quick morning meal. You can cut the recipe in half if you're eating solo.

Preparation time: 2 minutes ● **Cooking time: 2 minutes**

- 1 whole grain English muffin
- ¼ cup 1% dry-curd cottage cheese
  Ground cinnamon
- 6 apple slices (about 1½ ounces)
- 1 teaspoon maple syrup

1. Split the muffin and place on a broiler pan or sheet of heavy-duty aluminum foil. Spread the cottage cheese evenly over the muffin halves. Sprinkle to taste with cinnamon. Cover with the apple slices in a single layer. Drizzle ½ teaspoon syrup over the apples on each half.

2. Broil 6" from the heat source for about 2 minutes, or until the apples start to sizzle. Serve right away.

MAKES 2 SERVINGS

Per serving: 110 calories, 19 g carbohydrate, 8 g protein, 1 g fat, 0 g saturated fat, 2 mg cholesterol, 124 mg sodium, 3 g fiber

Carbohydrate Choices: 1

Dietary Exchanges: 1 starch, 1 meat

NOTE: It's hard to beat low-fat cottage cheese as a source of lean protein. Just ½ cup contains a mere 81 calories, 1 gram of fat, and 14 grams of protein.

FILL UP ON WHOLE FOODS

Grains of Truth

Whole grains, the seeds of various grass plants, provide important nutrients and fiber. Each of the three parts of a seed plays a role in nourishing you.

- **Bran.** The outer layer or the skin of the wheat seed is a rich source of niacin, thiamine, riboflavin, magnesium, phosphorus, iron, zinc, and fiber.

- **Germ.** A concentrated source of energy, the germ is designed to nourish the new wheat plant after it sprouts. It includes niacin, thiamine, riboflavin, vitamin E, magnesium, phosphorus, iron, zinc, protein, and some fat.

- **Endosperm.** The biggest part, containing most of the protein and carbohydrate but the fewest vitamins and minerals. All-purpose flour is mostly the endosperm.

STRAWBERRY-BANANA TOPPED FRENCH TOAST

This meal is so decadent, you'll think you're eating dessert!

Preparation time: 5 minutes ● **Cooking time: 6 minutes**

1   **egg**
¼   **cup fat-free milk**
¼   **teaspoon ground cinnamon**
1   **slice (1 ounce) whole grain bread**
1   **teaspoon Better Butter (page 323) or trans-fat free spread**
¼   **cup sliced strawberries**
¼   **cup sliced banana**

1. In a shallow bowl, beat the egg with the milk and cinnamon. Dip both sides of the bread in the milk mixture.

2. Melt the Better Butter or spread in a non-stick skillet over medium heat. Place the bread in the pan. Cook for about 2 to 3 minutes per side, or until golden and cooked through. Cut in half diagonally. Place half on a plate. Top with half of the strawberries and bananas. Cover with the other toast half and the remaining strawberries and bananas.

MAKES 1 SERVING

Per serving: 250 calories, 31 g carbohydrate, 12 g protein, 10 g fat, 3 g saturated fat, 210 mg cholesterol, 290 mg sodium, 4 g fiber

Carbohydrate Choices: 2

Dietary Exchanges: 1 starch, 1 fruit, ½ milk, 1 meat, 1 fat

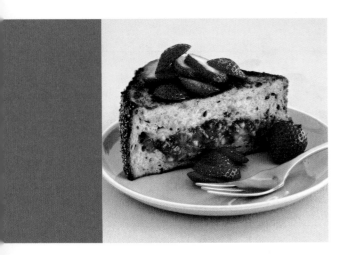

CINNAMON BUCKWHEAT PANCAKES
WITH HONEYED STRAWBERRIES

These classic fruit-topped flannel cakes are a special treat on the weekend, but you can also prepare just the pancakes and store them individually wrapped in the freezer to toast for a quicker weekday breakfast.

Preparation time: 5 minutes ● **Cooking time: 15 minutes**

STRAWBERRIES

- 1½ tablespoons honey
- 1 tablespoon water
- 2 teaspoons cornstarch
- 1½ cups fresh strawberries, sliced, or frozen strawberries, thawed and sliced

PANCAKES

- 1 cup buckwheat flour
- 1 tablespoon sugar
- 1 teaspoon baking powder
- 1 teaspoon baking soda
- ¼ teaspoon ground cinnamon
  Pinch of salt
- 1 egg
- ¾ cup reduced-fat buttermilk

1. To prepare the strawberries: In a saucepan, combine the honey, water, and cornstarch. Mix until blended. Add the strawberries. Cook over medium heat, stirring gently, for about 4 minutes, or until the mixture bubbles. Remove from the heat. Cover to keep warm.

2. To prepare the pancakes: Coat a nonstick griddle with vegetable oil spray and preheat over medium-high heat.

Meanwhile, in a mixing bowl, combine the flour, sugar, baking powder, baking soda, cinnamon, and salt. Stir with a fork to combine. In another bowl, beat the egg with a fork until smooth. Add the buttermilk. Beat to blend. Add to the dry ingredients. Stir just until combined (don't overmix).

3. Ladle the batter in ¼-cup dollops onto the hot griddle. (The batter is sticky, so some of it will stick to the ladle.) Cook for about 2 minutes, or until browned on the bottom. Flip and cook for 1 to 2 minutes, or until cooked through. Continue, adjusting the heat higher or lower as needed and coating the griddle with vegetable oil spray, until all the pancakes are cooked. Top with the reserved strawberries.

MAKES 8 SERVINGS (1 PANCAKE PER SERVING)

Per serving: 93 calories, 17 g carbohydrate, 4 g protein, 1 g fat, 0.5 g saturated fat, 27 mg cholesterol, 270 mg sodium, 3 g fiber

Carbohydrate Choices: 1

Dietary Exchanges: ½ starch

CORNMEAL AND WALNUT WAFFLES

Treat yourself to these delicious nutty, grainy waffles to enjoy with your Sunday newspaper or crossword puzzle—on the deck or by the fire—it works either way!

Preparation time: 11 minutes ● **Cooking time: 8 minutes**

---

    1 cup stone-ground cornmeal
    ½ cup whole wheat pastry flour
    2 tablespoons finely chopped toasted
       walnuts
    2 tablespoons brown sugar
    1½ teaspoons baking powder
    ½ teaspoon baking soda
    2 eggs, separated
       Pinch of salt
    1½ cups reduced-fat buttermilk
    10 teaspoons cream cheese
    10 teaspoons maple syrup

1. Lightly coat the top and bottom of a waffle iron, preferably nonstick, with vegetable oil spray and preheat.

2. In a mixing bowl, combine the cornmeal, flour, walnuts, sugar, baking powder, and baking soda. Stir with a fork to mix. In the bowl of an electric mixer, combine the egg whites and salt. Beat on medium speed for about 1 minute, or until foamy. Increase the speed to high. Beat for about 2 minutes, or until peaks form. In a small bowl, whisk the buttermilk with the egg yolks. Add to the reserved dry ingredients. Mix just until combined (don't overmix). Fold in the beaten whites.

3. Ladle some of the batter onto the waffle iron so it spreads to within 1" of all sides. Cook according to the manufacturer's directions, until crisp. Remove the waffles. Recoat the iron with vegetable oil spray. Continue until all the waffles are cooked.

4. Top each waffle with 1 teaspoon cream cheese and drizzle with 1 teaspoon maple syrup.

MAKES 10 SERVINGS

Per serving: 146 calories, 22 g carbohydrate, 5 g protein, 5 g fat, 2 g saturated fat, 49 mg cholesterol, 438 mg sodium, 2 g fiber

Carbohydrate Choices: 1½

Dietary Exchanges: ½ starch, ½ fat

PUMPKIN WALNUT CRANBERRY QUICK BREAD

The perfect treat to have on hand for unexpected company or for that first chilly day of autumn. The contrast of flavors and textures is great—the sweetness of the pumpkin with the tartness of the cranberries; the crunch of the walnuts with the moistness of the bread.

Preparation time: 20 minutes ● **Baking time: 30 minutes**

1¼ cups oat bran

½ cup whole wheat flour, preferably white whole wheat

⅓ cup brown sugar

2 teaspoons baking powder

1 teaspoon pumpkin pie spice

⅛ teaspoon salt

1 egg

1 cup canned pumpkin

½ cup fat-free milk

2 tablespoons canola oil

¼ cup chopped walnuts

¼ cup dried cranberries

1. Preheat the oven to 375°F. Lightly coat a 9" × 5" nonstick loaf pan with vegetable oil spray.

2. In a mixing bowl, combine the oat bran, flour, sugar, baking powder, spice, and salt.

Stir with a fork to mix. In another bowl, beat the egg with a fork until smooth. Add the pumpkin, milk, and oil. Stir to mix. Add to the dry ingredients. Stir just until no dry remains. Add the walnuts and cranberries. Stir to mix. Transfer to the pan.

3. Bake for about 30 minutes, or until a tester inserted into the center comes out clean. Remove from the oven and let cool for 10 minutes before turning out onto a rack. Let cool. Cut into 18 slices.

MAKES 18 SERVINGS (1 SLICE PER SERVING)

Per serving: 84 calories, 14 g carbohydrate, 3 g protein, 4 g fat, 0.5 g saturated fat, 12 mg cholesterol, 80 mg sodium, 2 g fiber

Carbohydrate Choices: 1

Dietary Exchanges: ½ starch, ½ fat

LOOSEN UP/GET MOVING

Move to Improve

Need some good reasons to get physical? Physical activity can help you control your blood glucose, weight, and blood pressure. It can raise your "good" cholesterol and lower your "bad" cholesterol. It can help prevent heart and bloodflow problems, reducing your risk of heart disease and nerve damage.

ALMOND AND MIXED BERRY MUFFINS WITH FLAXSEED

These warm and tasty quick breads make getting out of bed worthwhile. The flaxseed contains soluble fiber like the kind found in beans and oat bran.

Preparation time: 12 minutes ● **Baking time: 24 minutes**

2¼ cups whole grain or wheat pastry flour

4 teaspoons baking powder

¼ cup ground flaxseed

½ teaspoon salt

⅔ cup fresh blueberries

⅔ cup fresh raspberries

1 cup 2% milk

2 eggs

⅔ cup sugar

⅓ cup canola oil

1 teaspoon almond extract

1. Preheat the oven to 400°F. Line a 12-cup muffin pan with paper liners.

2. In a large bowl, combine the flour, baking powder, flaxseed, and salt. Whisk to mix. Add the berries and stir to coat.

3. In another bowl, combine the milk, eggs, sugar, oil, and almond extract. With a fork, beat until smooth.

4. Pour the egg mixture into the berry mixture and gently mix with a fork to moisten the dry ingredients. Don't overmix (a few lumps in the batter are normal). Dollop the batter into the prepared muffin cups.

5. Bake for 20 to 24 minutes, or until a wooden pick inserted into the center of a muffin comes out clean. Let stand for 5 minutes on a rack before serving.

MAKES 12 SERVINGS

Per serving: 210 calories, 28 g carbohydrate, 5 g protein, 9 g fat, 1 g saturated fat, 35 mg cholesterol, 280 mg sodium, 3 g fiber

Carbohydrate Choices: 2

Dietary Exchanges: 1½ starch, 1½ fat

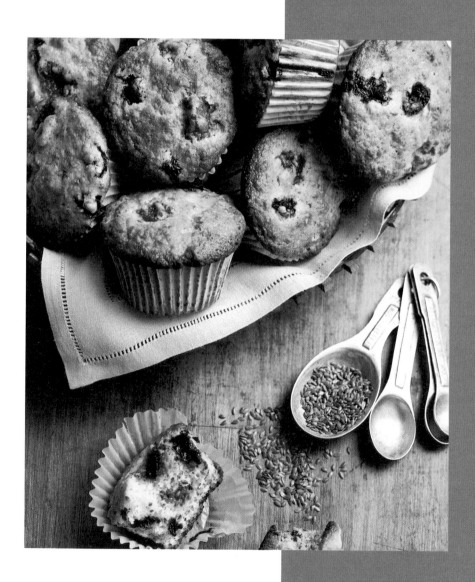

WESTERN CORNBREAD

A delightful alternative to hot cereal, this savory cornbread is a whole grain treat. Be sure to use 100 percent stone-ground cornmeal for the best texture, flavor, and nutrition.

Preparation time: 15 minutes ● **Baking time: 15 minutes**

---

3 tablespoons canola oil

¼ cup finely chopped scallions, all parts

¼ cup finely chopped bell pepper, any color

2 slices (2 ounces) finely chopped Canadian bacon

1 cup stone-ground cornmeal

¾ cup whole wheat pastry flour

½ cup all-purpose flour

2 teaspoons baking powder

1 teaspoon baking soda

¼ teaspoon salt

1 egg

1⅓ cups buttermilk

1. Preheat the oven to 425°F. Heat the oil in a 9" heavy skillet, preferably cast iron, over medium-high heat for 30 seconds. Add the scallions, bell pepper, and bacon. Cook, stirring, for about 1 minute, or until the scallions are wilted. Remove from the heat.

2. In a mixing bowl, combine the cornmeal, flours, baking powder, baking soda, and salt. Stir with a fork or pastry blender to mix. In a small bowl, beat the egg with a fork. Add the egg and the buttermilk to the dry ingredients. Stir just until no dry ingredients are visible. Add the skillet mixture to the bowl. Stir to mix. Pour the batter into the skillet.

3. Bake for about 15 minutes, or until a tester inserted in the center comes out clean. Serve warm, cut into wedges.

MAKES 8 SERVINGS

Per serving: 174 calories, 21 g carbohydrate, 6 g protein, 8 g fat, 1 g saturated fat, 33 mg cholesterol, 483 mg sodium, 2 g fiber

Carbohydrate Choices: 1

Dietary Exchanges: 1 starch, 1 fat

NOTE: Any extra wedges can be frozen individually. Reheat in a toaster oven.

BREAK THE BREAKFAST RULES

Who decided that breakfast can only be cereal, pancakes, and eggs? With these nutritious and filling options for daybreak meals, you can be a morning maverick.

"Refried" Bean Quesadillas (page 144). With the "Refried" Beans ready-made in the refrigerator or freezer, this stuffed flatbread takes just minutes. The lean protein filling will stick with you until snacktime.

Green Split Pea Soup (page 182). Pack and freeze in single-size servings. It's warm and satisfying, particularly when the weather's cold or wet.

Easy Couscous Salad (page 194). Pretend you're breakfasting on a Greek isle with a leftover serving of this whole grain, chickpea, and feta cheese combo. It's a refreshing way to start the day in warm weather.

Portobello Mushroom Barley (page 223). Think barley in place of oats and mushrooms instead of fruit, and you have the makings of a breakfast that's far from ho-hum.

Provençal Lentil Ragout (page 313). Prepare a batch of this tasty legume stew to freeze in single-size servings to reheat in the microwave. Top with a dollop of fat-free plain yogurt.

Black Bean Patties (page 317). When you don't have time to sit down to a proper breakfast, microwave a frozen Black Bean Patty and head out the door armed with a lean protein, saturated-fat-free, complex-carb meal-on-the-go.

Broccoli Pizza (page 151). As any college sophomore will attest, leftover cold pizza is a fine way to start the day. With our leftovers, however, you can kiss the extra fat and calories good-bye. And you'll be starting your day right with some green veggie and a serving of whole grains in the crust.

Garden Vegetable Soup with Grilled Chicken (page 183). Chicken, vegetables, pasta, and herbs simmered in a savory broth—what a delightful entry into your workday.

CHEESE AND PEPPER FRITTATA

The frittata, a flat Italian omelet, is one of the most versatile of egg dishes. You can improvise fillings by using bits of leftover cooked vegetables, meats, or poultry.

Preparation time: 10 minutes ● **Cooking time: 35 minutes**

---

1 teaspoon olive oil, preferably extra virgin

¾ cup chopped red bell pepper

¾ cup chopped green bell pepper

¾ cup (3 ounces) shredded reduced-fat Monterey Jack cheese

2 tablespoons chopped fresh basil

5 eggs + 2 egg whites, lightly beaten

¼ teaspoon salt

Ground black pepper

1. Preheat the oven to 375°F. Coat a 9" oven-proof skillet with vegetable oil spray. Place over medium-high heat. Add the oil. Heat for 30 seconds. Add the bell peppers. Cook, stirring occasionally, for about 5 minutes, or until just soft. Sprinkle the cheese and basil into the pan. Add the eggs, egg whites, salt, and pepper.

2. Bake for about 30 minutes, or until the eggs are set. Let stand to cool slightly. Cut into wedges.

MAKES 4 SERVINGS

Per serving: 180 calories, 5 g carbohydrate, 15 g protein, 12 g fat, 4.5 g saturated fat, 285 mg cholesterol, 440 mg sodium, 1 g fiber

Carbohydrate Choices: ½

Dietary Exchanges: ½ vegetable, 2 meat, 1½ fat

LOOSEN UP/GET MOVING

Cumulative Effect

"The physical activity recommendation for improving health is to accumulate 30 minutes of moderate-intensity physical activity on most, if not all, days of the week," advises exercise physiologist Richard Weil, MEd, CDE, director of the New York Obesity Research Center weight-loss program at St. Luke's–Roosevelt Hospital Center. "The key words in this recommendation are 'accumulate,' which means you can do it in three bouts of 10 minutes, two bouts of 15 minutes, or one bout of 30 minutes, and 'moderate-intensity,' which means the work should leave you feeling warm and slightly out of breath but not exhausted."

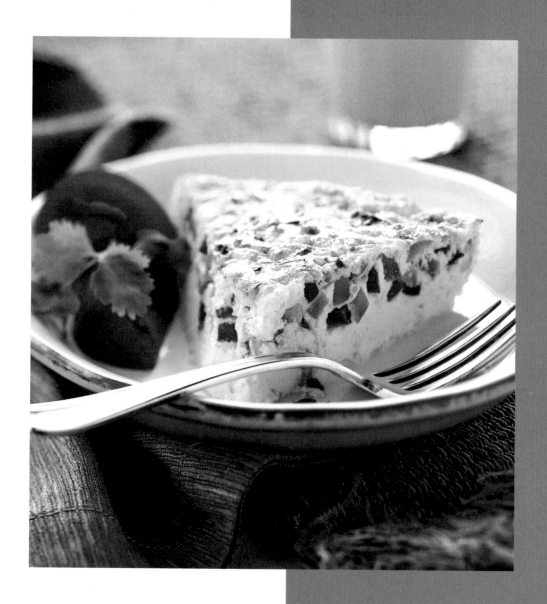

BACON, SPINACH, AND TOMATO SCRAMBLED EGGS

If you have some fresh basil leaves on hand, they make an aromatic addition to this dish.

Preparation time: 4 minutes ● **Cooking time: 5 minutes**

---

4   eggs + 2 egg whites

½   teaspoon salt-free seasoning blend

1   teaspoon olive oil

2   slices (2 ounces) Canadian bacon, cubed

1   cup packed baby spinach leaves, chopped

½   cup grape or cherry tomatoes, chopped

Ground black pepper (optional)

1. In a bowl, combine the eggs, egg whites, and seasoning blend. Beat with a fork until smooth.

2. Heat the oil in a nonstick skillet over medium heat. Add the bacon, spinach, and tomatoes. Cook, stirring, for about 2 minutes, or until the spinach is wilted.

3. Add the egg mixture. Cook, stirring, for about 2 minutes, or until the eggs are set. Season with pepper, if desired.

MAKES 4 SERVINGS

Per serving: 120 calories, 2 g carbohydrate, 11 g protein, 7 g fat, 2 g saturated fat, 220 mg cholesterol, 310 mg sodium, 0 g fiber

Carbohydrate Choices: 0

Dietary Exchanges: ½ vegetable, 2 meat, 1 fat

NIPS AND TATS HAM HASH

A poached egg perched atop this hash makes a delightful start to the day.

Preparation time: 5 minutes ● **Cooking time: 15 minutes**

---

2 medium Yukon Gold potatoes (about 12 ounces)

1 large turnip (about 8 ounces)

1 tablespoon canola oil

2 slices (2 ounces) Canadian bacon, cut into small cubes

⅓ cup sliced scallions

2 tablespoons finely chopped parsley

⅛ teaspoon salt

Ground black pepper

1. Pierce the potatoes and turnips several times with a small sharp knife. Place on a microwaveable dish. Cover with waxed paper. Microwave on high power, rotating once, for about 6 minutes, or until tender when pierced with a knife. Let stand until cool enough to touch. Peel the turnips. Chop the turnips and potatoes into small pieces.

2. Heat the oil in a nonstick skillet over medium-high heat. Add the potatoes, turnips, bacon, and scallions. Cook, tossing, for about 1 minute, or until the scallions soften. Cover and cook for 2 minutes, or until starting to brown on the bottom. Flip the mixture with a spatula. Press it down. Cover and cook, flipping the mixture and scraping the pan bottom occasionally, for about 6 minutes, or until the vegetables are browned on the outside and soft in the center. Reduce the heat if the mixture is browning too quickly. Add the parsley, salt, and pepper to taste just before serving.

MAKES 4 SERVINGS

Per serving: 139 calories, 19 g carbohydrate, 6 g protein, 5 g fat, 0.5 g saturated fat, 7 mg cholesterol, 288 mg sodium, 3 g fiber

Carbohydrate Choices: 1

Dietary Exchanges: 1 starch, 1 vegetable, ½ meat, 1 fat

NOTE: The hash can be prepared in advance and refrigerated. Reheat individual servings in the microwave.

GARDEN BREAKFAST WRAP

Wraps are so versatile and portable, too. If you can't find spinach tortillas, replace them with 100 percent whole wheat tortillas.

Preparation time: 3 minutes ● **Cooking time: 5 minutes**

---

4   **spinach-flavored flour tortillas (12" diameter)**

2   **teaspoons Better Butter (page 323) or trans-fat free spread**

4   **eggs + 4 egg whites, beaten**

½   **cup (2 ounces) crumbled reduced-fat lemon, garlic, and herb feta cheese or ¼ cup (1 ounce) grated Parmesan cheese**

4   **cups (4 ounces) baby arugula or baby spinach**

   Hot-pepper sauce (optional)

1. Preheat a grill pan over medium-high heat. Lightly toast 1 tortilla in the pan about 20 seconds, flip, and cook 10 seconds longer. Set aside on a plate and cover with a slightly damp paper towel. Repeat with the remaining tortillas.

2. Melt the Better Butter or spread in a large nonstick skillet over medium heat. Pour in the eggs, egg whites, and cheese. Cook, stirring, for 2 minutes. Add the greens. Continue cooking, stirring, for about 1 minute longer, or until the eggs are set and the greens are wilted.

3. Mound one-quarter of the mixture on the bottom half of 1 tortilla, flap up the 2 sides, and roll into a tube. Repeat with the remaining tortillas and filling. Cut the wraps diagonally in half and serve with hot-pepper sauce, if desired.

MAKES 4 SERVINGS

Per serving: 300 calories, 33 g carbohydrate, 19 g protein, 11 g fat, 3.5 g saturated fat, 210 mg cholesterol, 470 mg sodium, 1 g fiber

Carbohydrate Choices: 2

Dietary Exchanges: 1½ meat, 1 fat

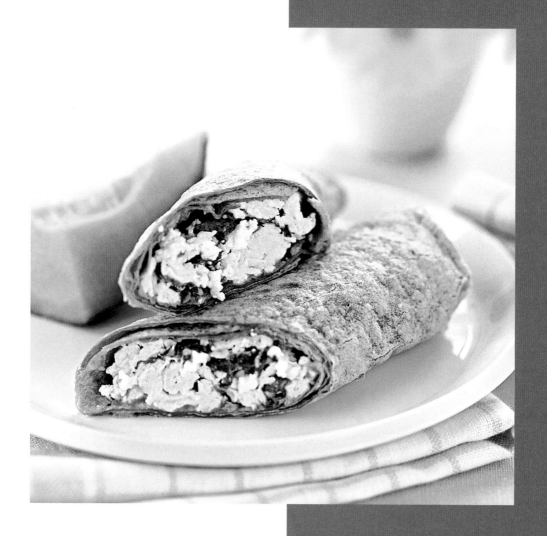

MONTEREY STRATA

This savory bread pudding could just be the ideal entertaining dish—you can put it together and refrigerate it the night before. Just pop it into the oven before serving. Serve with grilled Canadian bacon and a citrus salad.

Preparation time: 10 minutes ● **Baking time: 45 minutes**

---

8 ounces broccoli florets, cut into bite-size chunks

2 eggs + 2 egg whites

2 cups fat-free milk

2 teaspoons salt-free seasoning blend

¼ teaspoon salt

4 slices (5 ounces) 7-grain sourdough whole wheat bread, cut into ½" cubes

¼ cup minced scallions or onion

½ cup (2 ounces) shredded Swiss or Gruyère cheese

1. Preheat the oven to 325°F. Coat a 12" × 8" baking dish with vegetable oil spray.

2. Fill a skillet with ½" water. Cover and bring to a boil. Add the broccoli. Cover and cook for 1 to 2 minutes, or until crisp-tender. Drain.

3. In the baking dish, combine the eggs and egg whites. Beat with a fork until smooth. Add the milk, seasoning blend, and salt. Stir to blend. Add the bread, scallions or onion, and broccoli. Press with the back of a fork to submerge. Let stand for 5 minutes, or until the bread is soaked. Sprinkle on the cheese.

4. Bake for about 45 minutes, or until puffed and golden.

MAKES 6 SERVINGS

Per serving: 168 calories, 18 g carbohydrate, 12 g protein, 5 g fat, 2 g saturated fat, 81 mg cholesterol, 306 mg sodium, 3 g fiber

Carbohydrate Choices: 1

Dietary Exchanges: 1 starch, ½ milk, ½ vegetable, 1 meat, 1 fat

NOTE: Any type of 100 percent whole grain bread can replace the 7-grain sourdough whole wheat bread.

PORK AND APPLE BREAKF[A]

This recipe makes a big batch so you can [...]eezer to cook a serving whenever the mood strike[...]

Preparation time: 15 minutes ● **Cooking time: 5[...]**

1 **pound pork tenderloin, cut into 1" chunks**
½ **apple, cut into 1" chunks**
¾ **teaspoon poultry seasoning**
½ **teaspoon paprika**
½ **teaspoon salt**

1. In the bowl of a food processor fitted with a metal blade, combine the pork, apple, poultry seasoning, paprika, and salt. Process for about 1 minute, or until finely chopped. With clean hands, shape the mixture into 24 patties. Coat the tops lightly with vegetable oil spray.

2. Heat a nonstick skillet over medium-high heat. Place the patties, sprayed side down, in the pan. Cook for about 5 minutes, turning as needed, or until browned and no pink remains. (Check by cutting a patty in half.) Reduce the heat if the patties are browning too quickly.

MAKES 8 SERVINGS (3 PATTIES PER SERVING)

Per serving: 73 calories, 1 g carbohydrate, 12 g protein, 2 g fat, 1 g saturated fat, 37 mg cholesterol, 174 mg sodium, 0 g fiber

Carbohydrate Choices: 0

Dietary Exchanges: 2 meat

NOTE: The patties may be cooled, packed into a resealable plastic freezer bag, and refrigerated for up to 4 days or frozen for up to 6 weeks. To reheat, place on a microwaveable plate. Cover loosely with waxed paper. Microwave on medium power for 1 minute, or until heated through.

LET YOURSELF GO/STRESS LESS

Strength in Numbers

Support groups—also known as self-help groups or mutual-aid groups—are tremendous resources for busting stress. Good support groups help people feel less isolated, better about themselves, more comfortable with their diabetes, and more able to do the right thing when it comes to their self-care, advises Richard R. Rubin, PhD, CDE, of the Johns Hopkins Medical School, in his book *Psyching Out Diabetes: A Positive Approach to Your Negative Emotions.* In addition, support groups are free or, at most, require a small contribution. To locate a group in your area, consult your physician, certified diabetes educator, or local hospital. For online support with particular issues, check out the message boards at the American Diabetes Association Web site www.diabetes.org.

CHAPTER 7

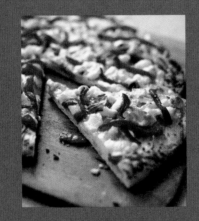

APPETIZERS, SANDWICHES, AND SNACKS

EDAMAME HUMMUS

Fresh soybeans called edamame are a popular snack in Japan that is catching on in the States, too. Serve as a party dip or snack with toasted pita or seasonal vegetables such as cucumber, squash, or orange bell pepper.

Preparation time: 9 minutes ● **Cooking time: 6 minutes**

---

1 package (16 ounces) shelled, frozen edamame
3 tablespoons tahini
¼ cup olive oil
3 tablespoons lemon juice
1 large clove garlic, smashed
½ teaspoon salt
⅓–½ cup cold water

1. In a large pot, bring 2 quarts of water to a rapid boil. Pour in the edamame. Return to a boil and cook for about 6 minutes, or until the beans are creamy inside and easy to smash with a fork. Drain the edamame and dunk in a large bowl of cold water, about 3 minutes. Drain when cool.

2. In a food processor fitted with a metal blade or in a blender, combine the edamame, tahini, oil, lemon juice, garlic, and salt. Pulse, scraping down the sides of the bowl occasionally, until the mixture is pureed smooth. Add cold water, a little at a time, until the mixture is creamy.

MAKES 8 SERVINGS (¼ CUP PER SERVING)

Per serving: 170 calories, 9 g carbohydrate, 7 g protein, 12 g fat, 1.5 g saturated fat, 0 mg cholesterol, 170 mg sodium, 3 g fiber

Carbohydrate Choices: ½

Dietary Exchanges: ½ starch, ½ meat, 2 fat

NOTE: Tahini is prepared ground sesame seeds. Look for it in the gourmet cheese section of the supermarket.

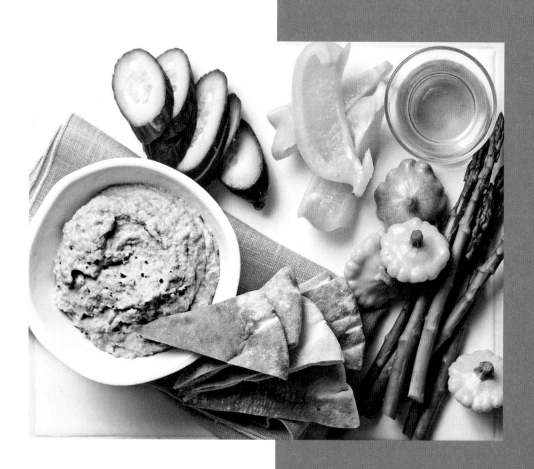

BRUSCHETTA WITH TUSCAN WHITE BEANS

The bean topping can be prepared and refrigerated several days in advance of serving. Reheat in a microwaveable dish for about 2 minutes on high power before spreading on the toast or crackers.

Preparation time: 10 minutes ● **Cooking time: 6 minutes**

---

1 tablespoon + 2 teaspoons olive oil, preferably extra virgin

1 teaspoon minced garlic

½ teaspoon crumbled dried sage

Pinch of salt

Pinch of ground red pepper

1 cup cooked cannellini beans

½ cup canned diced tomatoes in juice

20 thinly sliced rounds whole wheat baguette, toasted, or whole wheat crackers

1. In a nonstick skillet, combine the oil, garlic, sage, salt, and pepper. Cook over low heat for 1 minute, or until sizzling. Add the beans and tomatoes. Increase the heat to medium. Simmer for 5 minutes, mashing occasionally with a fork, or until thickened.

2. Spread the mixture on the baguette slices or crackers. Serve right away.

MAKES 10 SERVINGS (2 BRUSCHETTA PER SERVING)

Per serving: 84 calories, 10 g carbohydrate, 2 g protein, 4 g fat, 0.5 g saturated fat, 0 mg cholesterol, 96 mg sodium, 1 g fiber

Carbohydrate Choices: 1

Dietary Exchanges: ½ starch, ½ fat

SALSA FRESCA

This fresh and feisty salsa might just become a staple condiment in your refrigerator, replacing bottled salsas that are extremely high in sodium. When it's prepared from ripe garden tomatoes, no commercial salsa can match its flavor.

Preparation time: 12 minutes ● **Standing time: 30 minutes**

---

2 pints cherry or grape tomatoes, finely chopped

½ cup minced white onion

½ cup chopped cilantro

2 jalapeño or 4 serrano chile peppers, seeded and minced (wear plastic gloves when handling), or more to taste

1 tablespoon lime juice or sherry wine vinegar

2 teaspoons minced garlic

¼ teaspoon salt

In a glass jar or a plastic food storage container, combine the tomatoes, onion, cilantro, chile peppers, lime juice or vinegar, garlic, and salt. Stir to mix. Serve right away or let stand for at least 30 minutes to allow the flavors to blend.

MAKES 20 SERVINGS (2 TABLESPOONS PER SERVING)

Per serving: 5 calories, 2 g carbohydrate, 0 g protein, 0 g fat, 0 g saturated fat, 0 mg cholesterol, 30 mg sodium, 0 g fiber

Carbohydrate Choices: 0

Dietary Exchanges: ½ vegetable

NOTES: Fresh chile peppers can vary in heat intensity. Add fewer or more chile peppers depending on your personal heat tolerance. The cilantro and lime juice or vinegar can also be adjusted to taste.

The salsa can be refrigerated for up to 1 week.

CHUNKY GUACAMOLE WITH JICAMA STICKS

Even though the fat in avocado is primarily healthy monounsaturated and polyunsaturated fats, you don't want to eat too much of a good thing or the calories will add up fast. In this version of the popular avocado dip, we've added crunchy fresh vegetables for added texture and less fat.

Preparation time: 10 minutes

½ large jicama (8 ounces), peeled

1 ripe avocado, pitted and peeled

1 tablespoon lime juice

½ teaspoon hot-pepper sauce

2 tablespoons finely chopped bell pepper

2 tablespoons chopped red onion

1 tablespoon finely chopped cilantro

1. Cut the jicama into thick 1"-long sticks. Arrange on a serving plate.

2. Cut the avocado into chunks. Place in a bowl with the lime juice and hot-pepper sauce. Mash with a fork until chunky. Add the pepper, onion, and cilantro. Stir to mix. Serve right away with the jicama for dipping.

MAKES 12 SERVINGS (1 TABLESPOON GUACAMOLE WITH 2 JICAMA STICKS PER SERVING)

Per serving: 33 calories, 3 g carbohydrate, 0 g protein, 2 g fat, 0.5 g saturated fat, 0 mg cholesterol, 3 mg sodium, 2 g fiber

Carbohydrate Choices: 0

Dietary Exchanges: ½ vegetable, ½ fat

LET YOURSELF GO/STRESS LESS

Numerous studies conducted at Duke University by Richard S. Surwit, PhD, have proven that practicing relaxation on a regular basis will improve blood sugar control. Progressive muscle relaxation is a technique that is easy to learn and the one that has been tested most often in patients with diabetes. The technique works by tensing and then relaxing muscles systematically as a means of releasing pent-up stress that manifests itself in symptoms such as rapid heart rate, elevated blood pressure, and heightened stress hormone levels. This method of consciously relieving muscle tension leads to decreased levels of stress hormones. You can find easy-to-follow instructional CDs at fitness and wellness centers and some bookstores.

FIESTA DIP

Serve homemade Chili Tortilla Chips (page 122) or bagged baked tortilla chips for dipping.

Preparation time: 4 minutes

---

1 cup "Refried" Beans (page 145)

⅓ cup reduced-fat sour cream

¾ cup drained Salsa Fresca (page 119)

Spoon the beans into an 8"-wide dish (such as a pasta bowl) that has sides at least 1½" high. Spread to smooth. Spread on the sour cream. Cover with the salsa. Serve right away or refrigerate for up to 24 hours.

MAKES 8 SERVINGS

Per serving: 79 calories, 6 g carbohydrate, 2 g protein, 5 g fat, 2.5 g saturated fat, 12 mg cholesterol, 45 mg sodium, 1 g fiber

Carbohydrate Choices: ½

Dietary Exchanges: 1 fat

CHILI TORTILLA CHIPS

Although good-tasting 100 percent whole grain baked tortilla chips are now sold in some supermarkets, it's fun to create your own chips where you control the seasoning.

Preparation time: 4 minutes ● **Baking time: 10 minutes**

---

4 **whole wheat tortillas (8" diameter)**
Vegetable oil spray
Chili powder

1. Preheat the oven to 350°F. Spread the tortillas on a work surface. Coat lightly with vegetable oil spray. Sprinkle lightly with chili powder. Flip the tortillas and repeat with the spray and chili powder.

2. Place the tortillas in a stack. With a serrated knife, cut the stack into 8 equal wedges. Spread the triangles out on a baking sheet or sheets so they are not touching. Bake for about 10 minutes, or until crisp and starting to puff. Let stand to cool. Serve right away or store in an airtight container.

MAKES 8 SERVINGS (4 CHIPS PER SERVING)

Per serving: 53 calories, 9 g carbohydrate, 1 g protein, 1 g fat, 0 g saturated fat, 0 mg cholesterol, 115 mg sodium, 2 g fiber

Carbohydrate Choices: ½

Dietary Exchanges: ½ carbohydrate

ROASTED GARLIC DIP

Garlic is sweet, mellow, and utterly irresistible when it's slow-roasted with a bit of olive oil. Here, we've mixed it with ricotta cheese and seasonings to create a delectable dip. It's also a wonderful spread for sandwiches or a garnish for grilled meats.

Preparation time: 10 minutes ● **Roasting time: 50 minutes**

---

1   **head garlic (10 good-size cloves), peeled**

2   **teaspoons olive oil, preferably extra virgin**

¾   **cup part-skim ricotta cheese**

1   **tablespoon minced parsley**

Ground black pepper

1. Preheat the oven to 350°F. Place the garlic in the center of an 8" sheet of heavy-duty aluminum foil. Drizzle on the oil. Seal the packet tightly. Set in a small baking dish.

2. Roast the garlic for about 50 minutes, or until very tender. Remove and let stand to cool completely.

3. In a small food processor fitted with a metal blade or in a blender, combine the cheese and garlic. Process for about 2 minutes, scraping down the sides of the bowl as needed, or until smooth. Add the parsley. Season to taste with pepper. Pulse to mix.

MAKES 6 SERVINGS (2 TABLESPOONS PER SERVING)

Per serving: 65 calories, 3 g carbohydrate, 4 g protein, 4 g fat, 2 g saturated fat, 10 mg cholesterol, 40 mg sodium, 0 g fiber

Carbohydrate Choices: 0

Dietary Exchanges: ½ meat, ½ fat

NOTES: Garlic can be roasted according to these recipe directions in larger batches. Cool and then store, just covered with olive oil, in a jar in the refrigerator for up to 2 weeks. It makes a tasty spread for sandwiches or a flavoring for stews or soups.

Peeling the garlic before roasting makes it much simpler to deal with after it's roasted. Gadgets called garlic peelers are silicone tubes in which you insert the clove and roll it lightly to release the skin. You can also set the clove on a work surface and tap lightly with the blunt side of a heavy knife. The skin will pop right off.

NEW MEXICAN PUMPKIN SEED DIP

Serve raw bell pepper chunks or sliced jicama for scooping this rustic dip. It also makes a delicious filling for warm corn tortillas.

Preparation time: 10 minutes ● **Cooking time: 9 minutes**

---

1 teaspoon + 1 tablespoon olive oil, preferably extra virgin

2 teaspoons minced garlic

1 teaspoon ground cumin

1¾ cups cooked chickpeas or 1 can (15½ ounces) chickpeas, rinsed and drained

¾ cup chicken or vegetable broth, divided

1 teaspoon minced fresh red chile pepper (wear plastic gloves when handling)

1 tablespoon lime juice

¼ teaspoon salt

2 tablespoons toasted pumpkin seed kernels, coarsely chopped

1. In a skillet, combine 1 teaspoon oil, garlic, and cumin. Cook over low heat for 1 minute, or until sizzling and fragrant. Do not brown the garlic. Add the chickpeas, ½ cup broth, and 1 teaspoon chile pepper. Cook, smashing the chickpeas occasionally with a fork, for about 8 minutes, or until scant liquid remains.

2. Transfer the mixture to the bowl of a food processor fitted with a metal blade or to a blender. Add the lime juice, salt, and remaining 1 tablespoon oil. Process for about 30 seconds, scraping down the sides of the bowl as needed, until the mixture is the consistency of chunky peanut butter. Add up to ¼ cup more broth and process to make a moist but not runny consistency. Taste and add more chile pepper, if desired.

3. Transfer to an 8"-wide dish (such as a pasta bowl) that has sides at least 1½" high. Spread to smooth. Scatter the seeds evenly on the top. Cover and refrigerate for at least 1 hour (or as long as 1 day) to allow the flavors to develop.

MAKES 10 SERVINGS (2 TABLESPOONS PER SERVING)

Per serving: 79 calories, 9 g carbohydrate, 3 g protein, 4 g fat, 0.5 g saturated fat, 0 mg cholesterol, 71 mg sodium, 2 g fiber

Carbohydrate Choices: ½

Dietary Exchanges: 1 starch, ½ fat

NOTE: To toast the seeds, place them in a cold skillet. Cook over medium-high heat, stirring, for about 3 minutes, or until browned and crackling.

SPINACH ARUGULA DIP

No one would ever guess that this festive dip is so low in fat. Serve it with raw vegetables or whole grain crackers. It also makes a delicious sandwich spread on whole grain toast.

Preparation time: 4 minutes

---

1 cup 1% dry-curd cottage cheese
½ cup packed baby spinach leaves
¼ cup packed arugula leaves
2 tablespoons (½ ounce) grated Romano cheese
½ teaspoon salt-free lemon-pepper seasoning

In the bowl of a food processor fitted with a metal blade, combine the cottage cheese, spinach, arugula, Romano cheese, and seasoning blend. Pulse about 12 times, or until the greens are chopped. Serve right away or refrigerate in an airtight container for up to 3 days.

MAKES 5 SERVINGS (¼ CUP PER SERVING)

Per serving: 49 calories, 2 g carbohydrate, 7 g protein, 2 g fat, 1 g saturated fat, 5 mg cholesterol, 279 mg sodium, 0 g fiber

Carbohydrate Choices: 0

Dietary Exchanges: 1 meat

NOTE: Fresh basil, cilantro, or mint leaves may replace the arugula, if desired.

NOW YOU KNOW

Keep snack calories and dessert calories at 200 calories or fewer. It makes it easy to quantify how much you should have.

GOLDEN PEPPER DIP

Prepare this well in advance of serving. It improves in flavor. It's special enough for a gathering and satisfying enough for a daily snack. Enjoy it with sticks of raw jicama, Chili Tortilla Chips (page 122), or 100 percent whole grain crackers.

Preparation time: 10 minutes ● Cooking time: 9 minutes

½ **tablespoon olive oil**

8 **ounces orange or yellow bell peppers, cut into large chunks**

⅓ **cup chopped onion**

2 **teaspoons minced garlic**

½ **teaspoon paprika**

⅛ **teaspoon salt**

½ **cup water, divided**

1 **tablespoon raw almonds**

¼ **cup canned pumpkin**

1. Heat a large skillet over medium heat. Add the oil. Let stand for 30 seconds. Add the peppers, onion, garlic, paprika, and salt. Toss to combine. Cover and cook, tossing occasionally, over medium-high heat for 8 minutes, or until the peppers are softened. Add a few tablespoons of water occasionally, if the pan bottom is browning too fast.

2. Meanwhile, place the almonds in the bowl of a food processor fitted with a metal blade. Process for about 1 minute, or until finely ground. Add the pepper mixture. Process, scraping down the sides of the bowl as needed, for about 4 minutes, or until coarsely pureed. Add the pumpkin. Pulse to mix.

MAKES 4 SERVINGS (¼ CUP PER SERVING)

Per serving: 70 calories, 9 g carbohydrate, 2 g protein, 3 g fat, 0 g saturated fat, 0 mg cholesterol, 5 mg sodium, 2 g fiber

Carbohydrate Choices: 1

Dietary Exchanges: 1 vegetable, ½ fat

NOTE: This dip keeps well, and actually improves in flavor, in the refrigerator for up to 5 days. It makes a delicious condiment for wraps and sandwiches.

SIX NEW STICKS

If the mention of celery and carrot sticks screams "diet" to you, trade them for any of a half-dozen healthful munchies you can keep handy in resealable refrigerator bags.

- Jicama
- Fennel
- Broccoli stems
- Turnips, baby if available
- Kohlrabi
- Bok choy

ZESTY DILL SPREAD ON WHOLE GRAIN CRACKERS

This dip makes a good anytime snack even without the tomato wedge on top. Store the dip in a tightly covered container in the refrigerator for up to 1 week. Spread on the crackers just before eating.

Preparation time: 12 minutes

½ cup 1% cottage cheese

1 teaspoon horseradish

1½ teaspoons finely chopped fresh or dried dill

Ground black pepper

24 7-grain snack crackers

6 grape tomatoes, quartered

1. In a bowl, combine the cottage cheese, horseradish, and dill. Stir to mix. Add more horseradish to taste if desired. Season to taste with pepper.

2. Spread evenly on the crackers. Top each cracker with a piece of tomato. Serve right away.

MAKES 6 SERVINGS (4 CRACKERS PER SERVING)

Per serving: 52 calories, 7 g carbohydrate, 3 g protein, 1 g fat, 0 g saturated fat, 0 mg cholesterol, 123 mg sodium, 1 g fiber

Carbohydrate Choices: ½

Dietary Exchanges: ½ meat

CREAMY CHIPOTLE SPREAD ON CUCUMBER SLICES

This simple appetizer or snack makes an exciting flavor play on the tongue with its contrast of cool, crisp vegetable and spicy cream topping.

Preparation time: 5 minutes

---

  1 **teaspoon olive oil, preferably extra virgin**

⅛–¼ **teaspoon ground chipotle chile or ground red pepper**

  ½ **teaspoon minced garlic**

  ½ **cup fat-free soft cream cheese**

  1 **English cucumber, cut into ½"-thick rounds**

  2 **tablespoons minced chives or scallion greens (optional, for garnish)**

1. In a microwaveable bowl, combine the oil, ⅛ teaspoon chipotle or red pepper, and garlic. Cover with waxed paper. Cook on high power for 45 seconds, or until sizzling. Add the cream cheese. Stir until well blended. Taste for heat and add up to ⅛ teaspoon chipotle or red pepper to taste.

2. To serve, spread the chipotle cream on the cucumber rounds. Sprinkle on the chives or scallions, if using.

MAKES 7 SERVINGS (3 PIECES PER SERVING)

Per serving: 30 calories, 2 g carbohydrate, 3 g protein, 1 g fat, 0 g saturated fat, 5 mg cholesterol, 115 mg sodium, 0 g fiber

Carbohydrate Choices: 0

Dietary Exchanges: ½ vegetable, ½ meat

NOTE: The chipotle cream can be covered and refrigerated for up to 1 week if desired. Spread onto the cucumbers just before serving. It also makes a delicious dip for raw vegetables or whole grain tortilla chips.

BLUE CHEESE–WALNUT SPREAD ON ASIAN PEAR SLICES

By pairing reduced-fat ricotta cheese with a relatively small amount of delectable full-fat blue cheese, we're able to capture the lush flavor and rich texture while keeping the total fat low.

Preparation time: 10 minutes

---

1 large Asian pear (8 ounces)

¼ cup crumbled blue cheese

¼ cup part-skim ricotta cheese

2 tablespoons finely chopped toasted walnuts

1. Cut the pear in ʰters through the stem end. Lay the qⁱ ˙ut side down, on a work surfaˊ ˃r into ¼"-thick slices. Arˈ

too dry!

2. Inˈ ʰeese anˑ ˑ. Stir iⁱ slices. Seₗ

MAKES 4 SERVˑ SERVING)

Per serving: 100 calories, ˏ 4 g protein, 6 g fat, 3 g saturateₗ ˳holesterol, 135 mg sodium, 3 g fiber

Carbohydrate Choices: ½

Dietary Exchanges: ½ fruit, ½ meat, 1 fat

NOTES: Toasting brings out the flavor and crispness in nuts. Spread walnut halves on a dry baking sheet. Bake in a preheated 350°F oven, stirring occasionally, for about 10 minutes, or until sizzling and fragrant. Be careful not to burn. Let stand to cool. Store in an airtight tin for several weeks.

If desired, the cheese spread can be refrigerated in a tightly sealed container for up to a week. Slice the pear just before serving.

The spread can also top apples or whole grain crackers.

If serving the Asian pear slices as a party appetizer, sprinkle the nuts over the spread instead of mixing them in.

SUMMER SHRIMP ROLLS

By wrapping the savory ingredients into lettuce leaves instead of egg roll wrappers, the carb count remains moderate. In summer, the fresh lettuce rolls make a refreshing light meal.

Preparation time: 9 minutes   ●   **Cooking time: 6 minutes**

3	ounces Asian-style rice noodles
1	pound large peeled, cooked frozen shrimp, tails removed
12	large green leaf lettuce leaves
¼	ounce fresh mint or basil leaves
2	medium carrots, grated
⅓	cup bottled peanut dipping sauce

1. Bring 4 cups of water to a boil in a medium saucepan. Submerge the noodles and turn off the heat. Let the noodles soften for 3 minutes, then drain in a strainer over a large bowl, saving the hot water. Submerge the shrimp in the hot water for 3 minutes to thaw. Drain.

2. Meanwhile, rinse, dry, and stack the lettuce and mint or basil leaves on a plate. Put the carrots, noodles, and shrimp in separate dishes.

3. Lay 1 large lettuce leaf on one hand. Top with noodles and carrots, 2 mint or basil leaves, and 3 or 4 shrimp. Roll the leaf around the contents to make a cylinder. Repeat with the remaining lettuce leaves. Serve with peanut sauce in individual bowls for dipping.

MAKES 4 SERVINGS (3 ROLLS PER SERVING)

Per serving: 281 calories, 27 g carbohydrate, 30 g protein, 5 g fat, 2.5 g saturated fat, 229 mg cholesterol, 519 mg sodium, 2 g fiber

Carbohydrate Choices: 2

Dietary Exchanges: 1 starch, ½ vegetable, 4 meat

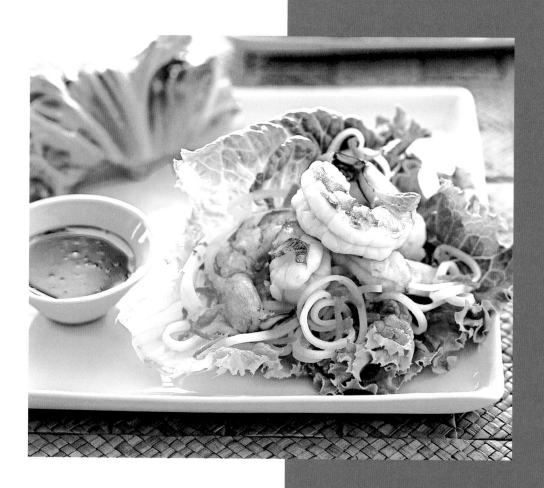

SEAFOOD COCKTAIL CARIBE

This first course is as refreshing as an island breeze. Navel oranges or clementines can take the place of the grapefruit if you prefer them.

Preparation time: 5 minutes ● **Standing time: 30 minutes**

½ pink grapefruit

4 ounces cooked sea bass, cut into small chunks

4 ounces peeled cooked medium shrimp

¼ cup finely chopped yellow or red bell pepper

¼ cup finely chopped celery heart

2 tablespoons minced cilantro

Pinch of salt

Hot-pepper sauce

4 lettuce or radicchio leaves

1. Over a small bowl, use a serrated knife to cut the sections from the grapefruit. Squeeze the juice into the bowl. Add the sea bass, shrimp, pepper, celery, cilantro, salt, and a few drops of hot-pepper sauce. Stir.

2. Cover with plastic and refrigerate for about 30 minutes to allow the flavors to blend.

3. Stir the mixture. Spoon onto lettuce-lined appetizer plates.

MAKES 4 SERVINGS

Per serving: 84 calories, 5 g carbohydrate, 13 g protein, 1 g fat, 0 g saturated fat, 58 mg cholesterol, 110 mg sodium, 1 g fiber

Carbohydrate Choices: 0

Dietary Exchanges: 2 meat

RADICCHIO-WRAPPED GRILLED TILAPIA

This distinctive sit-down appetizer can also serve as a main dish. Allow 2 bundles per main dish serving.

Preparation time: 6 minutes ● **Cooking time: 5 minutes**

6 large radicchio leaves
12 ounces tilapia
1 teaspoon ground fennel
Pinch of salt
Ground black pepper
Olive oil in a spray bottle
Balsamic vinegar

1. Preheat a grill or stove-top griddle.

2. Place the radicchio leaves on a work surface. Cut the fish into 6 equal pieces. Set a piece in the center of each leaf. Sprinkle evenly with the fennel. Season lightly with salt and pepper to taste. Spritz lightly with olive oil. Wrap each leaf into a bundle. Spritz the outsides lightly with oil.

3. Place the bundles on the grill or griddle over direct heat. Cook for 3 minutes, or until lightly browned. Move to indirect heat or lower the heat on the grill pan. Cook for about 2 minutes, or until the fish flakes easily. (Check by peeking inside one bundle.) Serve drizzled with vinegar.

MAKES 6 SERVINGS

Per serving: 50 calories, 1 g carbohydrate, 11 g protein, 1 g fat, 0 g saturated fat, 28 mg cholesterol, 22 mg sodium, 0 g fiber

Carbohydrate Choices: 0

Dietary Exchanges: ½ meat

SICILIAN SARDINE ANTIPASTO

The addition of naturally sweet raisins in a nondessert dish is typical of Sicilian cooking. Use either dark or golden raisins.

Preparation time: 5 minutes

1 tablespoon balsamic vinegar

2 teaspoons olive oil, preferably extra virgin

Pinch of salt

1 cup very thinly sliced fresh fennel + some finely chopped fennel greens for garnish

½ cup very thinly sliced red or yellow bell pepper

½ cup very thinly sliced red onion

1 can (4.375 ounces) water-packed sardines, drained and patted dry

Ground black pepper

In a bowl, combine the vinegar, oil, and salt. Whisk to blend. Add the fennel, bell pepper, onion, and sardines. Toss gently. Season to taste with black pepper. Serve garnished with fennel greens.

MAKES 4 SERVINGS

Per serving: 87 calories, 5 g carbohydrate, 6 g protein, 5 g fat, 1 g saturated fat, 17 mg cholesterol, 242 mg sodium, 1 g fiber

Carbohydrate Choices: 0

Dietary Exchanges: 1 vegetable, 1 meat, ½ fat

TOMATOES STUFFED WITH TUNA-BEAN SALAD

These tasty morsels are a little bit fussy—but fun when you want to do something different for a party. For everyday eating, you can simply halve the cherry tomatoes and stir them into the tuna-bean mixture as a luncheon dish served on spinach or romaine.

Preparation time: 25 minutes

---

24 cherry tomatoes (12 ounces)

¼ cup home-cooked cannellini beans or canned cannellini beans, rinsed and drained

¼ cup pouch-packed tuna

1 teaspoon olive oil

1 teaspoon lemon juice

½ teaspoon minced garlic (optional)

Ground black pepper

Finely chopped parsley

1. Cut off the tops of the tomatoes and discard. With a small sharp knife or kitchen scissors, snip the center membrane in each tomato. With a finger or small spoon, scoop out the seeds and juice. Discard. Set the tomatoes, cut side up, on a plate.

2. In a bowl, combine the beans, tuna, oil, lemon juice, and garlic, if using. Season to taste with pepper. Stir to mix, mashing the beans and tuna with the back of a spoon. With a tiny spoon, transfer the mixture into the tomatoes. Serve right away or cover and refrigerate for up to several hours. Sprinkle with parsley just before serving.

MAKES 12 SERVINGS (2 TOMATOES PER SERVING)

Per serving: 21 calories, 2 g carbohydrate, 2 g protein, 1 g fat, 0 g saturated fat, 2 mg cholesterol, 4 mg sodium, 0 g fiber

Carbohydrate Choices: 0

Dietary Exchanges: 0

STUFFED CAJUN EGGS

Whether served as a party appetizer or on-the-go snack, these stuffed eggs have far less fat than the classic version. You can vary the flavor if you like by replacing the Cajun seasoning with curry powder or sodium-free seasoning blend.

Preparation time: 5 minutes

4   hard-cooked eggs, chilled
¼   cup 1% dry-curd cottage cheese
¼   teaspoon salt-free Cajun seasoning
1   tablespoon minced scallion

1. Cut the eggs in half lengthwise. Remove the yolks and discard half of them or reserve for another recipe. Place the remaining yolks in a small bowl. Mash with a fork. Add the cottage cheese and the seasoning. Mash to mix completely. Stir in the scallion.

2. Arrange the egg white shells, hollow side up, on a plate. Mound the egg yolk mixture into each hollow. Sprinkle lightly with Cajun seasoning, if desired. Serve right away or cover and refrigerate for up to 24 hours.

MAKES 8 SERVINGS

Per serving: 44 calories, 1 g carbohydrate, 4 g protein, 3 g fat, 1 g saturated fat, 106 mg cholesterol, 62 mg sodium, 0 g fiber

Carbohydrate Choices: 0

Dietary Exchanges: ½ meat, ½ fat

SHANGHAI CHICKEN MEATBALLS

Peeled fresh ginger can be stored, tightly wrapped in plastic, in the freezer to prevent spoilage if you don't use it regularly. There's no need to thaw before grating.

Preparation time: 12 minutes ● **Baking time: 10 minutes**

8 ounces boneless, skinless chicken breast

½ teaspoon reduced-sodium soy sauce

½ teaspoon minced garlic

½ teaspoon grated fresh ginger

2 tablespoons finely chopped scallions or onion

2 teaspoons minced parsley

1. Preheat the oven to 375°F. Coat a baking sheet with vegetable oil spray.

2. Cut the chicken into 1" chunks. Coat the inside of a food processor work bowl and the metal blade with vegetable oil spray. Transfer the chicken to the work bowl. Pulse 6 times until coarsely chopped. In a small dish, combine the soy sauce, garlic, and ginger. Stir to blend. Add to the work bowl along with the scallions or onion and the parsley. Pulse 3 or 4 times just to mix.

3. With 2 forks or clean hands, shape the mixture into 32 marble-size balls. Place on the baking sheet. Continue until all the meatballs are shaped. Spritz lightly with vegetable oil from a spray bottle. Roll gently to coat.

4. Bake for about 10 minutes, or until no longer pink and the juices run clear.

MAKES 8 SERVINGS (4 MEATBALLS PER SERVING)

Per serving: 33 calories, 0 g carbohydrate, 7 g protein, 1 g fat, 0 g saturated fat, 16 mg cholesterol, 31 mg sodium, 0 g fiber

Carbohydrate Choices: 0

Dietary Exchanges: 1 meat

TURKEY COUSCOUS ROLL-UPS

Break the wrap mold by using cooked grain instead of a tortilla. It's a fun alternative.

Preparation time: 4 minutes

½ cup cooked whole wheat couscous, chilled

1 tablespoon lemon juice

3 sun-dried tomatoes (jarred in extra virgin olive oil), minced

¼ cup finely chopped celery

2 tablespoons coarsely chopped scallions

3 thick slices cracked-pepper deli turkey (¾ ounce each)

In a medium bowl, combine the couscous, lemon juice, tomatoes, celery, and scallions. Stir to mix. Fill the center of each turkey slice with the mixture and roll up.

MAKES 1 SERVING

Per serving: 315 calories, 54 g carbohydrate, 23 g protein, 3 g fat, 0 g saturated fat, 23 mg cholesterol, 601 mg sodium, 9 g fiber

Carbohydrate Choices: 3½

Dietary Exchanges: 2½ starch, 1 vegetable, 2 meat, ½ fat

LOOSEN UP/GET MOVING

Water Works

Ask your physician or physical trainer if non-weight-bearing swimming pool workouts could help your weight loss and fitness efforts. You don't even have to know how to swim to work out in water—you can do shallow-water or deep-water exercises without swimming. Benefits include:

- Increased flexibility—bending and moving your body in water is easier than on land.

- Enhanced strength from working against the water.

- Decreased risk of injury. Water makes your body float. This keeps your joints from being pounded or jarred and helps prevent sore muscles and injury.

- Refreshment—you can keep cooler in water, even when you are working hard.

ROSEMARY-GARLIC PORK KEBABS

Chicken breast can take the place of pork in these hearty appetizers. If eating as a main dish, double the servings.

Preparation time: 12 minutes ● **Marinating time: 30 minutes** ● **Cooking time: 8 minutes**

---

12 **ounces pork tenderloin**
2 **teaspoons fresh or dried rosemary**
2 **teaspoons olive oil**
1 **teaspoon minced garlic**
Pinch of salt
Ground black pepper

1. Soak 6 bamboo skewers (6" long) in cold water for 30 minutes. (If using metal skewers, there's no need to soak.)

2. Cut the pork into ½" cubes. Thread the cubes onto the skewers. Transfer to a 12" × 8" baking dish. Add the rosemary, oil, garlic, and salt. With clean hands, rub the mixture onto the pork cubes. Cover and refrigerate, turning occasionally, for 30 minutes.

3. Preheat a grill, stove-top griddle, or oven broiler. Grill or broil the skewers, turning occasionally, for about 8 minutes total, or until well browned and no pink remains in the center. Season to taste with pepper.

MAKES 6 SERVINGS

Per serving: 84 calories, 0 g carbohydrate, 12 g protein, 4 g fat, 1 g saturated fat, 37 mg cholesterol, 28 mg sodium, 0 g fiber

Carbohydrate Choices: 0

Dietary Exchanges: 2 meat, ½ fat

STUFFED BABY BELLO MUSHROOMS

Wonderful as pass-around appetizers for a party, these mushrooms can be stuffed in the morning and baked just before serving. Leftovers make tasty snacks.

Preparation time: 15 minutes ● **Cooking time: 20 minutes**

24	baby portobello mushrooms (10 ounces)
2	teaspoons olive oil
2	tablespoons minced tomato
1	tablespoon minced onion
¼	teaspoon minced garlic
½	teaspoon herbes de Provence
	Pinch of salt
1	tablespoon dry whole wheat bread crumbs
2	teaspoons finely chopped parsley
2	tablespoons grated Swiss or Gruyère cheese
	Ground black pepper

1. Preheat the oven to 375°F. Lightly coat a 12" × 8" baking dish with vegetable oil spray.

2. Carefully remove the stems from the mushroom caps. Set the caps, hollow side up, in the dish. Transfer the stems to a cutting board. Chop finely.

3. Heat the oil in a nonstick skillet over medium heat. Add the chopped mushrooms, tomato, onion, garlic, herbes de Provence, and salt. Cook, stirring, for 2 minutes, or until the liquid from the mushrooms evaporates. Stir in the bread crumbs, parsley, and cheese. Season to taste with pepper. Stir to mix.

4. Spoon the mixture into the reserved caps, pressing gently to adhere. Bake for 20 minutes, or until heated through.

MAKES 8 SERVINGS (3 MUSHROOMS PER SERVING)

Per serving: 28 calories, 2 g carbohydrate, 1 g protein, 2 g fat, 0.5 g saturated fat, 2 mg cholesterol, 46 mg sodium, 1 g fiber

Carbohydrate Choices: 0

Dietary Exchanges: ½ vegetable

NOTE: Herbes de Provence is a blend of dried herbs that are characteristic of southern French cooking. The mixture typically contains basil, fennel, lavender, marjoram, rosemary, sage, savory, and thyme. If unavailable, replace with dried thyme, rosemary, and sage.

CAULIFLOWER ITALIANO

Cooked vegetables in a vinaigrette dressing are a popular item in traditional Italian antipasto spreads.

Preparation time: 8 minutes ● **Cooking time: 4 minutes**

1 pound cauliflower florets, cut into marble-size pieces

1 tablespoon olive oil, preferably extra virgin

2 teaspoons red wine vinegar
Pinch of salt

1 ounce aged Provolone, thinly shaved
Red-pepper flakes

1. Fill a skillet with ½" water. Cover and set over high heat. Bring to a boil. Add the cauliflower. Cover and cook, stirring occasionally, for 4 minutes, or until crisp-tender. Drain.

2. Meanwhile, in a bowl, combine the oil, vinegar, and salt. Whisk to blend. Add the drained cauliflower. Toss to combine. Serve on appetizer plates topped with cheese and red-pepper flakes to taste.

MAKES 8 SERVINGS

Per serving: 42 calories, 3 g carbohydrate, 2 g protein, 3 g fat, 1 g saturated fat, 2 mg cholesterol, 66 mg sodium, 1 g fiber

Carbohydrate Choices: 0

Dietary Exchanges: ½ vegetable. ½ fat

CORN AND LENTIL FRITTERS

Be sure the lentils are cooked until very soft so they mash easily. These sweet morsels are divine topped with a dab of sour cream.

Preparation time: 10 minutes ● **Cooking time: 5 minutes**

¾ cup cooked lentils or leftover Provençal Lentil Ragout (page 313)

3 tablespoons stone-ground cornmeal

1 egg yolk

½ teaspoon baking powder

½ teaspoon minced garlic

⅛ teaspoon salt

Pinch of ground red pepper

¼ cup corn kernels, fresh or (thawed) frozen

2 tablespoons minced scallions

2 teaspoons finely chopped parsley

1. In the bowl of a food processor, combine the lentils or Provençal Lentil Ragout, cornmeal, egg yolk, baking powder, garlic, salt, and pepper. Pulse about 6 times, scraping down the sides of the bowl as needed, until a coarse puree forms. Add the corn, scallions, and parsley. Pulse once or twice just to mix.

2. Heat a griddle or heavy skillet over medium-high heat. Take off the heat to coat with vegetable oil spray and return to stovetop. Dollop the batter in level tablespoonfuls onto the griddle. Press lightly with the back of a spoon to make a tiny pancake. Cook for about 1 minute, or until browned on the bottom. Flip and cook for 1 to 2 minutes, or until cooked through. Remove and set aside on a platter. Continue until all the batter is cooked.

MAKES 16 SERVINGS (1 FRITTER PER SERVING)

Per serving: 22 calories, 4 g carbohydrate, 1 g protein, 1 g fat, 0 g saturated fat, 13 mg cholesterol, 35 mg sodium, 1 g fiber

Carbohydrate Choices: 0

Dietary Exchanges: 0

VEGGIE CRUST MUSHROOM QUICHE

Replacing a flour-butter crust for one made from vegetables not only boosts the fiber and nutrients, it dramatically cuts the fat, calories, and carbs.

Preparation time: 20 minutes ● Baking time: 40 minutes ● Standing time: 15 minutes

CRUST

- 1 **pound zucchini, shredded**
- ½ **cup shredded carrots**
- ¼ **cup sliced scallions**
- 2 **tablespoons dry whole wheat bread crumbs**
- ⅛ **teaspoon salt**
  Ground black pepper

FILLING

- 2 **eggs + 1 egg white**
- 1½ **cups whole milk**
- ¼ **teaspoon grated nutmeg**
- ¼ **cup (1 ounce) grated Swiss or Gruyère cheese**
- 2 **tablespoons crumbled dried porcini mushrooms**
- 1 **tablespoon grated Romano cheese**

1. Preheat the oven to 400°F. Coat a 9" pie pan or 8" x 8" baking dish with vegetable oil spray.

2. Combine the zucchini, carrots, and scallions in a large cold skillet. Set over high heat. Cook, tossing frequently, for 5 minutes, or until the vegetables shrink significantly. Drain any excess water through a colander. Transfer the vegetables to a bowl. Add the bread crumbs, salt, and pepper to taste. Toss with a fork. Transfer to the prepared pan or dish. Press to evenly cover the bottom and sides of the pan or dish.

3. Bake the crust for 10 minutes, or until golden.

4. Meanwhile, in a mixing bowl, beat the eggs and egg white with a fork. Add the milk and nutmeg and stir to combine. Remove the crust from the oven. Sprinkle the Swiss or Gruyère, mushrooms, and Romano evenly in the bottom of the pan. Gently pour in the milk mixture.

5. Reduce the oven temperature to 350°F. Bake the quiche for about 30 minutes, or until a knife inserted in the center comes out clean. Let stand for 15 minutes before cutting.

MAKES 8 SERVINGS

Per serving: 90 calories, 7 g carbohydrate, 6 g protein, 4 g fat, 2 g saturated fat, 62 mg cholesterol, 117 mg sodium, 1 g fiber

Carbohydrate Choices: ½

Dietary Exchanges: 1 vegetable, ½ meat ½ fat

NOTE: Other dried mushrooms can replace the porcini. Do not reconstitute the mushrooms before using in this recipe. Place the dried mushrooms in a small food processor fitted with a metal blade or in a blender. Process into a coarse powder.

"REFRIED" BEAN QUESADILLAS

Traditional Mexican fried beans are prepared with lard. Here, we use a scant amount of olive oil to bring out the flavor of the seasonings before simmering the pink beans in broth.

Preparation time: 4 minutes ● **Cooking time: 12 minutes**

---

6 whole wheat flour tortillas
(8" diameter)

¾ cup "Refried" Beans (page 145)

1 cup Salsa Fresca (page 119) or
purchased fresh salsa

1. Preheat a heavy skillet or griddle over medium-high heat. Lay the tortillas on a work surface. Spread ¼ cup of the beans evenly over 3 tortillas. Cover with the other 3 tortillas.

2. Cook the quesadillas, one at a time, on the skillet or griddle for 2 minutes, or until browned on the bottom. Flip and cook for about 2 minutes, or until heated through. Continue until all of the quesadillas are cooked.

3. Cut each quesadilla into 8 wedges. Serve with salsa for topping.

MAKES 12 SERVINGS (2 WEDGES PER SERVING)

Per serving: 74 calories, 12 g carbohydrate, 2 g protein, 2 g fat, 0 g saturated fat, 0 mg cholesterol, 140 mg sodium, 2 g fiber

Carbohydrate Choices: 1

Dietary Exchanges: 1 starch, ½ meat

LET YOURSELF GO/STRESS LESS

Don't Play the Blame Game

Feeling guilty about excess weight and its relationship to diabetes can take the form of negative self-talk like "I'm a bad person." Such thoughts can actually deter positive efforts to change. In his book *Psyching Out Diabetes*, Richard R. Rubin, PhD, CDE, of the Johns Hopkins Medical School in Baltimore, advises that a shift from feeling guilty to feeling responsible can actually set up a pattern that will aid in weight reduction. "*Feeling guilty* involves negative judgments about yourself, and it focuses on the past in a way that tends to paralyze. *Feeling responsible* involves no judgments, and it focuses on the present and future in a way that tends to motivate," Rubin explains.

"Refried" Beans

These beans are a convenient ingredient to have on hand to make "Refried" Bean Quesadillas (page 144), vegetarian-style tortilla wraps or burritos, or huevos rancheros (sunny-side up eggs with beans).

Preparation time: 5 minutes ● **Cooking time: 18 minutes**

---

2 tablespoons olive oil

2 tablespoons minced garlic

1½ teaspoons ground cumin

1½ teaspoons dried oregano

⅛ teaspoon salt

1¾ cups home-cooked pink beans or 1 can (15½ ounces) pink beans, rinsed and drained

1 cup vegetable broth or water

1. In a saucepan, combine the oil, garlic, cumin, oregano, and salt. Cook over low heat for 3 minutes, or until fragrant (do not brown the garlic). Add the beans and stir to coat with the seasonings. Add the broth or water. Increase the heat to medium.

2. Cook at a medium simmer for 15 minutes, or until the liquid reduces and the beans squash easily with the back of a spoon.

3. Transfer to a blender or food processor fitted with a metal blade, or use an immersion blender, and process for about 2 minutes, scraping down the sides of the bowl as needed, until smooth.

MAKES 12 SERVINGS (¼ CUP PER SERVING)

Per serving: 66 calories, 8 g carbohydrate, 2 g protein, 3 g fat, 0.5 g saturated fat, 0 mg cholesterol, 26 mg sodium, 2 g fiber

Carbohydrate Choices: ½

Dietary Exchanges: ½ starch, ½ fat

NOTE: To store, cool the mixture completely. Refrigerate in an airtight container for up to 1 week or freeze in recipe-ready portions in resealable plastic freezer bags for up to 3 months.

MOLDED GAZPACHO SALAD

Try a dollop of mayonnaise on this cool summer first course. It also makes a good salad for a picnic.

Preparation time: 10 minutes ● **Chilling time: 6 hours**

½ cup cold water

1 tablespoon unflavored gelatin

2 cups reduced-sodium tomato juice

⅓ cup finely chopped celery

⅓ cup finely chopped red or yellow bell pepper

¼ cup finely chopped scallions

2 tablespoons finely chopped cilantro

2 tablespoons lime juice

¼ teaspoon hot-pepper sauce

Lettuce leaves (optional)

1. Pour the water into a microwaveable bowl. Sprinkle on the gelatin. Let stand for 5 minutes to soften. Microwave on high power for 1 minute, or until hot. Stir until the gelatin is completely dissolved.

2. In an 8" x 8" glass or ceramic baking dish, combine the juice and gelatin liquid. Whisk thoroughly to combine. Add the celery, pepper, scallions, cilantro, lime juice, and hot-pepper sauce. Stir to blend. Cover and refrigerate for about 6 hours, or until set.

3. Cut into squares. Serve on lettuce leaves, if desired.

MAKES 6 SERVINGS

Per serving: 26 calories, 5 g carbohydrate, 2 g protein, 0 g fat, 0 g saturated fat, 0 mg cholesterol, 170 mg sodium, 1 g fiber

Carbohydrate Choices: 0

Dietary Exchanges: 1 vegetable

NOTE: To serve as a decorative mold for a party, transfer the tomato juice mixture into a nonstick 3-cup decorative mold. Cover and refrigerate for several hours, or until solid. To unmold, remove from the refrigerator and dip the mold up to the rim in a pan of hot water. Loosen the edges of the mold with a wet knife. Rinse a serving plate with cold water; shake off excess. Place the serving plate on top of the mold. Using both hands, flip the mold onto the plate. Lift the mold away from the plate.

HOT AND SWEET MELON SALAD

An Asian play of sweet melon and hot chile pepper makes an interesting addition to a cocktail buffet. The dish also pairs nicely with grilled pork tenderloin or chicken breast.

Preparation time: 4 minutes ● **Chilling time: 30 minutes**

---

6 ounces cantaloupe balls

6 ounces honeydew melon balls

1 small serrano or jalapeño chile pepper, cut into strips (wear plastic gloves when handling)

1 tablespoon slivered fresh basil leaves

2 teaspoons lemon or lime juice

1 teaspoon sugar

1. In a bowl, combine the cantaloupe, honeydew melon, pepper, basil, lemon or lime juice, and sugar. Toss to mix. Cover and refrigerate for 30 minutes.

2. Toss before serving. If desired, pick out and discard the pepper strips before serving.

MAKES 7 SERVINGS (3 PIECES PER SERVING)

Per serving: 20 calories, 5 g carbohydrate, 0 g protein, 0 g fat, 0 g saturated fat, 0 mg cholesterol, 8 mg sodium, 1 g fiber

Carbohydrate Choices: ½

Dietary Exchanges: 0

UNLEASH NUTRIENTS

Oh, Say, Can You "C"?

If you have diabetes, you'll want to get your daily dose of foods rich in vitamin C to protect the health of your eyes, nerves, and blood vessels. But did you also know that it might help your body use insulin better? A study conducted in Italy found that diabetes patients who took 1 gram of vitamin C daily for 4 months significantly improved their bodies' ability to use insulin. We all know that citrus is a great source, but just 1 cup of either broccoli, cantaloupe, or red bell peppers all exceed the Daily Value (DV) for vitamin C.

PIZZA BIANCA

"White pizza" is a delightful alternative to the classic tomato-topped pie. It's especially good with steamed kale or broccoli on the side.

Preparation time: 10 minutes ● **Rising and resting time: 1 hour 10 minutes**
Baking time: 12 minutes

Easy Pizza Crust (page 149)

1 tablespoon olive oil, preferably extra virgin

¾ cup chopped onion

2 teaspoons minced garlic

½ teaspoon dried oregano

Pinch of salt

½ cup (2 ounces) shredded Swiss or Gruyère cheese

1. Prepare the dough for the crust. Coat a 14" round pizza pan with vegetable oil spray. Punch down the dough. Transfer to a lightly floured work surface. Let stand for 5 minutes. With floured hands or a rolling pin, pat or roll into a 14" circle. Transfer to the prepared pan. Cover with plastic wrap and let stand for 15 minutes.

2. Preheat the oven to 375°F. Set a skillet over high heat for 1 minute. Add the oil and swirl to coat the pan. Heat for 30 seconds. Add the onion, garlic, oregano, and salt. Reduce the heat to medium-low. Cook, stirring occasionally, for about 5 minutes, or until golden. Spread the mixture evenly over the prepared crust. Sprinkle on the cheese.

3. Bake for about 12 minutes, or until golden and bubbly. Cut into 8 slices.

MAKES 8 SERVINGS (1 SLICE PER SERVING)

Per serving: 170 calories, 24 g carbohydrate, 6 g protein, 5 g fat, 2 g saturated fat, 5 mg cholesterol, 110 mg sodium, 4 g fiber

Carbohydrate Choices: 1½

Dietary Exchanges: 1½ starch, ½ vegetable, ½ meat, 1 fat

Easy Pizza Crust

You can have pizza made from scratch, even for weeknight meals, by planning ahead. You may make the dough in the morning and refrigerate it for a slow rise. Or make several crusts on a weekend and freeze them to bake (no need to thaw) for a quick weeknight meal.

Preparation time: 10 minutes ● **Rising and resting time: 1 hour 10 minutes**

⅔ cup warm water (105° to 115°F)

1 envelope (¼ ounce) active dry yeast (2¼ teaspoons)

1¾–2 cups whole wheat flour, preferably white whole wheat, divided

¼ teaspoon salt

2 teaspoons olive oil, preferably extra virgin

1. Coat a large bowl with vegetable oil spray; set aside. In a glass measuring cup, mix the water and the yeast to dissolve. In the bowl of a food processor, combine 1¾ cups flour and the salt. Pulse to mix. Add the oil to the yeast water. With the machine running, add the yeast water through the feed tube. Process for 1 to 2 minutes, or until the mixture forms a moist ball.

2. Transfer the dough to a work surface lightly floured with some of the remaining ¼ cup flour. With your hands, knead for about 1 minute, or until the dough is smooth. Use scant amounts of any remaining flour only to prevent surface sticking. Some flour may not be needed. Place the dough in the prepared bowl. Coat lightly with vegetable oil spray. Cover with plastic wrap. Set aside to rise for about 30 minutes, or until doubled in size.

3. Punch down the dough. Shape into a ball and transfer to a work surface. Let stand for 5 minutes. Shape, add toppings, and bake according to recipe directions.

MAKES 8 SERVINGS (1 THIN PIZZA CRUST—14" DIAMETER)

Per serving: 120 calories, 21 g carbohydrate, 4 g protein, 2 g fat, 0 g saturated fat, 0 mg cholesterol, 75 mg sodium, 4 g fiber

Carbohydrate Choices: 1

Dietary Exchanges: 1½ starch

NOTES: The dough can be prepared in a bread dough machine according to the manufacturer's directions.

To freeze the pizza dough after the first rise: Punch down the dough and shape into a ball. Coat well with vegetable oil spray. Place in a freezer-quality plastic bag. Squeeze out all air and close tightly. Store in the freezer for up to 1 month. To thaw, place in the refrigerator overnight. With scissors, cut away the plastic bag. Place the dough on a lightly floured work surface. Shape according to the recipe directions.

To freeze the unbaked pizza crust: Roll or pat the dough according to the recipe directions. Place on a pizza pan dusted with cornmeal. Cover tightly with plastic wrap, then wrap in aluminum foil. Store in the freezer for up to 1 month. To bake, remove from the freezer (no need to thaw). Remove wrappings. Top and bake according to the recipe directions.

DOUBLE-CHEESE DOUBLE-STUFFED PIZZA POCKETS

Whole wheat pitas are handy to have on hand for impromptu individual pizzas. This recipe can be halved or quartered to make 1 or 2 pizzas.

Preparation time: 10 minutes ● **Cooking time: 20 minutes**

1   medium zucchini, chopped

¼   cup chopped red bell pepper

4   whole wheat pitas (6½" diameter)

¼   cup fat-free chunky garden-style pasta sauce

¼   cup part-skim ricotta cheese

⅓   cup shredded reduced-fat mozzarella cheese

1   cup chopped plum tomatoes

1. Preheat the oven to 425°F.

2. Coat a medium nonstick skillet with vegetable oil spray and place over medium-high heat. Add the zucchini and pepper. Cook, stirring frequently, for about 10 minutes, or until the vegetables are softened.

3. Meanwhile, place the pitas on an ungreased baking sheet. Bake for 5 minutes, or until crisp.

4. Add the sauce to the skillet and mix well. Spread the sauce over the pitas. Dot with the ricotta. Sprinkle with the mozzarella and tomatoes.

5. Bake for 7 to 10 minutes, or until the cheese is melted.

MAKES 4 SERVINGS

Per serving: 240 calories, 42 g carbohydrate, 12 g protein, 5 g fat, 2 g saturated fat, 10 mg cholesterol, 480 mg sodium, 6 g fiber

Carbohydrate Choices: 3

Dietary Exchanges: 2 starch, 1 vegetable, ½ meat

BROCCOLI PIZZA

If you have a homemade Easy Pizza Crust in the freezer, this savory pie can be on the table in only 25 minutes.

Preparation time: 10 minutes ● **Rising and resting time: 1 hour 10 minutes**
Baking time: 15 minutes

Easy Pizza Crust (page 149)

1 tablespoon olive oil, preferably extra virgin

8 ounces broccoli florets and stems, cut into marble-size pieces

2 teaspoons minced garlic

⅛ teaspoon salt

1 can (14½ ounces) diced tomatoes, well drained

¾ cup (3 ounces) shredded provolone cheese

Red-pepper flakes

1. Prepare the dough for the crust. Coat a 14" round pizza pan with vegetable oil spray. Punch down the dough. Transfer to a lightly floured work surface. Let stand for 5 minutes. With floured hands or a rolling pin, pat or roll into a 14" circle. Transfer to the prepared pan. Pinch the edges to make a border. Cover with plastic wrap and let stand for 15 minutes.

2. Preheat the oven to 375°F. Set a heavy skillet over medium-high heat for 1 minute. Add the oil and swirl to coat the pan bottom. Heat for 30 seconds. Add the broccoli, garlic, and salt. Toss to mix. Cover and cook for about 2 minutes, tossing occasionally, or until the broccoli turns bright green. Add the tomatoes. Reduce the heat to medium. Cook, tossing frequently, for about 2 minutes, or until any liquid from the tomatoes is cooked away.

3. Sprinkle a few tablespoons of the cheese over the crust. Spoon the broccoli mixture evenly over the crust. Sprinkle on the remaining cheese. Bake for about 15 minutes, or until golden and bubbly. Cut into 8 slices. Serve with red-pepper flakes.

MAKES 8 SERVINGS (1 SLICE PER SERVING)

Per serving: 185 calories, 24 g carbohydrate, 7 g protein, 6 g fat, 2 g saturated fat, 8 mg cholesterol, 254 mg sodium, 5 g fiber

Carbohydrate Choices: 1½

Dietary Exchanges: 1½ starch, ½ vegetable, ½ meat, 1 fat

NOTE: Any extra slices can be placed on a tray and frozen for 24 hours. Wrap individual slices in aluminum foil. To reheat, bake the frozen slices in a 350°F oven for about 15 minutes, or until hot.

GOAT CHEESE AND RED PEPPER PIZZA

Add a side spinach salad for extra fiber. A ready-made whole wheat crust may replace the from-scratch Easy Pizza Crust, but it will add considerably more sodium.

Preparation time: 10 minutes ● **Rising and resting time: 1 hour 10 minutes**
Baking time: 12 minutes

Easy Pizza Crust (page 149)

5 ounces low-fat soft goat cheese

1 large clove garlic, minced

½ teaspoon chopped fresh oregano leaves or ¼ teaspoon dried

Ground black pepper

1 cup (10 ounces) roasted sweet red bell pepper strips or jarred, roasted sweet red bell peppers, drained and cut lengthwise into thin strips

Slivered fresh basil leaves, for garnish

1. Prepare the dough for the crust. Coat a 14" round pizza pan with vegetable oil spray. Punch down the dough. Transfer to a lightly floured work surface. Let stand for 5 minutes. With floured hands or a rolling pin, pat or roll into a 14" circle. Transfer to the prepared pan. Cover with plastic wrap and let stand for 15 minutes.

2. Preheat the oven to 375°F. In a small bowl, combine the cheese, garlic, and oregano. Season with black pepper to taste.

3. Dapple the crust with the crumbled cheese mixture. Scatter the red pepper strips on top of the cheese.

4. Bake for about 12 minutes, or until golden and bubbly.

5. Remove the pizza from the oven and garnish with basil. Cut into eighths and serve at once.

MAKES 4 SERVINGS (2 SLICES PER SERVING)

Per serving: 300 calories, 47 g carbohydrate, 11 g protein, 7 g fat, 3 g saturated fat, 5 mg cholesterol, 430 mg sodium, 8 g fiber

Carbohydrate Choices: 3

Dietary Exchanges: 3 starch, ½ meat, 1 fat

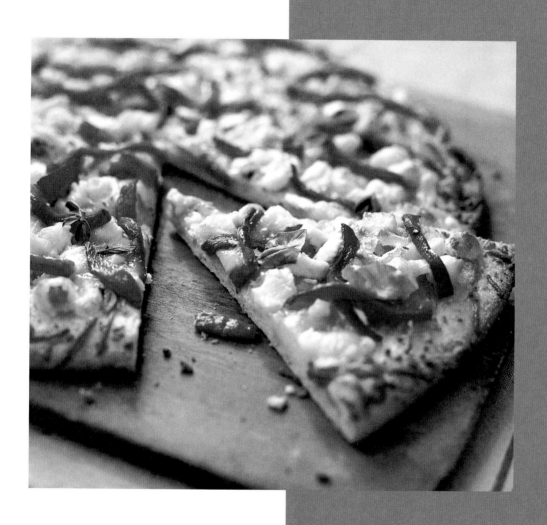

ITALIAN EGG AND PEPPER SANDWICH ON MULTIGRAIN BREAD

Even when the cupboard is almost bare, you can make this enjoyable sandwich. If no peppers are on hand, leave them out or substitute additional onion.

Preparation time: 6 minutes ● **Cooking time: 10 minutes**

1 teaspoon olive oil
¼ cup sliced onion
¼ cup sliced green bell pepper
  Pinch of dried oregano
  Pinch of salt
1 egg + 1 egg white
1 slice multigrain country bread, toasted

1. Heat the oil in a nonstick skillet over medium heat. Add the onion, pepper, oregano, and salt. Toss. Cook, tossing occasionally, for 5 minutes, or until softened.

2. In a small bowl, beat the egg and egg white with a fork. Add to the skillet. Cook for 3 minutes, or until set on the bottom. Flip the mixture. Fold if necessary to make the egg mixture the same size as the bread slice. Cook for about 2 minutes, or until cooked through. Set atop the toast.

MAKES 1 SERVING

Per serving: 227 calories, 18 g carbohydrate, 14 g protein, 11 g fat, 2 g saturated fat, 212 mg cholesterol, 262 mg sodium, 5 g fiber

Carbohydrate Choices: 1

Dietary Exchanges: 1 starch, 1 vegetable, 1½ meat, 1½ fat

MEDITERRANEAN VEGGIE BURGER

Try these vegetarian sandwiches at your next cookout. You'll be surprised how quickly they disappear.

Preparation time: 15 minutes ● **Cooking time: 3 minutes**

2 large red leaf lettuce leaves

2 grilled-vegetable soy burgers

2 tablespoons goat cheese

1 bottled roasted red pepper, halved

½ cup BroccoSprouts

½ cup baby spinach leaves

1. Place the lettuce leaves onto a work surface, with the long sides facing you. With your fingers, press lightly to flatten the center of each.

2. Prepare the burgers per the package directions for the microwave. Place one on the center of each lettuce leaf. Top each with 1 tablespoon of the cheese, ½ red pepper, and ¼ cup each of the sprouts and spinach. Fold up the bottom and sides of each lettuce leaf to enclose the burgers. Serve immediately.

MAKES 2 SERVINGS

Per serving: 140 calories, 8 g carbohydrate, 16 g protein, 5 g fat, 3 g saturated fat, 10 mg cholesterol, 460 mg sodium, 5 g fiber

Carbohydrate Choices: ½

Dietary Exchanges: ½ vegetable, ½ meat, ½ fat

NOTE: BroccoSprouts is a brand of sprouted broccoli seeds, created by scientists at Johns Hopkins University School of Medicine, that provide high levels of antioxidants. They are available in many supermarkets.

SKINNY MONTE CRISTO

A typical Monte Cristo is oozing with unnecessary fat, but our version satisfies with a mere 6 grams of fat. Cut the recipe in half if you need only one sandwich.

Preparation time: 2 minutes ● **Cooking time: 8 minutes**

---

4 slices 100 percent whole wheat thin-sliced bread, toasted

2 slices (¾ ounce) low-sodium deli ham

2 slices (¾ ounce) low-sodium deli turkey

2 slices Swiss cheese

Ground black pepper

2 pinches of ground nutmeg

2 egg whites

¼ teaspoon confectioners' sugar

1. On two slices of toast, layer the ham, turkey, and cheese. Season to taste with pepper. Top with the other slices of toast.

2. Coat a cast-iron skillet with vegetable oil spray and place over medium heat for 2 minutes. In a shallow bowl, slightly stir the nutmeg into the egg whites. Dip one side of a sandwich into the egg whites and let the excess drip off. Repeat on the other side. Repeat with the other sandwich.

3. Cook for about 3 minutes on each side, or until the meat is warmed through, the cheese is melting, and the egg is cooked. Slice diagonally. Dust with sugar and serve right away.

MAKES 2 SERVINGS

Per serving: 190 calories, 18 g carbohydrate, 17 g protein, 6 g fat, 3 g saturated fat, 30 mg cholesterol, 440 mg sodium, 5 g fiber

Carbohydrate Choices: 1

Dietary Exchanges: 1½ starch, 2 meat, 1 fat

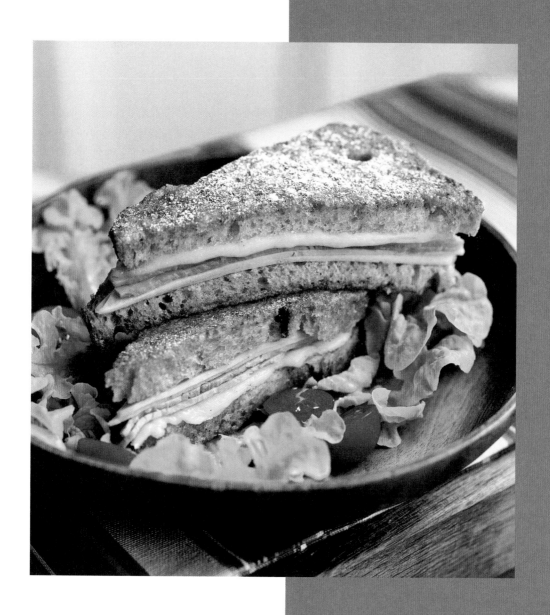

CHICKEN-CRANBERRY SANDWICH

During the Thanksgiving and Christmas holidays, replace the chicken with slices of leftover turkey breast.

Preparation time: 5 minutes

---

2   tablespoons reduced-fat cream cheese, at room temperature

2   slices whole grain bread, toasted if desired

2   tablespoons cranberry chutney, sauce, or relish

1   ounce thinly sliced reduced-fat Cheddar cheese

2   ounces thinly sliced cooked chicken breast

　 Apple slices

　 Trimmed watercress or baby spinach leaves

Smear the cream cheese onto 1 slice of bread. Spread the chutney, sauce, or relish onto the other slice. Fill the sandwich with the cheese, chicken, apple slices, and a handful of watercress or spinach leaves.

MAKES 1 SERVING

Per serving: 398 calories, 40 g carbohydrate, 33 g protein, 13 g fat, 7 g saturated fat, 85 mg cholesterol, 449 mg sodium, 12 g fiber

Carbohydrate Choices: 3

Dietary Exchanges: 1½ starch, 1 fruit, 4 meat, 2 fat

NOTE: To cut down the carbohydrates and sodium, replace the regular bread with 2 slices thin-sliced 100 percent whole wheat bread.

TURKEY IN THE SLAW SANDWICH

Enjoying your salad *on* your sandwich makes for a munching good lunch.

Preparation time: 5 minutes

---

1 teaspoon canola oil

2 teaspoons white wine vinegar

Pinch of celery seeds

½ cup finely shredded red or green cabbage

1 slice seeded rye bread, toasted

Honey mustard (optional)

2 ounces thinly sliced roasted turkey breast

Ground black pepper

1. In a bowl, whisk the oil, vinegar, and celery seeds. Add the cabbage; toss to coat.

2. Lay the toast on a work surface. Spread lightly with mustard, if using. Top with the turkey and slaw. Season with pepper to taste. Serve right away.

MAKES 1 SERVING

Per serving: 184 calories, 19 g carbohydrate, 13 g protein, 6 g fat, 0.5 g saturated fat, 25 mg cholesterol, 571 mg sodium, 3 g fiber

Carbohydrate Choices: 1

Dietary Exchanges: 1 starch, ½ vegetable, 1½ meat, 1 fat

A CUT ABOVE

While cured delicatessen meats are very convenient for snacks and lunches, they are high in sodium and unnecessary refined carbohydrates from add-ins such as high-fructose corn syrup. Avoid these unwanted additives by roasting fresh turkey breast on the weekend. It's a cinch, taking only about 5 minutes of hands-on time. Purchase boneless skinless turkey breast, often labeled turkey London broil. For a 1½-pound breast, rub with 1 teaspoon olive oil and 1 teaspoon poultry seasoning. Sprinkle very lightly with salt. Place in a small heavy pan or ovenproof skillet coated with vegetable oil spray. Roast in a preheated 350°F oven for about 45 minutes, or until an instant-read thermometer inserted in the center registers 165°F. Remove to a cutting board. Let stand to cool. Wrap well in plastic wrap or place in a resealable plastic storage bag. Refrigerate for up to 5 days, thinly slicing as needed. You can also thinly slice 2-ounce portions for sandwiches or salads and package them in small resealable storage bags. Freeze for up to 3 months.

SLOPPY TOM

It's really all the wonderful seasonings that give Sloppy Joes their flavor. We've kept those but subbed ground turkey breast for the high saturated fat ground beef.

Preparation time: 10 minutes ● **Cooking time: 21 minutes**

1½ teaspoons olive or canola oil
½ green bell pepper, finely chopped
¼ medium onion, finely chopped
1 teaspoon minced garlic
1 rib celery, finely chopped
8 ounces 99 percent lean ground turkey breast
1 tablespoon red wine vinegar
2 tablespoons tomato paste
1½ teaspoons brown sugar (optional)
⅓ cup chopped tomatoes
Dash of nutmeg
Pinch of salt
Ground black pepper
2 large whole wheat hamburger buns
Chopped scallions, for garnish

1. Preheat the broiler.

2. Heat the oil in a large skillet over low heat. Add the bell pepper, onion, garlic, and celery. Cover and cook, stirring occasionally, for about 7 minutes, or until the vegetables are softened and translucent.

3. Push the vegetables to one side of the skillet. Raise the heat to medium-high. Add the turkey to the side without vegetables. Cook, stirring, about 7 minutes, or until almost cooked through.

4. Combine the turkey and vegetables. Add the vinegar and stir. Add the tomato paste and sugar, if desired. Cook, stirring occasionally, about 4 minutes, or until lightly browned.

5. Add the tomatoes, nutmeg, and salt. Season to taste with black pepper. Lower the heat and simmer for about 3 minutes, or until thickened.

6. Open the buns and toast in a broiler until golden brown. Divide the meat between the buns. Garnish with scallions.

MAKES 2 SERVINGS

Per serving: 306 calories, 30 g carbohydrate, 33 g protein, 7 g fat, 1 g saturated fat, 45 mg cholesterol, 492 mg sodium, 5 g fiber

Carbohydrate Choices: 2

Dietary Exchanges: 2 starch, 1 vegetable, 3½ meat, 1 fat

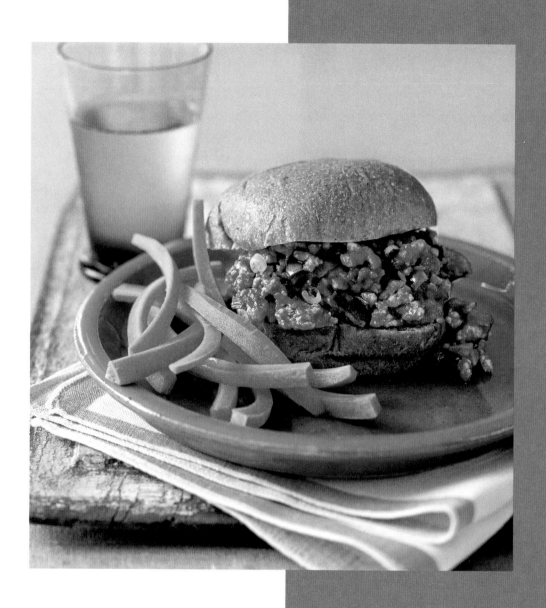

ROASTED VEGETABLE SANDWICH

This sophisticated sandwich is something you'd expect to order in a fancy café, but it's surprisingly easy to prepare at home.

Preparation time: 10 minutes ● **Cooking time: 30 minutes**

2 portobello mushroom caps

1 zucchini, cut in 3" segments, then sliced lengthwise

1 medium tomato, sliced

2 crusty multigrain rolls (4 ounces each), insides scooped out, or 2 slices whole grain bread

2 ounces fresh goat cheese

2 tablespoons Artichoke Tapenade (page 163)

1. Preheat the oven to 400°F. Arrange the mushrooms and zucchini on a nonstick baking sheet. Roast for 10 minutes. Arrange the tomato slices on the same baking sheet and continue roasting, flipping the vegetables halfway through cooking, for 20 minutes, or until sizzling and any liquid is cooked away.

2. Divide the sandwich fillings between the rolls, layering the mushrooms, then zucchini, cheese, tomato, and tapenade.

MAKES 2 SERVINGS

Per serving: 240 calories, 27 g carbohydrate, 13 g protein, 11 g fat, 6 g saturated fat, 22 mg cholesterol, 400 mg sodium, 9 g fiber

Carbohydrate Choices: 2

Dietary Exchanges: 1 starch, 2 vegetable, 1 meat, 1½ fat

Artichoke Tapenade

This vegetable condiment is nice to have on hand for a variety of sandwiches. It can be refrigerated in an airtight container for up to 3 days.

Preparation time: 3 minutes

---

1 cup canned (in water) artichoke hearts, drained

Juice of ½ lemon

1 tablespoon olive oil, preferably extra virgin

1 teaspoon minced garlic

1 teaspoon white wine vinegar

¼ teaspoon salt

Ground black pepper

In the bowl of a food processor fitted with a metal blade, combine the artichokes, lemon juice, oil, garlic, vinegar, and salt. Pulse about 8 times, scraping down the sides of the bowl as needed, or until the mixture is spreadable. Season to taste with pepper.

MAKES 6 SERVINGS (2 TABLESPOONS PER SERVING)

Per serving: 43 calories, 3 g carbohydrate, 1 g protein, 2 g fat, 0 g saturated fat, 0 mg cholesterol, 299 mg sodium, 1 g fiber

Carbohydrate Choices: 0

Dietary Exchanges: 1 vegetable, ½ fat

SALAD PITA

A folded lettuce leaf keeps things neat in this high-fiber, handheld meal. It's perfect for a meatless lunch.

Preparation time: 15 minutes

  3 red radishes, chopped
 ½ small seedless cucumber, peeled and chopped
 ½ green bell pepper, chopped
 ½ small red onion, finely chopped
 ¼ cup (2 ounces) crumbled feta cheese
 ½ cup rinsed and drained canned chickpeas
  1 tablespoon tahini
  3 tablespoons fat-free plain yogurt
 ¼ teaspoon dried oregano
 ¼ teaspoon ground cumin
  2 whole wheat pitas (6" diameter)
  4 medium romaine lettuce leaves

1. In a medium bowl, combine the radishes, cucumber, pepper, and onion. Mix in the cheese.

2. In another bowl, use a fork to partially mash the chickpeas with the tahini, yogurt, oregano, and cumin. The mixture will be thick and coarse in texture.

3. Slice open each pita by cutting off a piece about 1½" from the edge. Insert your hand to open the pocket.

4. Cut off the bottom part of 2 lettuce leaves so when folded in half crosswise, they fit into the pitas. Gently line each pita with 1 leaf. Finely shred the remaining lettuce leaves and tuck ½ cup into each pita.

5. Divide the chopped vegetables between the pitas. Dollop the chickpea mixture on top.

MAKES 2 SERVINGS

Per serving: 370 calories, 57 g carbohydrate, 16 g protein, 10 g fat, 3.5 g saturated fat, 17 mg cholesterol, 590 mg sodium, 9 g fiber

Carbohydrate Choices: 4

Dietary Exchanges: 2 starch, 1 vegetable, 1 meat, 1½ fat

NOTES: Tahini is prepared ground sesame seeds. Look for it in the gourmet cheese section of the supermarket.

The stuffed sandwiches can be slipped into resealable plastic bags and refrigerated for up to 24 hours.

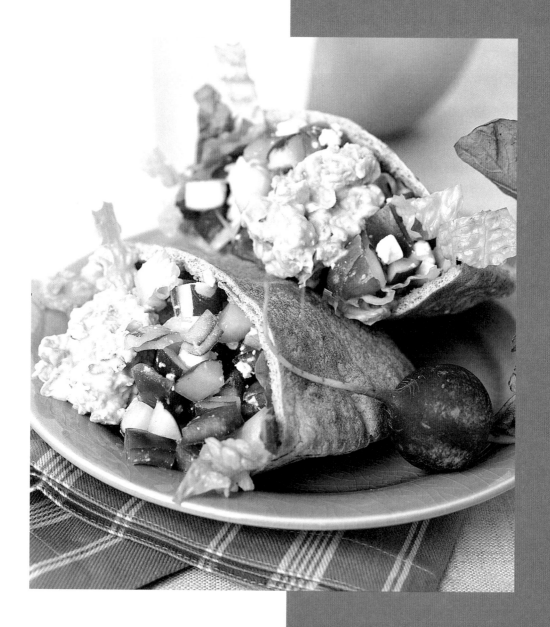

ROAST BEEF AND CREAMY HORSERADISH SANDWICH ON RYE

Prepared horseradish is a good condiment to keep in the refrigerator. It adds plenty of zip to foods but has virtually no fat or sodium.

Preparation time: 5 minutes

2 teaspoons mayonnaise

½ teaspoon prepared horseradish

1 slice 100 percent rye bread, toasted

2 ounces thinly sliced lean roast beef

1 large red romaine lettuce leaf

Spread the mayonnaise and horseradish on the toast. Top with the beef and lettuce.

MAKES 1 SERVING

Per serving: 216 calories, 16 g carbohydrate, 14 g protein, 10 g fat, 2 g saturated fat, 35 mg cholesterol, 588 mg sodium, 2 g fiber

Carbohydrate Choices: 1

Dietary Exchanges: 1 starch, 1½ meat, 1½ fat

BETTER-FOR-YOU BURRITOS

If you don't have the homemade Salsa Fresca on hand for this recipe, replace it with prepared refrigerated salsa found in the produce section of the supermarket. It generally contains less sodium than the bottled salsa.

Preparation time: 25 minutes ● Cooking time: 18 minutes

---

8 100 percent whole wheat flour tortillas (8" diameter)

12 ounces ground turkey breast

¾ cup chopped green bell pepper

½ cup chopped scallions

2 cups seeded and chopped plum tomatoes, divided

⅓ cup shredded carrot

¼ cup Salsa Fresca (page 119) or low-sodium salsa

1 teaspoon mild chili powder

8 romaine lettuce leaves

¼ cup (1 ounce) shredded reduced-fat Cheddar cheese

¼ cup fat-free sour cream

1. Preheat the oven to 200°F. Wrap the tortillas in aluminum foil and heat in the oven.

2. Meanwhile, coat a large nonstick skillet with vegetable oil spray and place over medium-high heat. Add the turkey, pepper, and scallions. Cook, breaking up the meat with a wooden spoon, for 8 minutes, or until the turkey is no longer pink. Drain the fat.

3. Add 1 cup of the tomatoes and the carrot, salsa, and chili powder. Reduce the heat to medium-low. Cover and simmer for 10 minutes, stirring occasionally. Remove the cover and continue to cook until any liquid is evaporated.

4. Trim the lettuce leaves so they are about 6" long. Place a leaf onto the center of a warm tortilla. Press lightly to flatten the center. Spoon one-eighth of the turkey mixture over the leaf. Sprinkle with some of the cheese and some of the remaining tomatoes. Top with a dollop of sour cream. Roll up the tortilla to cover the filling and then fold in the ends. Repeat with the remaining tortillas.

MAKES 4 SERVINGS (2 BURRITOS PER SERVING)

Per serving: 380 calories, 48 g carbohydrate, 30 g protein, 8 g fat, 1 g saturated fat, 40 mg cholesterol, 600 mg sodium, 9 g fiber

Carbohydrate Choices: 3

Dietary Exchanges: 3 starch, 1½ vegetable, 3 meat

TUNA SALAD WRAP

Canned tuna is an inexpensive, easy way to get your omega-3 fats. We like wrap bread because it's satisfying without being too filling.

Preparation time: 25 minutes

---

2   scallions (white and green parts), cut into 1" pieces
⅔   cup broccoli florets
½   cup packed parsley leaves
¼   Granny Smith apple with skin, cored and coarsely chopped
1   can (6½ ounces) water-packed albacore tuna
1½ tablespoons reduced-fat mayonnaise
    Ground black pepper
2   100 percent whole wheat tortillas (10" diameter)
2   large plum tomatoes, seeded and thinly sliced vertically

1. Place the scallions and broccoli into the bowl of a food processor fitted with a metal blade. Pulse 6 times to chop coarsely. Add the parsley and apple. Pulse 4 times to finely chop. The mixture should be moist but still crunchy. Scoop into a bowl. Wipe out the food processor bowl with a paper towel.

2. In the food processor bowl, combine the tuna and mayonnaise. Process until the mixture is a spreadable paste, about 45 seconds, scraping down the sides of the bowl as needed. Season to taste with pepper.

3. Divide the tuna between the tortillas, spreading firmly with a rubber spatula to cover all but ¾" along the outer edge of each wrap. Heap half of the chopped vegetables in the center of each wrap. Using your hand, spread them to cover the tuna, pressing lightly. Arrange the tomatoes evenly over the vegetables.

4. Roll the tortillas from the bottom, pulling toward you slightly to make them tight. Trim off the ends, cutting them on a diagonal in the same direction. Cut each wrap diagonally in half. Wrap pieces in plastic wrap and refrigerate 2 hours, or up to 24 hours, before serving.

MAKES 2 SERVINGS

Per serving: 300 calories, 28 g carbohydrate, 26 g protein, 12 g fat, 2 g saturated fat, 40 mg cholesterol, 590 mg sodium, 5 g fiber

Carbohydrate Choices: 2

Dietary Exchanges: 1 starch, 1 vegetable, 3 meat, 2 fat

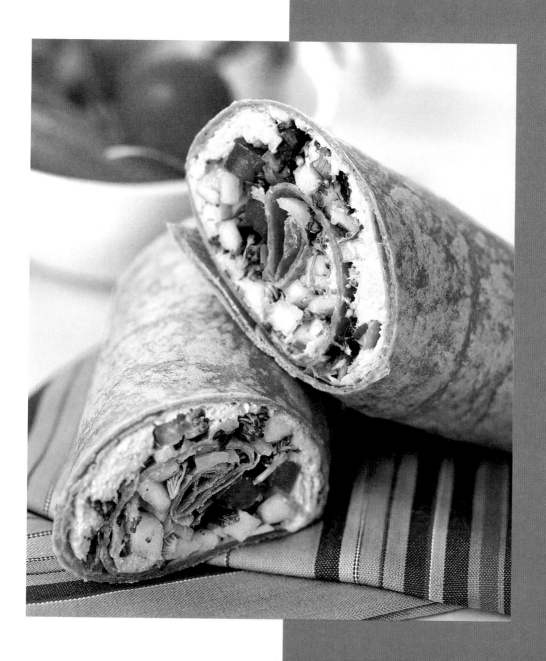

CHILI-ROASTED PEANUTS WITH CILANTRO

For more heat with the spice, add up to ⅛ teaspoon ground red pepper along with the chili powder.

Preparation time: 4 minutes ● **Cooking time: 15 minutes**

1 egg white
1 tablespoon water
1 cup dry-roasted unsalted peanuts
½ teaspoon sugar
¼ teaspoon chili powder
½ teaspoon minced garlic
⅛ teaspoon salt
2 tablespoons minced fresh cilantro

1. Preheat the oven to 350°F. In a small bowl, beat the egg white and water with a fork. Add the peanuts and toss to coat. Drain the nuts through a fine sieve. Pick up a few nuts at a time (so any remaining clumps of egg white drip off) and transfer to a large nonstick baking sheet. Sprinkle on the sugar, chili powder, garlic, and salt. Toss with the fork to coat with the seasoning mixture. Spread the peanuts out in a single layer so they are not in clumps.

2. Bake for 5 minutes. Stir the peanuts. Bake for 10 minutes more, stirring occasionally, or until sizzling and browned. Remove from the oven. Toss with the cilantro. Serve hot.

MAKES 32 SERVINGS (1 TABLESPOON PER SERVING)

Per serving: 55 calories, 2 g carbohydrate, 2 g protein, 5 g fat, 0.5 g saturated fat, 0 mg cholesterol, 22 mg sodium, 1 g fiber

Carbohydrate Choices: 0

Dietary Exchanges: ½ meat, 1 fat

NOTE: Any leftover peanuts can be refrigerated in an airtight container. To serve, spread a portion on a microwaveable plate. Microwave on high power for 30 seconds, or until heated.

CHOCOLATE-DIPPED ALMOND APRICOT POUCHES

These fruit and nut treats are the snack to have when you crave something distinctive. They also make a delightful alternative sweet to Christmas cookies.

Preparation time: 15 minutes ● Baking time: 10 minutes ● Chilling time: 30 minutes

½ teaspoon sugar

¼ teaspoon apple pie spice

1 egg white

1 tablespoon water

1 ounce raw whole almonds
(30 almonds)

1 bag (7 ounces) dried apricots
(30 apricots)

2 ounces bittersweet chocolate,
coarsely chopped

¹⁄₁₆ teaspoon almond extract

1. Preheat the oven to 350°F. Coat a small baking sheet with vegetable oil spray. In a small bowl, combine the sugar and spice mixture. Stir to mix. In another small bowl, beat the egg white and water with a fork. Add the almonds to the egg white mixture and toss to coat. Drain the nuts through a fine sieve. Pick up a few nuts at a time (so any remaining clumps of egg white drip off) and add to the sugar mixture. Toss with the fork to coat with the sugar mixture. Spread the almonds on the prepared pan. Spread out the nuts so they are separated.

2. Bake for 10 minutes, stirring occasionally, or until sizzling. Let stand to cool.

3. With a small sharp knife or kitchen scissors, cut a sideways pouch in the middle of each apricot. Insert an almond into each pouch. Press the opening to seal. (It's okay if some of the almond shows as long as it sticks to the apricot.)

4. Place the chocolate in a small microwaveable dish. Microwave on high power for about 90 seconds, or until melted. Add the extract. Stir until smooth. One at a time, dip the open side of the apricot pouch into the chocolate to coat about one-third of the apricot. Place on a plate. Continue until all the apricots are dipped. Refrigerate for about 30 minutes for the chocolate to set. Eat right away or store in an airtight tin in the refrigerator for up to 2 weeks.

MAKES 15 SERVINGS (2 PER SERVING)

Per serving: 70 calories, 11 g carbohydrate, 1 g protein, 3 g fat, 1 g saturated fat, 0 mg cholesterol, 0 mg sodium, 1 g fiber

Carbohydrate Choices: 1

Dietary Exchanges: ½ fruit, ½ fat

PEANUT BUTTER AND RAISIN PORCUPINES

A tasty nibble for peanut butter lovers. These keep well in an airtight container in the refrigerator for up to 1 week.

Preparation time: 15 minutes

½ cup 100 percent bran cereal with extra fiber

¼ cup raisins

2 tablespoons fat-free milk powder

¼ cup + 1 tablespoon part-skim ricotta cheese

3 tablespoons natural peanut butter

1. Place the cereal in a shallow dish. With your hands, crumble into smaller pieces. In the work bowl of a food processor fitted with a metal blade, combine the raisins and milk powder. Process for about 2 minutes, or until the raisins are finely chopped. Remove to a bowl. Add the ricotta and peanut butter. Stir until smooth.

2. Lightly oil your hands with vegetable oil spray. One at a time, shape the raisin mixture into small balls (2 level teaspoons each). Roll each ball into the cereal to coat lightly. Press to adhere with bits of cereal. Continue with the remaining mixture. Set the balls in a plastic storage container. If there is more than one layer, separate them by waxed paper.

MAKES 7 SERVINGS (3 PER SERVING)

Per serving: 90 calories, 10 g carbohydrate, 4 g protein, 5 g fat, 1 g saturated fat, 0 mg cholesterol, 70 mg sodium, 3 g fiber

Carbohydrate Choices: ½

Dietary Exchanges: ½ fruit, ½ meat, 1 fat

FILL UP ON WHOLE FOODS

Pure and Simple Popcorn

Popcorn is fun! It's also a whole grain snack that's a source of fiber and very low in fat. Keep it that way by purchasing the best-quality popcorn kernels you can find and popping them in a hot-air popper or microwaveable popcorn bowl. Spritz very lightly with olive oil or Better Butter (page 323) and season with your favorite sodium-free herb or spice blend.

CANDIED SPICED NUTS

When you've reached your goal weight and can afford a few more calories, a 1-ounce (2-tablespoon) serving of nuts several times a week makes an excellent snack. Although high in fat, walnuts and almonds are a good vegetable source of omega-3 fatty acids.

Preparation time: 15 minutes ● **Cooking time: 1 hour**

1   egg white
1   tablespoon water
½   pound shelled walnut halves
½   pound shelled almonds
½   cup sugar (preferably superfine)
1   tablespoon ground cinnamon
1   teaspoon ground ginger
1   teaspoon salt
½   teaspoon ground coriander
¼   teaspoon ground allspice
      Pinch of ground red pepper

1. Preheat the oven to 250°F.

2. In a medium bowl, whisk the egg white and water until frothy. Add the walnuts and almonds and stir to coat completely. Transfer the nuts to a strainer or sieve and allow to drain about 5 minutes.

3. In a large plastic bag, combine the sugar, cinnamon, ginger, salt, coriander, allspice, and pepper. Holding the open end tightly, shake vigorously to blend. Add half of the nuts to the bag and shake to coat thoroughly. Remove the nuts and place on a large nonstick baking sheet. Repeat with the remaining nuts and spread on the baking sheet.

4. Bake for 15 minutes and then stir, smoothing the nuts into a single layer. Lower the oven temperature to 200°F. Bake until the nuts are caramelized, about 45 minutes.

5. Allow the nuts to cool.

MAKES 18 SERVINGS (¼ CUP PER SERVING)

Per serving: 175 calories, 8 g carbohydrate, 5 g protein, 15 g fat, 1 g saturated fat, 0 mg cholesterol, 133 mg sodium, 3 g fiber

Carbohydrate Choices: ½

Dietary Exchanges: 1 meat, 2½ fat

NOTE: Store in an airtight container at room temperature for up to 2 weeks.

CHAPTER 8

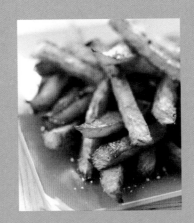

SOUPS, SALADS, AND SIDES

NEW ENGLAND CLAM CHOWDER

A warming bowl of soup as an appetizer not only prolongs the pleasure of a relaxing mealtime, but also may help you eat fewer calories for the remainder of the meal.

Preparation time: 25 minutes ● **Cooking time: 25 minutes**

---

  1 slice bacon
  2 teaspoons canola oil
  ½ cup chopped onion
  ½ cup chopped celery
  1 teaspoon minced garlic
  ½ teaspoon dried thyme
  1 bay leaf
1½ cups diced Yukon Gold potatoes (½" dice)
1½ cups clam juice
  ½ cup water (optional)
1½ cups 2% milk, divided
1½ tablespoons all-purpose flour
  3 cans (6½ ounces each) minced clams, drained
  ¼ cup chopped parsley
     Whole wheat crackers (optional)

1. Cook the bacon in the microwave, per package directions, until crisp. Crumble into small pieces and set aside.

2. In a large saucepan, heat the oil over medium-low heat. Add the onion, celery, and garlic and cook for 5 minutes. Add the thyme and bay leaf and continue to cook for 3 minutes, stirring occasionally, until the onion is softened but not browned. Add the potatoes and clam juice. The liquid should just cover the potatoes, so add the water if necessary. Bring the chowder to a simmer and cook the potatoes for about 10 minutes, or until tender but not mushy.

3. In a small bowl, whisk ¼ cup of the milk with the flour until smooth. Add to the chowder with the remaining 1¼ cups milk and increase the heat to bring to a boil, stirring constantly, until the soup has slightly thickened, about 3 minutes. Remove the pot from the heat and add the clams. Remove and discard the bay leaf. Divide into 4 bowls and sprinkle each serving with crumbled bacon and parsley. Garnish each serving with a crumbled whole wheat cracker, if using.

MAKES 4 SERVINGS

Per serving: 140 calories, 13 g carbohydrate, 10 g protein, 5 g fat, 1.5 g saturated fat, 25 mg cholesterol, 600 mg sodium, 1 g fiber

Carbohydrate Choices: 1

Dietary Exchanges: ½ milk, ½ vegetable, 1 meat, 1 fat

NOTE: To reduce the sodium in this soup, replace the bottled clam juice with no-sodium-added vegetable broth or half canned vegetable broth and half water.

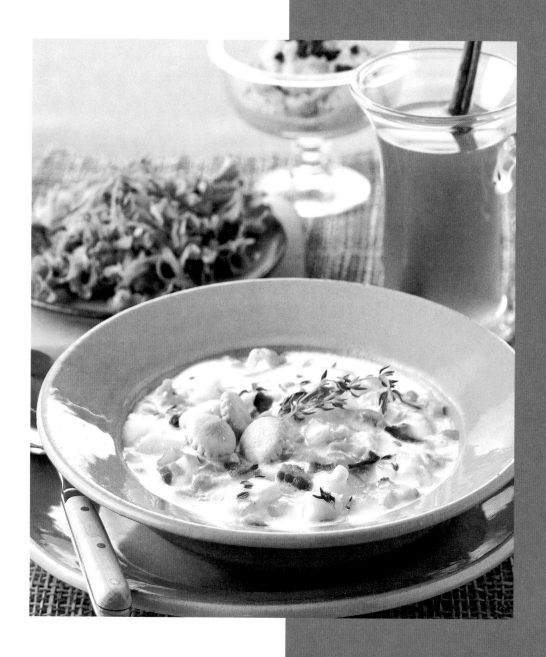

AUTUMN HARVEST MINESTRONE

The slow cooker is perfect for simmering dried beans to tender perfection. You just combine all the ingredients and let time do all the work.

Preparation time: 20 minutes ● **Cooking time: 7–9 hours**

---

2 cans (15 ounces each) cannellini beans, rinsed and drained

2 cans (14½ ounces each) chicken broth

3 cups (½" chunks) butternut squash (1 pound)

1 can (14½ ounces) diced tomatoes

2 medium turnips, peeled and cut into ½" chunks

1 medium parsnip, peeled, quartered, and sliced ¼" thick

2 cups bagged coleslaw mix

1 large leek (white and light green parts), sliced

1 tablespoon minced garlic, divided

1 cup (packed) fresh basil

⅓ cup chopped parsley

¼ cup grated Parmesan cheese

3 tablespoons olive oil, preferably extra virgin

¼ teaspoon salt

¼ teaspoon ground black pepper

2 tablespoons water

1. In a 4-quart or larger slow cooker, mix the beans, broth, squash, tomatoes (with juice), turnips, parsnip, coleslaw, leek, and 1½ teaspoons of the garlic. Cover and cook on the low setting for 7 to 9 hours, or until the vegetables are tender.

2. In the bowl of a food processor fitted with a metal blade or in a blender, combine the basil, parsley, cheese, oil, salt, pepper, water, and the remaining 1½ teaspoons garlic. Process for about 2 minutes, scraping down the sides of the bowl as needed, or until smooth. Transfer to a small bowl and refrigerate.

3. To serve, ladle the soup into serving bowls and top with a heaping tablespoon of basil sauce.

MAKES 6 SERVINGS

Per serving: 280 calories, 41 g carbohydrate, 11 g protein, 10 g fat, 2 g saturated fat, 5 mg cholesterol, 570 mg sodium, 9 g fiber

Carbohydrate Choices: 3

Dietary Exchanges: 4 vegetable, ½ meat, 1½ fat

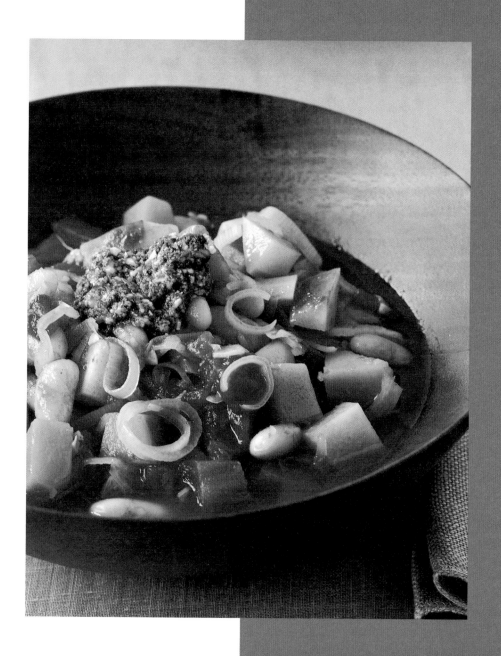

HEARTY CHICKPEA SOUP

The spicy, pungent mix of cinnamon and ginger is a warming backdrop for this healthy, colorful soup.

Preparation time: 15 minutes ● **Cooking time: 35 minutes**

2 tablespoons olive oil

1 rib celery, finely chopped

1 medium carrot, chopped

1 medium onion, chopped

2 teaspoons minced garlic

1 teaspoon ground cinnamon

¼ teaspoon ground turmeric

¼ teaspoon ground ginger or 1 teaspoon grated fresh ginger

Pinch of saffron (optional)

2 cups vegetable broth

1 can (15 ounces) chickpeas, rinsed and drained

1 can (14½ ounces) diced or stewed tomatoes with no salt added

2 cups baby spinach leaves

Lemon wedges (optional)

1. In a medium saucepan, heat the oil over medium heat. Add the celery, carrot, onion, and garlic. Cook, stirring occasionally, for 3 to 5 minutes, or until starting to soften. Add the cinnamon, turmeric, ginger, and saffron, if desired. Cook 1 to 2 minutes longer, or until the spices are fragrant.

2. Add the broth, chickpeas, and tomatoes (with juice). Bring to a boil. Reduce the heat to simmer. Cook, partially covered, for 25 minutes, or until the vegetables are tender.

3. Stir in the spinach and cook for about 2 minutes, or until wilted. Garnish with the lemon wedges, if desired.

MAKES 4 SERVINGS

Per serving: 196 calories, 24 g carbohydrate, 6 g protein, 9 g fat, 1 g saturated fat, 0 mg cholesterol, 394 mg sodium, 6 g fiber

Carbohydrate Choices: 1½

Dietary Exchanges: 1 starch, 2 vegetable, 1½ fat

YELLOW SPLIT PEA–CAULIFLOWER SOUP

Yellow split peas are a sunny addition to this soup. While not as well known as green split peas, they are every bit as good.

Preparation time: 12 minutes ● **Cooking time: 50 minutes**

2 tablespoons olive oil

8 ounces cauliflower florets, coarsely chopped (3 cups)

½ cup chopped onion

½ cup chopped celery

¼ cup chopped carrot

1½ teaspoons ground cumin

2 teaspoons minced garlic

2 bay leaves

Pinch + ⅛ teaspoon salt

1 pound yellow split peas

8 cups chicken broth or vegetable broth

Ground black pepper

10 tablespoons fat-free plain yogurt

Paprika (optional)

1. Heat the oil in a large pot set over high heat. Add the cauliflower, onion, celery, carrot, cumin, garlic, bay leaves, and a pinch of salt. Stir. Cover and cook over medium-high heat, stirring occasionally, for 5 minutes, or until golden. Add the split peas. Stir for 2 minutes to coat with the seasonings. Add the broth and ⅛ teaspoon salt. Bring almost to a boil.

2. Reduce the heat so the mixture simmers. Cook for 35 to 40 minutes, or until the peas are very tender. Remove and discard the bay leaves. Ladle 3 cups of the soup into the bowl of a food processor fitted with a metal blade or into a blender. Process the mixture until smooth. Return to the pot. Season with pepper to taste. Stir to combine. Garnish each bowlful with 1 tablespoon yogurt and a dusting of paprika, if desired.

MAKES 10 SERVINGS

Per serving: 227 calories, 35 g carbohydrate, 16 g protein, 3 g fat, 1 g saturated fat, 4 mg cholesterol, 165 mg sodium, 1 g fiber

Carbohydrate Choices: 2

Dietary Exchanges: 2 starch, ½ vegetable, ½ meat, ½ fat

GREEN SPLIT PEA SOUP

For a snack, lunch, or light dinner, keep this hearty soup on hand in individual-serving containers in the freezer. It's low in fat and filled with nutrients and fiber.

Preparation time: 12 minutes ● **Cooking time: 2 hours 10 minutes**

---

1 tablespoon canola oil
½ cup chopped turnip
½ cup chopped celery
½ cup chopped onion
½ teaspoon dried thyme
2 bay leaves
1 pound green split peas
8 cups chicken or vegetable broth
¼ teaspoon salt
1 teaspoon hot-pepper sauce

1. Set a pot over medium-high heat for 1 minute. Add the oil and swirl to coat the bottom. Heat for 30 seconds. Add the turnip, celery, onion, thyme, and bay leaves. Stir. Cook, stirring occasionally, for 4 minutes, or until softened. Add the peas and broth. Bring almost to a boil.

2. Reduce the heat to medium-low. Cover partially and simmer for about 2 hours, or until the peas are very soft. Remove the bay leaves and discard.

3. In the bowl of a food processor fitted with a metal blade, in a blender, or with an immersion blender, puree the mixture until smooth. Add the salt and hot-pepper sauce. If the mixture is too thick, add water if desired.

MAKES 8 SERVINGS

Per serving: 253 calories, 41 g carbohydrate, 19 g protein, 2 g fat, 1 g saturated fat, 4 mg cholesterol, 211 mg sodium, 0 g fiber

Carbohydrate Choices: 3

Dietary Exchanges: 2½ starch, ½ vegetable, ½ meat, ½ fat

GARDEN VEGETABLE SOUP WITH GRILLED CHICKEN

If you plan ahead to grill some extra chicken at your next outdoor cooking session, you can have the makings of this delightful soup.

Preparation time: 12 minutes ● **Cooking time: 30 minutes**

1⅓ cups vegetable or multicolored rotini pasta

1 teaspoon olive oil, preferably extra virgin

¾ cup coarsely chopped red onion

2 cloves garlic, quartered

1 teaspoon chopped fresh oregano or ¼ teaspoon dried

4 cups chicken broth

1 can (14½ ounces) reduced-sodium diced tomatoes, drained

½ cup chopped carrots

8 ounces grilled chicken breast, chopped

½ cup chopped fresh basil

Ground black pepper

1. Prepare the pasta according to the package directions. Drain. Rinse with cold water and set aside.

2. Meanwhile, in a medium saucepan over medium heat, combine the oil with the onion, garlic, and oregano. Cook, stirring frequently, for about 7 minutes, or until the onion and garlic are tender.

3. Add the broth and bring the mixture to a boil. Add the tomatoes and carrots. Lower the heat and simmer for about 15 minutes, or until the vegetables are tender.

4. Stir in the chicken and pasta. Simmer for about 2 minutes, or until the chicken is heated through. Stir in the basil. Season with pepper to taste.

MAKES 4 SERVINGS

Per serving: 160 calories, 19 g carbohydrate, 16 g protein, 3 g fat, 0 g saturated fat, 30 mg cholesterol, 320 mg sodium, 3 g fiber

Carbohydrate Choices: 1

Dietary Exchanges: ½ starch, 1½ vegetable, 2 meat, ½ fat

SUMMER TOMATO SOUP WITH FRESH DILL

This is the dish to prepare in late August when home gardens and farmers' markets are bursting with ripe and ready tomatoes.

Preparation time: 12 minutes ● **Cooking time: 45 minutes** ● **Chilling time: 2 hours**

1 tablespoon olive oil

1 medium onion, finely chopped

1 tablespoon water

2 cloves garlic, minced

1½ pounds tomatoes, peeled and chopped

4 tablespoons stemmed and chopped fresh dill + 4 fronds for garnish

3 cups chicken or vegetable broth

Salt

Ground black pepper

1. In a medium pot over low heat, combine the oil, onion, and water. Cook, stirring occasionally, for 12 minutes, or until soft. Add the garlic and cook 5 minutes longer.

2. Increase the heat to medium. Add the tomatoes, dill, and broth. Simmer for 25 minutes, or until the tomatoes are very soft. Season with salt and pepper to taste.

3. Chill in the refrigerator for 2 hours. Serve garnished with dill fronds.

MAKES 4 SERVINGS

Per serving: 92 calories, 10 g carbohydrate, 5 g protein, 5 g fat, 1 g saturated fat, 0 mg cholesterol, 61 mg sodium, 2 g fiber

Carbohydrate Choices: 1

Dietary Exchanges: 2 vegetable, ½ meat, 1 fat

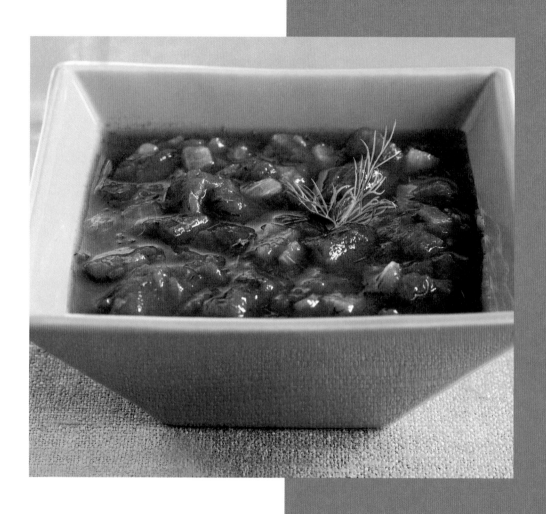

CHILLED CARROT AND SUMMER SQUASH SOUP

Don't limit your soup choices to steaming cold-weather options. A cool smooth vegetable puree can be utterly refreshing in hot weather.

Preparation time: 12 minutes ● **Cooking time: 27 minutes** ● **Chilling time: 1 hour**

2 cups sliced carrots

3 cups chicken broth

¼ cup chopped red onion

1 clove garlic

¾ teaspoon ground cumin

½ teaspoon salt

¼ teaspoon ground coriander

¼ teaspoon ground black pepper

1 large yellow summer squash, chopped

¾ cup low-fat plain yogurt

Fresh chives, cut in ¼" lengths (optional)

1. In a large saucepan, combine the carrots and broth. Cover and bring to a boil. Reduce the heat to medium and simmer about 7 minutes, or until the carrots begin to soften.

2. Add the onion, garlic, cumin, salt, coriander, pepper, and all but 4 tablespoons of squash. Cover, raise heat to high, and bring to a boil. Reduce the heat to low and simmer, covered, for 15 to 20 minutes, or until the vegetables are very tender and the flavors are blended.

3. In the bowl of a food processor fitted with a metal blade, in a blender, or with an immersion blender, puree the soup until smooth. Pour into a bowl, cover, and refrigerate for 1 hour.

4. Stir the yogurt into the soup until combined. Divide into 4 bowls and garnish each with a tablespoon of reserved squash and chives, if desired.

MAKES 4 SERVINGS

Per serving: 104 calories, 16 g carbohydrate, 8 g protein, 2 g fat, 0.8 g saturated fat, 3 mg cholesterol, 425 mg sodium, 3 g fiber

Carbohydrate Choices: 1

Dietary Exchanges: 2 vegetable, ½ meat

FARMERS' MARKET PASTA SALAD

This salad comes together so quickly that you can easily prepare it the night before and carry it to work for lunch. Or, have it on hand in the refrigerator for evenings when you're too conked to cook.

Preparation time: 5 minutes ● **Cooking time: 8 minutes**

1   package (9 ounces) refrigerated
      tricolor cheese tortellini
2   cups trimmed sugar snap peas
2   tablespoons refrigerated pesto
1   cup cherry tomatoes, halved
¼   teaspoon ground black pepper
      Fresh basil (optional)

1. Place the tortellini into a large pot of boiling water. Cook for 5 minutes, stirring occasionally. Add the sugar snap peas and cook for 3 minutes, or until tender but still crisp.

2. Drain the pasta and peas, and rinse with cold water. Place into a large bowl and toss with the pesto. Gently fold in the tomatoes and pepper. Garnish with basil, if using.

MAKES 4 SERVINGS

Per serving: 280 calories, 40 g carbohydrate, 13 g protein, 8 g fat, 3 g saturated fat, 29 mg cholesterol, 354 mg sodium, 4 g fiber

Carbohydrate Choices: 3

Dietary Exchanges: 2½ starch, ½ vegetable, 1½ fat

FILL UP ON WHOLE FOODS

V for Vegan

Could eating only vegetable foods be an effective treatment for controlling diabetes symptoms? That was the conclusion of a study reported in the August 2006 issue of *Diabetes Care*, a journal published by the American Diabetes Association. Study participants who followed a low-fat vegan (all plant foods) diet showed dramatic improvement in four disease markers: blood sugar control, cholesterol reduction, weight control, and kidney function as compared to those who followed a standard diabetes diet. The vegan diet represents a major departure from current diabetes diets in that it places no limits on calories, carbohydrates, or portions. "The diet appears remarkably effective, and all the side effects are good ones— especially weight loss and lower cholesterol," says lead researcher Neal D. Barnard, MD, PCRM president and adjunct associate professor of medicine at George Washington University in Washington, DC. "I hope this study will rekindle interest in using diet changes first rather than prescription drugs."

FRESH PEA SOUP WITH MINT

Green peas are a fresh member of the legume family (related to dried beans), so they are a good source of lean protein and fiber. If you have access to fresh garden peas in early summer, this soup will be a sweet revelation.

Preparation time: 7 minutes ● **Cooking time: 15 minutes** ● **Chilling time: 1 hour**

---

1 tablespoon olive oil

2 scallions, green parts only, cut into 4" lengths

1 rib celery, trimmed and cut into 2" lengths

½ medium onion, finely chopped

3 cups chicken or vegetable broth

4 cups peas, fresh or (thawed) frozen

⅓ cup fresh mint leaves + extra for garnish

Ground black pepper

½ cup low-fat plain yogurt

1. Place the oil in a large pot over medium-high heat. Add the scallions, celery, and onion. Cook, stirring, about 5 minutes, or until the vegetables soften.

2. Add the broth and bring to a boil. Add the peas and simmer for 10 minutes.

3. Carefully transfer the mixture to the bowl of a food processor fitted with a metal blade or a blender (in batches, if necessary). Add the mint. Season to taste with pepper. Puree until smooth. Chill 1 hour. Serve with yogurt in center, and garnish with mint leaves if desired.

MAKES 4 SERVINGS

Per serving: 198 calories, 27 g carbohydrate, 13 g protein, 5 g fat, 1 g saturated fat, 1 mg cholesterol, 258 mg sodium, 7 g fiber

Carbohydrate Choices: 2

Dietary Exchanges: 1½ starch, ½ vegetable, ½ meat

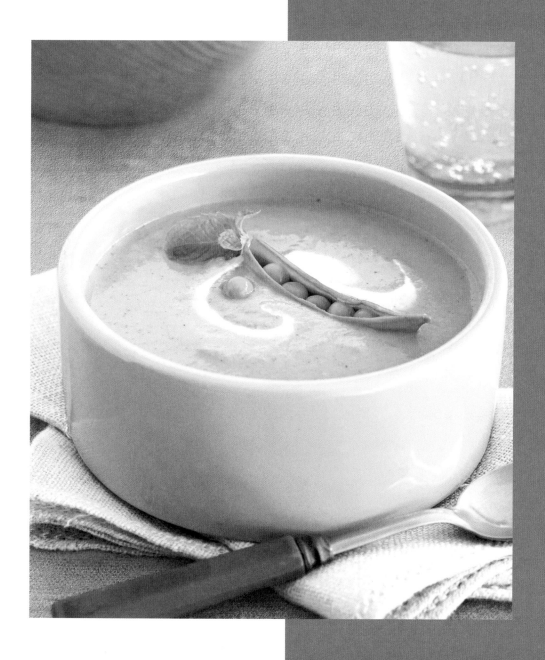

SPINACH-ENDIVE SALAD WITH VINTNER'S DRESSING

Spinach is an excellent source of folate as well as one of the leading sources of vitamin K. Pairing it with endive and grapes gives it a sweet, sophisticated taste.

Preparation time: 20 minutes

---

1 tablespoon rice wine or white wine vinegar

1 tablespoon olive oil

¼ teaspoon salt

⅛ teaspoon ground black pepper

1½ cups small red seedless grapes, divided

2 Belgian endives (12 ounces), sliced crosswise

3 cups baby spinach

¼ cup crumbled Gorgonzola or other blue cheese

3 tablespoons chopped smoked, lightly salted almonds

1. Using a blender or immersion blender, process the vinegar, oil, salt, pepper, and ¾ cup of the grapes until smooth. Set aside for dressing.

2. In a salad bowl, combine the endives, spinach, and the remaining ¾ cup grapes. When ready to serve, toss with dressing, and top with cheese and almonds.

MAKES 4 SERVINGS

Per serving: 186 calories, 18 g carbohydrate, 6 g protein, 11 g fat, 3 g saturated fat, 6 mg cholesterol, 377 mg sodium, 5 g fiber

Carbohydrate Choices: 1

Dietary Exchanges: 1 fruit, 1 vegetable, 1 fat

LET YOURSELF GO/STRESS LESS

A positive attitude is essential in dealing with the stress of diabetes, according to Richard R. Rubin, PhD, CDE, of the Johns Hopkins Medical School and author of *Psyching Out Diabetes: A Positive Approach to Your Negative Emotions.* With his colleague Joseph Napora, PhD, Rubin has developed seven frames to help people turn their negative mental pictures of diabetes into positive ones.

Frame 1—Partializing. Breaks a seemingly insurmountable problem into manageable pieces.

Frame 2—Letting Go. Focus your energy on what you can change, not on what you can't.

Frame 3—Love. Cherish yourself.

Frame 4—Faith and Hope. Identify a higher power or internal strength and call upon it.

Frame 5—Humor. Looking for the absurdity of a situation helps promote relaxation.

Frame 6—Sharing Information. Communicate with those around you to foster openness.

Frame 7—Celebration. Recognize your successes, no matter how small.

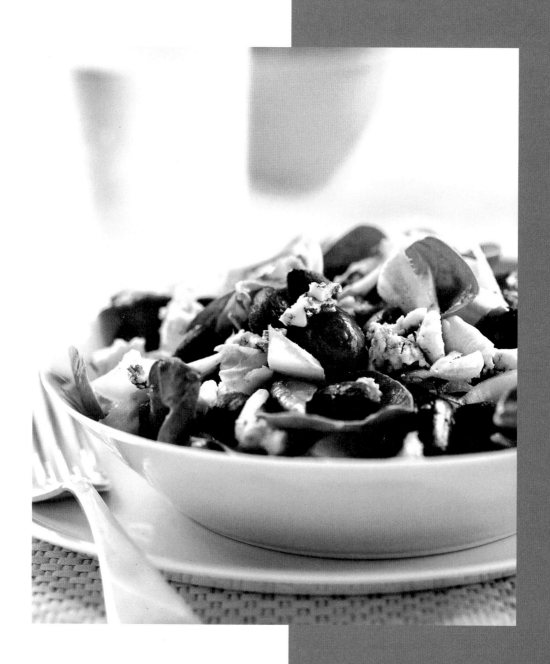

BARLEY, BUTTERNUT, AND BLACK BEAN SALAD

If you like pasta salads, you'll enjoy exploring options for cooked and cooled whole grain salads like this one made with barley.

Preparation time: 20 minutes ● **Cooking time: 35 minutes**

1 cup barley

3 tablespoons olive oil, divided

1 leek, white and light green parts only, thinly sliced

2 cups peeled, chopped butternut squash (about ½ medium)

¼ cup water

3 tablespoons chopped fresh parsley, divided

1¼ cups cooked black beans (see page 312) or 1 can (15 ounces) black beans, rinsed and drained

½ teaspoon salt

2 tablespoons lemon juice

¼ teaspoon ground black pepper

Grated lemon peel (garnish)

1. Cook the barley according to the package directions. Rinse and set aside.

2. Meanwhile, heat 2 tablespoons of the oil in a large nonstick skillet over medium-high heat. Add the leek and squash and cook, tossing or stirring, until slightly softened and lightly browned, about 10 minutes. Add the water and 1½ tablespoons of the parsley and cook 2 to 3 minutes longer. Transfer the vegetables to a large bowl.

3. Add the barley, black beans, salt, and the remaining 1 tablespoon oil and remaining 1½ tablespoons parsley. Stir to combine. Season with lemon juice and pepper. Garnish with lemon peel, if desired.

MAKES 6 SERVINGS

Per serving: 264 calories, 44 g carbohydrate, 7 g protein, 7 g fat, 1 g saturated fat, 0 mg cholesterol, 204 mg sodium, 9 g fiber

Carbohydrate Choices: 3

Dietary Exchanges: 2 starch, 1½ vegetable, 1½ fat

NOTE: Some supermarkets sell peeled butternut squash.

SPRING ORZO SALAD

Orzo looks like plump grains of rice, but it's actually pasta. If you like, you can replace the orzo with cooked barley or wheat berries.

Preparation time: 10 minutes ● **Cooking time: 9 minutes**

⅔ cup orzo

⅓ cup finely chopped red bell pepper

⅓ cup finely chopped orange bell pepper

⅓ cup finely chopped and seeded tomatoes

¼ cup quartered dry-packed sun-dried tomatoes

¼ cup chopped scallions

¼ cup chopped watercress

1 teaspoon minced garlic

2 teaspoons olive oil, preferably extra virgin

⅓ cup crumbled reduced-fat feta cheese

2 teaspoons fresh lemon juice

Ground black pepper

1. Prepare the orzo according to the package directions.

2. Meanwhile, in a medium bowl, combine the bell peppers, tomatoes, sun-dried tomatoes, scallions, watercress, garlic, oil, cheese, and lemon juice.

3. Mix the orzo with the vegetable mixture until well combined. Season to taste with black pepper.

MAKES 2 SERVINGS

Per serving: 343 calories, 53 g carbohydrate, 14 g protein, 9 g fat, 3 g saturated fat, 7 mg cholesterol, 461 mg sodium, 4 g fiber

Carbohydrate Choices: 3½

Dietary Exchanges: 3 starch, 2 vegetable, 1 meat, 1 fat

EASY COUSCOUS SALAD

Who says whole grains take too long to cook? Whole wheat couscous takes just 5 minutes to steam.

Preparation time: 8 minutes ● **Cooking time: 5 minutes**

1¼ cups whole wheat couscous

⅓ cup lemon juice

1 tablespoon olive oil, preferably extra virgin

2 medium bell peppers, 1 red and 1 orange, chopped

1 can (15 ounces) chickpeas, rinsed and drained

½ cup crumbled feta cheese

   Basil, cilantro, or parsley (garnish)

1. Bring 1¾ cups of hot water to a boil in a medium saucepan. Add the couscous, cover, and turn off heat. Let stand 5 minutes, then fluff with a fork or salad tongs and transfer to a large bowl.

2. Add the lemon juice to the couscous and toss. Add the oil and toss again to coat. Mix in the peppers, chickpeas, and cheese. Garnish with herbs, such as basil, cilantro, or parsley, if desired. Serve immediately, at room temperature, or chill.

MAKES 4 SERVINGS

Per serving: 394 calories, 44 g carbohydrate, 12 g protein, 9 g fat, 3.5 g saturated fat, 17 mg cholesterol, 420 mg sodium, 8 g fiber

Carbohydrate Choices: 3

Dietary Exchanges: 2 starch, ½ vegetable, 1 meat, 1½ fat

SUMMER TOMATO DINNER SALAD

Canned chickpeas and other dried beans are the kinds of items you'll want to have on hand for quick meals. Look for low-sodium brands of canned beans or rinse and drain regular canned beans to eliminate much of the salt.

Preparation time: 25 minutes

6 red radishes, trimmed and thinly sliced

4 scallions, trimmed and thinly sliced

2 cans (15½ ounces each) chickpeas, rinsed and drained

2 large tomatoes, cut into bite-size wedges

1 pint cherry or grape tomatoes, halved

1 avocado, peeled, pitted, and chopped

½ cup chopped fresh dill

3 tablespoons lemon juice

2 tablespoons Dijon mustard

2 tablespoons garlic-flavored olive oil

2 cups garlic-onion fat-free croutons

3 ounces goat cheese, crumbled

6 cups mesclun greens

1. In a large bowl, combine the radishes, scallions, chickpeas, tomatoes, cherry or grape tomatoes, avocado, and dill.

2. In a small bowl, whisk the lemon juice and mustard. Slowly whisk in the oil. Set aside.

3. Just before serving, add the croutons and cheese to the tomato mixture. Add the oil dressing and toss lightly.

4. To serve, arrange 1 cup mesclun on each of 6 dinner plates and top with 1⅔ cups tomato salad.

MAKES 6 SERVINGS

Per serving: 310 calories, 33 g carbohydrate, 12 g protein, 16 g fat, 4.5 g saturated fat, 10 mg cholesterol, 540 mg sodium, 9 g fiber

Carbohydrate Choices: 2

Dietary Exchanges: 1½ starch, 1½ vegetable, ½ meat, 2½ fat

WHEAT BERRY SALAD WITH RED PEPPER, EGGPLANT, AND ZUCCHINI

The seeds of the wheat plant are called wheat berries. Look for them in natural food stores or bulk food stores. The three parts of the berry—the bran, germ, and endosperm—are all intact.

Soaking time: Overnight ● **Preparation time: 15 minutes** ● **Cooking time: 1 hour 45 minutes**

1 cup wheat berries

1 red bell pepper, quartered

2 tablespoons olive oil, preferably extra virgin, divided

4 slices (½" thick) eggplant

4 slices (¼" thick) sweet onion

1 medium zucchini, cut into 4 thick diagonal slices

1 medium yellow crookneck squash, cut into 4 thick diagonal slices

¼ teaspoon salt, divided

¼ teaspoon ground black pepper, divided

3 tablespoons red wine vinegar

1 tablespoon chopped parsley + parsley sprigs (garnish)

1 teaspoon chopped fresh oregano leaves + oregano sprigs (garnish)

1 teaspoon minced garlic

1. Place the wheat berries in a medium bowl, fill the bowl with water, cover, and soak in the refrigerator overnight. Drain. Place in a medium saucepan, cover with water, and heat to a boil. Simmer, uncovered, until wheat berries are tender, about 1 hour.

2. Meanwhile, preheat the oven to 400°F. Arrange the bell pepper in a single layer on a large sheet pan or baking sheet. Measure 1 tablespoon oil. Lightly brush the pepper with some of the tablespoon. Roast for 20 minutes. Turn the pepper. Add the eggplant, onion, zucchini, and squash to the pan. Brush with what remains of the 1 tablespoon oil. Roast for about 25 minutes longer, or until browned. Let the vegetables stand to cool. Season with ⅛ teaspoon of the salt and the pepper. Set half of the vegetables aside. Cut the remaining vegetables into ½" pieces.

3. In a large bowl, combine the vinegar, chopped parsley, chopped oregano, garlic, the remaining 1 tablespoon oil, and the remaining ⅛ teaspoon salt and pepper. Add the wheat berries and cut-up vegetables. Toss to coat. Spoon onto a serving platter. Arrange the remaining vegetables around the edges. Garnish with herb sprigs.

MAKES 4 SERVINGS

Per serving: 280 calories, 44 g carbohydrate, 9 g protein, 8 g fat, 1 g saturated fat, 0 mg cholesterol, 160 mg sodium, 8 g fiber

Carbohydrate Choices: 3

Dietary Exchanges: 2 starch, 2 vegetable, 1½ fat

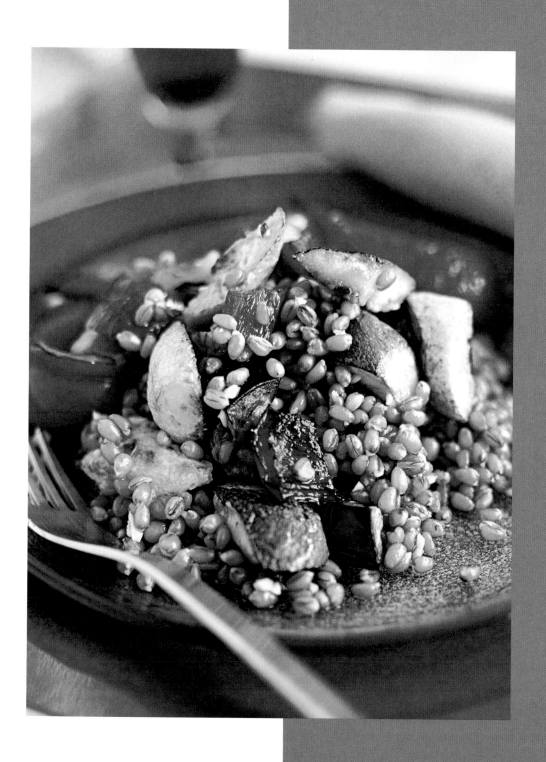

WARM QUINOA SALAD

Quinoa is a grain from South America that packs a low-fat, high-protein punch. It's a great food to incorporate into your diet if you're looking for nonmeat sources of protein.

Preparation time: 8 minutes ● **Cooking time: 10 minutes**

---

1 cup quinoa, rinsed and drained

2 cups water

1 cup chopped radicchio (about ½ head) + leaves for garnish

½ cup chopped cilantro

½ cup golden raisins

½ cup fat-free honey mustard dressing
Ground black pepper

1. In a medium pot, combine the quinoa and water and bring to a boil. Reduce the heat to a simmer, cover, and cook for about 5 minutes, or until all the liquid is absorbed. Transfer the quinoa to a medium serving bowl.

2. Combine the radicchio, cilantro, and raisins with the quinoa. Toss with the dressing. Season with pepper to taste, and serve on radicchio leaves.

MAKES 4 SERVINGS

Per serving: 247 calories, 50 g carbohydrate, 6 g protein, 3 g fat, 0.3 g saturated fat, 0 mg cholesterol, 140 mg sodium, 4 g fiber

Carbohydrate Choices: 3

Dietary Exchanges: 2½ starch, 1 fruit

LOOSEN UP/GET MOVING

Research in the United States and Australia has shown that resistance training (working with weights) can significantly reduce high blood sugar and improve heart health.

Lifting weights helps cells throughout your body become more sensitive to insulin. Plus, weight training increases a compound, called Glut-4, that binds to the cell membrane and then helps ease glucose into muscle cells. People with high blood sugar have suboptimal levels of glucose transporters like Glut-4. Weight training can increase their number, helping muscles absorb sugar and remove sugar from the blood.

All it takes is two or three at-home sessions a week. You can even break up the sessions into smaller workouts. Best of all, you will see dramatic changes in your body in about a month, and most women get a big energy boost right away. Of course, you should consult with your physician—and perhaps work initially with an exercise physiologist—when starting any new exercise program.

CURRIED BARLEY AND SHRIMP SALAD

The barley salad keeps well in an airtight container in the refrigerator for several days. It makes a great lunch with or without the lettuce leaves.

Preparation time: 20 minutes ● **Cooking time: 45 minutes**

---

3 cups water

1 teaspoon curry powder

½ teaspoon turmeric

1 cup barley

1 pound frozen peeled and deveined small cooked shrimp, thawed and drained

1½ cups seeded and diced tomatoes

½ cup chopped green bell pepper

½ cup chopped peeled cucumber

5 tablespoons lime juice

3 tablespoons canola oil

2 teaspoons seeded, finely chopped jalapeño chile pepper (wear plastic gloves when handling)

1 clove garlic, minced

¼ teaspoon salt

Romaine lettuce leaves

¼ cup chopped fresh basil or cilantro

1 lime, cut into sixths (garnish)

1. In a large saucepan, combine the water, curry powder, and turmeric. Bring to a boil. Stir in the barley. Cover and cook over low heat for about 45 minutes, or until the water is absorbed and the barley is tender. Transfer to a colander to drain any excess water.

2. Place the barley in a large bowl. Add the shrimp, tomatoes, bell pepper, and cucumber. In a small bowl, whisk the lime juice, oil, chile pepper (to taste), garlic, and salt until blended. Pour over the barley mixture and toss.

3. Spoon barley salad on top of lettuce and sprinkle with basil or cilantro. Garnish with lime.

MAKES 6 SERVINGS

Per serving: 287 calories, 33 g carbohydrate, 20 g protein, 9 g fat, 2 g saturated fat, 115 mg cholesterol, 263 mg sodium, 7 g fiber

Carbohydrate Choices: 2

Dietary Exchanges: 1½ starch, 1 vegetable, 2 meat, 1½ fat

HERB AND MESCLUN SALAD WITH GRILLED SHRIMP

Plan ahead and save time preparing this main dish salad. Cook the shrimp when you have the grill lighted for another meal. Or, feel free to adapt by using salmon or chicken breast instead of the shrimp.

Preparation time: 30 minutes ● Marinating time: 20 minutes ● Cooking time: 4 minutes

¼ cup lime juice, divided
½ teaspoon ground cumin, divided
¼ teaspoon salt, divided
¼ teaspoon red-pepper flakes, divided
1 pound large shrimp, peeled and deveined
6 cups mesclun or other mixed baby greens
1 cup fresh mint leaves
1 cup cilantro leaves
1 cup flat-leaf parsley leaves
1 small red onion, thinly sliced
2 tablespoons canola oil

1. In a medium bowl, whisk 2 tablespoons of the lime juice, ¼ teaspoon cumin, ⅛ teaspoon salt, and a pinch of pepper flakes. Stir in the shrimp. Let stand to marinate at room temperature, stirring occasionally, for 20 minutes.

2. Meanwhile, in a serving bowl, combine the mesclun, mint, cilantro, parsley, and onion. Refrigerate until ready to serve.

3. In a small bowl, whisk together the oil and the remaining 2 tablespoons lime juice, ¼ teaspoon cumin, ⅛ teaspoon salt, and the remaining pepper flakes.

4. Lightly oil a grill pan and preheat over medium heat. Grill the shrimp for about 2 minutes on each side, or until bright pink and just opaque throughout. Do not overcook. Toss the shrimp with the greens and dressing.

MAKES 4 SERVINGS

Per serving: 202 calories, 9 g carbohydrate, 23 g protein, 9 g fat, 1 g saturated fat, 150 mg cholesterol, 326 mg sodium, 3 g fiber

Carbohydrate Choices: 1

Dietary Exchanges: 1 vegetable, 3 meat, 1½ fat

NOTE: Shrimp may be broiled for the same amount of time, if desired.

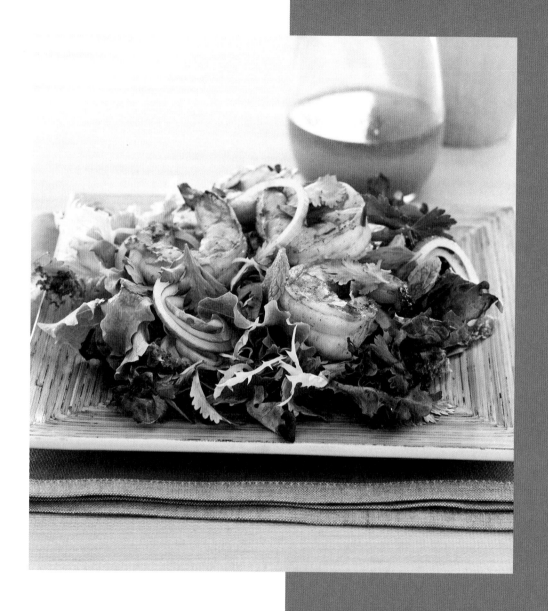

TOASTED MILLET SALAD WITH SALMON

Healthful omega-3 fatty acids are found in oily fish such as sardines, mackerel, and bluefish, so if you like, you can replace the salmon in this dish with one of these fish.

Preparation time: 20 minutes ● **Cooking time: 35 minutes**

2½ cups water
1 teaspoon + 2 tablespoons canola oil
1 cup millet
8 ounces boneless, skinless salmon fillets
1 teaspoon + 1 tablespoon reduced-sodium soy sauce
2 cups snow peas, trimmed
¼ cup rice wine vinegar
2 tablespoons water
1 tablespoon toasted sesame oil
2 teaspoons grated fresh ginger
1 teaspoon minced garlic
¼ teaspoon salt
½ cup minced scallions
½ cup finely chopped red bell pepper

1. In a medium saucepan, bring 2½ cups of water to a boil. Meanwhile, coat the bottom of a large skillet with 1 teaspoon of the canola oil. Add the millet and cook, stirring, over medium-low heat, for about 10 minutes, or until it gives off a toasted aroma. Add the boiling-hot water. Cover and cook over medium-low heat for about 25 minutes, or until the water is absorbed and the millet is tender. Uncover and cool.

2. Meanwhile, coat the salmon with 1 teaspoon of the soy sauce. Set a large nonstick skillet over high heat for 1 minute. When hot,

add the fish. Reduce the heat to medium, and cook for about 3 minutes, or until browned. Turn and cook 3 to 5 minutes longer, or until the fish is cooked through. Remove from the heat. Cool in the pan. Break into 1" chunks.

3. Bring a small saucepan of water to a boil. Add the peas and cook 1 minute. Drain, rinse, then blot dry.

4. In a large bowl, whisk the vinegar, 2 tablespoons water, sesame oil, ginger, garlic, salt, and remaining 2 tablespoons canola oil and 1 tablespoon soy sauce. Reserve 1 tablespoon of the mixture. Toss the reserved millet with the dressing. In a small bowl, toss the scallions, pepper, peas, and reserved dressing. Add half the vegetables and the salmon to the millet.

5. Spoon the millet salad onto a platter. Top with the remaining vegetables.

MAKES 4 SERVINGS

Per serving: 382 calories, 44 g carbohydrate, 19 g protein, 15 g fat, 2.5 g saturated fat, 29 mg cholesterol, 323 mg sodium, 6 g fiber

Carbohydrate Choices: 3

Dietary Exchanges: 2½ starch, 1 vegetable, 1½ meat, 2 fat

CHINESE CHICKEN SALAD WITH TOASTED ALMONDS

Kick the carry-out habit with this easy dish. The fat and sodium content are significantly lower than typical restaurant fare.

Preparation time: 12 minutes

SALAD

1½ pounds boneless, skinless chicken breast halves, grilled or roasted and sliced

1 large head romaine lettuce, torn into bite-size pieces (8 cups)

½ head red cabbage, shredded (4 cups)

8 scallions, sliced diagonally

½ cup chow mein noodles

½ cup chopped almonds, toasted

DRESSING

¼ cup vegetable broth

2½ tablespoons canola oil

¼ cup rice wine vinegar

2 tablespoons sugar

1 tablespoon reduced-sodium soy sauce

1 tablespoon toasted sesame oil

1. To prepare the salad: In a large bowl, combine the chicken, lettuce, cabbage, scallions, and noodles.

2. To prepare the dressing: In a small bowl, combine the broth, vinegar, sugar, soy sauce, and sesame oil. Whisk to blend.

3. Pour the dressing over the chicken salad. Toss to coat. Serve, sprinkled with the almonds.

MAKES 8 SERVINGS

Per serving: 300 calories, 13 g carbohydrate, 30 g protein, 14 g fat, 2 g saturated fat, 70 mg cholesterol, 180 mg sodium, 3 g fiber

Carbohydrate Choices: 1

Dietary Exchanges: ½ starch, 1 vegetable, 4 meat, 1½ fat

BROWN RICE AND SOY CHICKEN SALAD WITH MANGO

If you're pressed for time, just use ready-cooked brown rice (available in shelf-stable pouches) instead of cooking brown rice from scratch. Instant brown rice will also cut the cooking time.

Preparation time: 20 minutes ● Cooking time: 45 minutes

1 cup medium- or long-grain brown, red, or black rice

2 cups water

6 ounces green beans, trimmed and cut in half (about 2 cups)

12 ounces boneless, skinless chicken breast, cut into ½"-wide strips

1 tablespoon low-sodium soy sauce

4 tablespoons rice wine vinegar

2 tablespoons canola oil

1 teaspoon toasted sesame oil

1 teaspoon grated fresh ginger

¼ teaspoon salt

½ cup minced scallions, all parts

1 red bell pepper, cut into ¼" strips

1 mango, peeled and cut into ¼" dice, divided

¼ cup chopped cilantro

1. Combine the rice and 2 cups of water in a medium saucepan and heat to a boil. Cover and cook over low heat for about 45 minutes, or until the water is absorbed and the rice is tender. Transfer to a strainer, rinse with cold water, and drain well.

2. While the rice cooks, fill a small saucepan halfway with water and bring to a boil over high heat. Add the beans and cook until crisp-tender, about 3 minutes. Drain, rinse with cold water, and set aside.

3. Place the chicken in a small bowl. Add the soy sauce and toss to coat.

4. Lightly coat a nonstick skillet with vegetable oil spray and heat to medium. When hot, add the chicken. Cook, turning, for 1 to 2 minutes per side, or until evenly browned and cooked through. Transfer to a platter.

5. Whisk the vinegar, canola oil, sesame oil, ginger, and salt in a large bowl. Add the rice, beans, chicken, scallions, pepper, and half of the mango. Gently toss to combine. Spoon onto the platter and top with cilantro and the remaining mango.

MAKES 4 SERVINGS

Per serving: 384 calories, 50 g carbohydrate, 22 g protein, 12 g fat, 2 g saturated fat, 47 mg cholesterol, 292 mg sodium, 5 g fiber

Carbohydrate Choices: 3

Dietary Exchanges: 2 starch, ½ fruit, 1 vegetable, 2½ meat, 2 fat

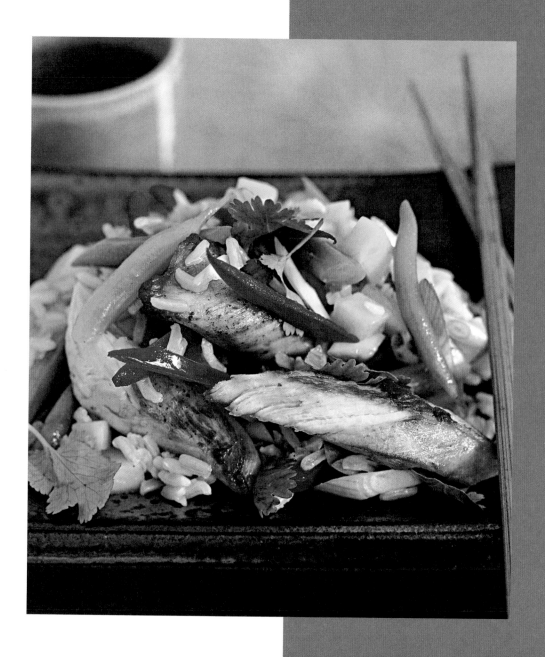

SPINACH SALAD TOPPED WITH ALMOND-ENCRUSTED CHICKEN BREAST

A tasty single-serving meal. If you'd like twice as much to serve two, there's no need to double the egg dip.

Preparation time: 8 minutes ● **Cooking time: 10 minutes**

CHICKEN

> **5** ounces boneless, skinless chicken breast
>
> **1** tablespoon cornstarch
>
> **1** egg beaten with 1 tablespoon water
>
> **1** tablespoon finely chopped almonds

SALAD

> **2** tablespoons balsamic vinegar
>
> **1** tablespoon olive oil
>
> **⅛** teaspoon ground black pepper
>
> **3** cups baby spinach leaves
>
> **¼** cup sliced mushrooms
>
> **¼** cup yellow or red grape tomatoes, halved
>
> **1** small red bell pepper, sliced into strips

1. To prepare the chicken: Sprinkle each side of the chicken with the cornstarch. Dip into the egg mixture to coat, allowing excess to drip off. Sprinkle both sides with the almonds.

2. Coat a small nonstick skillet with vegetable oil spray and heat over medium heat. Cook the chicken for 5 minutes on each side, or until no longer pink and the juices run clear. Remove from the pan and set aside.

3. To prepare the salad: In a medium bowl, whisk the vinegar, oil, and black pepper. Add the spinach, mushrooms, tomatoes, and bell pepper. Toss to coat. Transfer to a serving plate. Slice the reserved chicken diagonally and place on top.

MAKES 1 SERVING

Per serving: 489 calories, 29 g carbohydrate, 42 g protein, 23 g fat, 3.5 g saturated fat, 80 mg cholesterol, 533 mg sodium, 7 g fiber

Carbohydrate Choices: 2

Dietary Exchanges: 1 starch, 2½ vegetable, 6 meat, 4 fat

SOUTHWESTERN CHICKEN SALAD WITH CRISPY TORTILLA CHIPS

This dish is a complete meal providing whole grain carbs, lean protein, and vitamin- and antioxidant-rich vegetables.

Preparation time: 14 minutes ● **Cooking time: 5 minutes**

1   **whole wheat tortilla (9"–10" diameter)**
    Peel of 1 lime
½   **teaspoon minced garlic**
½   **teaspoon ground cumin**
⅛   **teaspoon red-pepper flakes**
1½   **cups cooked chicken breast, roasted or grilled**
1   **tablespoon lime juice**
1   **tablespoon olive oil**
1   **tablespoon chopped cilantro**
8   **cups mixed greens**
1   **red bell pepper, sliced**
¼   **avocado, sliced**

1. Preheat the oven to 400°F.

2. Cut the tortilla into quarters and each quarter into 2 wedges. Place on a baking sheet and bake until crisp, about 5 minutes. Remove from the oven and set aside.

3. Place the lime peel, garlic, cumin, and red-pepper flakes in a medium bowl and stir. Add the chicken and toss well to coat.

4. In a large salad bowl, combine the lime juice, oil, and cilantro. Add the greens, red bell pepper, and avocado and toss well.

5. Top the salad mix with chicken. Place the toasted tortilla wedges around the edge of the salad bowl.

MAKES 2 SERVINGS

Per serving: 383 calories, 22 g carbohydrate, 38 g protein, 16 g fat, 3 g saturated fat, 89 mg cholesterol, 253 mg sodium, 9 g fiber

Carbohydrate Choices: 1½

Dietary Exchanges: 2 vegetable, 5 meat, 2 fat

CRISP ROMAINE SALAD WITH CHICKEN AND MANGO

The more color that salad greens contain, the more nutritious they are. Choose regular or red romaine leaves for this dish.

Preparation time: 25 minutes ● **Cooking time: 15 minutes**

---

2 tablespoons olive oil, divided

3 boneless, skinless chicken breasts

½ teaspoon salt, divided

¼ teaspoon ground black pepper, divided

2 shallots, finely chopped

2 tablespoons balsamic vinegar, divided

4 cups shredded romaine lettuce

1 small bunch watercress, large stems discarded

½ cup finely shredded red cabbage

1 firm ripe mango, peeled, pitted, and cut into ½" pieces

1. Heat 1 tablespoon of the oil in a large non-stick skillet over medium heat. Season the chicken with ¼ teaspoon salt and ⅛ teaspoon pepper. Cook, turning, until golden brown and cooked through, about 6 minutes on each side. Transfer to a cutting board.

2. Add the shallots and 1 tablespoon of the vinegar to the skillet. Cook, stirring, about 3 minutes, or until the shallots are softened and the liquid is almost evaporated. Transfer the shallots to a small bowl. Whisk the remaining 1 tablespoon oil, 1 tablespoon vinegar, ¼ teaspoon salt, and ⅛ teaspoon pepper into the shallot mixture.

3. Place the romaine, watercress, cabbage, and mango in a serving bowl. Cut the chicken diagonally into long, thin strips. Add to the romaine mixture, toss with the dressing, and serve.

MAKES 4 SERVINGS

Per serving: 222 calories, 15 g carbohydrate, 22 g protein, 8 g fat, 1 g saturated fat, 51 mg cholesterol, 362 mg sodium, 2 g fiber

Carbohydrate Choices: 1

Dietary Exchanges: ½ fruit, 1 vegetable, 3 meat, 1½ fat

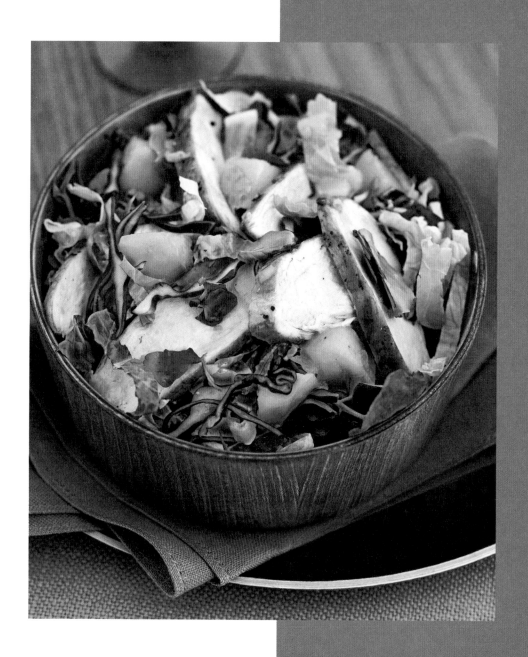

GRILLED BEEF AND ARUGULA SALAD

Arugula offers a peppery bite somewhat like watercress. For a milder flavor, replace half or all of the arugula with baby spinach leaves.

Preparation time: 8 minutes ● **Cooking time: 8 minutes** ● **Standing time: 5 minutes**

1 **scallion, thinly sliced**
2 **tablespoons olive oil, divided**
2 **tablespoons raspberry vinegar**
1 **tablespoon finely chopped parsley**
½ **teaspoon salt, divided**
¼ **teaspoon ground black pepper, divided**
4 **ripe apricots, halved, pits removed**
2 **¾"-thick filets mignons (4 ounces each)**
1 **bag (5 ounces) baby arugula**
3 **tablespoons crumbled blue cheese (optional)**

1. Prepare charcoal for grilling, preheat a gas grill, or heat a grill pan over medium heat.

2. In a large bowl, whisk together the scallion, 1⅔ tablespoons oil, vinegar, parsley, ¼ teaspoon salt, and ⅛ teaspoon pepper. Set aside.

3. Lightly brush the cut surface of the apricots with the remaining ⅓ tablespoon oil. Season the beef with the remaining ¼ teaspoon salt and ⅛ teaspoon pepper. Grill the beef and apricots, cut side down. Cook the apricots for about 6 minutes, or until soft. Turn the beef midway, a total of 8 minutes for medium-rare or longer for desired doneness. Remove from the heat and let stand 5 minutes. Cut the apricots into slices. Thinly slice beef against the grain.

4. In a medium bowl, toss the arugula with dressing to coat. Transfer to four serving plates. Top with slices of beef and 2 sliced apricot halves. Sprinkle with blue cheese, if desired.

MAKES 4 SERVINGS

Per serving: 153 calories, 7 g carbohydrate, 13 g protein, 9 g fat, 2 g saturated fat, 30 mg cholesterol, 329 mg sodium, 1 g fiber

Carbohydrate Choices: ½

Dietary Exchanges: ½ vegetable, 1½ meat, 1½ fat

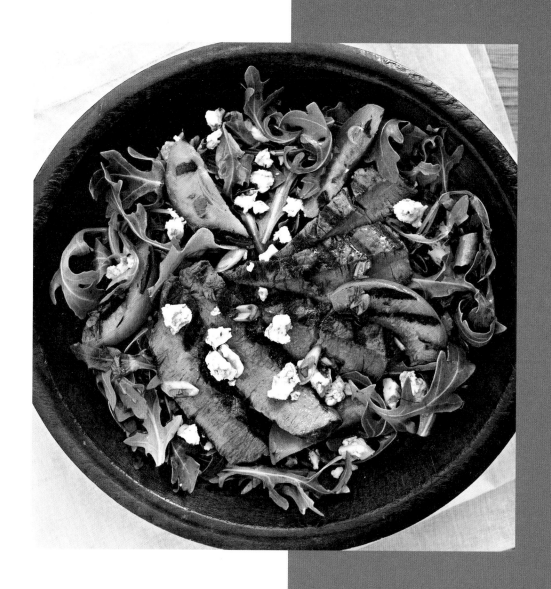

ASIAN ROASTED RUTABAGA "FRIES"

High in vitamins A and C, this root vegetable is a great substitute for potatoes. Asian spices bring out its natural sweetness.

Preparation time: 15 minutes ● **Cooking time: 42 minutes**

　1　small rutabaga (1¼ pounds), peeled
　2　tablespoons honey
　1　tablespoon hoisin sauce
1½　teaspoons grated fresh ginger
　1　teaspoon toasted sesame oil
　½　teaspoon red wine vinegar
　¼　teaspoon five-spice powder or ground cinnamon

1. Preheat the oven to 400°F. Line a jelly-roll pan with aluminum foil. Coat lightly with vegetable oil spray.

2. Slice the rutabaga ½" thick. Cut into ½"-wide strips. In a steamer basket set over simmering water, steam the rutabaga, covered, 12 minutes, or just until tender.

3. Meanwhile, in a large bowl, combine the honey, hoisin, ginger, oil, vinegar, and five-spice powder or cinnamon. Gently toss in the rutabaga until evenly coated.

4. Place the rutabaga mixture and liquids in the pan, and spread out in a single layer. Bake for 30 minutes, turning over after 20 minutes, or until tender and golden.

MAKES 4 SERVINGS

Per serving: 100 calories, 22 g carbohydrate, 2 g protein, 2 g fat, 0 g saturated fat, 0 mg cholesterol, 95 mg sodium, 4 g fiber

Carbohydrate Choices: 1½

Dietary Exchanges: ½ starch, 2 vegetable

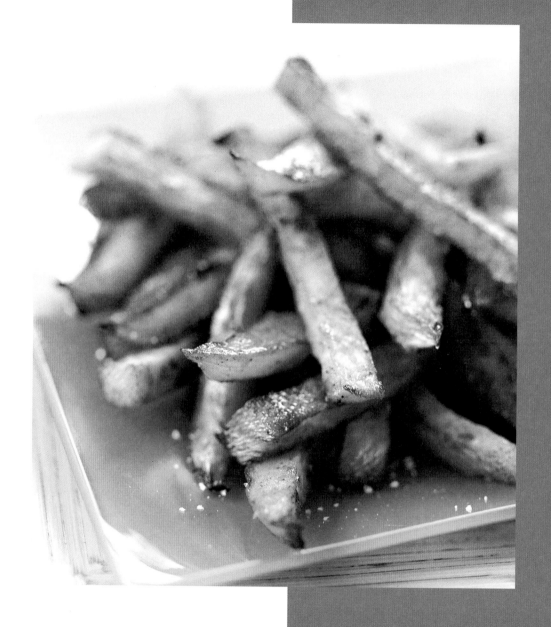

HONEY-GLAZED BRUSSELS SPROUTS WITH RED ONION

A bit of sweetness tames any harshness in the sprouts. This is a tasty side with roast pork tenderloin and sweet potato.

Preparation time: 5 minutes ● **Cooking time: 8 minutes**

---

 12 ounces Brussels sprouts, halved
 ½ small red onion, halved and sliced
 ½ cup water, divided
 1 tablespoon honey
 2 teaspoons canola oil
 ⅛ teaspoon salt
    Ground black pepper

In a skillet, combine the sprouts, onion, ¼ cup water, honey, oil, and salt. Stir to mix. Cover and set over medium-high heat. Cook, stirring occasionally, for about 8 minutes, or until the sprouts are crisp-tender and glazed. Add scant amounts of the remaining water, if needed, if the bottom of the skillet is browning too fast. Season to taste with pepper.

MAKES 4 SERVINGS

Per serving: 77 calories, 13 g carbohydrate, 3 g protein, 3 g fat, 0 g saturated fat, 0 mg cholesterol, 95 mg sodium, 4 g fiber

Carbohydrate Choices: 1

Dietary Exchanges: 1½ vegetable, ½ fat

CAULIFLOWER, GREEN BEAN, AND TOMATO GRATIN

All excuses not to eat your vegetables will disappear under the golden bread crumb and cheese topping on this easy oven dish.

Preparation time: 5 minutes ● **Cooking time: 25 minutes**

1 bag (16 ounces) frozen cauliflower florets

2 cups (half of 14-ounce bag) frozen cut Italian green beans, cut green beans, or sugar snap peas

2 cups cherry tomatoes

½ cup dried whole grain bread crumbs

⅓ cup grated Pecorino Romano cheese

1 tablespoon olive oil, preferably extra virgin

1 teaspoon minced garlic

1. Preheat the oven to 400°F. Coat a 13" × 9" baking dish with olive oil spray.

2. In a large saucepan, bring 1 cup of water to a boil. Add the cauliflower and beans, cover, and cook 3 minutes, then drain. Distribute the cauliflower, beans, and tomatoes evenly in the prepared dish.

3. In a small bowl, combine the bread crumbs, cheese, oil, and garlic. Stir with a fork until blended. Sprinkle the mixture evenly over the vegetables.

4. Bake for about 20 minutes, or until the crumbs are golden brown.

MAKES 8 SERVINGS

Per serving: 90 calories, 10 g carbohydrate, 5 g protein, 4 g fat, 1 g saturated fat, 5 mg cholesterol, 140 mg sodium, 4 g fiber

Carbohydrate Choices: 1

Dietary Exchanges: ½ starch, 1 vegetable, 1 fat

BULGUR WITH PINE NUTS

Once you get to know the nutlike flavor of bulgur (cracked and partially cooked wheat kernels), white rice will be too tame for your palate! Serve this recipe as a hot grain side dish or salad (cool the bulgur to room temperature) drizzled with balsamic vinegar.

Preparation time: 3 minutes ● **Cooking time: 25 minutes** ● **Standing time: 5 minutes**

½ cup coarse bulgur
1 cup chicken broth
¼ cup chopped green and red bell peppers
2 tablespoons pine nuts
2 tablespoons chopped parsley
Green leaf lettuce (optional)

1. In a saucepan, combine the bulgur and broth. Bring to a boil over high heat. Reduce the heat to low. Cover and cook for 20 to 25 minutes, or until the bulgur is tender.

2. Meanwhile, in a nonstick skillet coated with vegetable oil spray, cook the peppers over medium heat, stirring occasionally, for about 6 minutes, or until soft. Toast the nuts in a small skillet over medium heat until golden brown, about 3 minutes. Stir frequently to prevent burning.

3. When the bulgur is cooked, let stand 5 minutes. Transfer the bulgur to a serving plate. Add the peppers, nuts, and parsley. Toss to blend. Serve on a bed of green leaf lettuce, if desired.

MAKES 2 SERVINGS

Per serving: 195 calories, 29 g carbohydrate, 8 g protein, 6 g fat, 0.5 g saturated fat, 0 mg cholesterol, 79 mg sodium, 7 g fiber

Carbohydrate Choices: 2

Dietary Exchanges: 1½ starch, 1 fat

CHINESE ORANGE BROCCOLI

Broccoli deserves to appear on all of our tables much more of the time. Filled with antioxidants and flavor, it takes well to a host of seasonings.

Preparation time: 7 minutes ● **Cooking time: 6 minutes**

1 tablespoon canola oil

1 pound broccoli florets and stems, cut into walnut-size pieces

2 teaspoons minced garlic

¼ teaspoon salt

Juice of 1 navel orange

½ teaspoon grated orange peel

Set a wok or heavy skillet over medium-high heat for 1 minute. Add the oil and swirl to coat the pan bottom. Heat for 1 minute. Add the broccoli, garlic, salt, and about 1 table-spoon orange juice. Toss to mix. Cover and cook for about 2 minutes, tossing occasionally, or until the broccoli turns bright green. Add the peel and the remaining juice. Reduce the heat to medium. Cook, tossing frequently, for about 2 minutes, or until the broccoli starts to brown.

MAKES 4 SERVINGS

Per serving: 80 calories, 9 g carbohydrate, 4 g protein, 4 g fat, 0 g saturated fat, 0 mg cholesterol, 175 mg sodium, 4 g fiber

Carbohydrate Choices: 1

Dietary Exchanges: 1 vegetable, 1 fat

CAJUN BLACKENED ZUCCHINI

Who doesn't love a side dish that tends to itself? Slice and season the squash, spread onto a baking sheet, and pop into the oven.

Preparation time: 4 minutes ● **Cooking time: 20 minutes**

1 **pound zucchini**

Olive oil in a spray bottle, preferably extra virgin

2 **teaspoons salt-free Cajun seasoning**

⅛ **teaspoon salt**

½ **cup sliced scallions**

1. Preheat the oven to 400°F. Coat a large baking sheet with sides with vegetable oil spray.

2. Cut the zucchini in half through the middle. Cut each half into ¼"-thick lengthwise slices. Spread the zucchini on the sheet. Coat lightly with olive oil, then sprinkle with half of the seasoning and salt. Flip the slices and repeat. Spread out in a single layer.

3. Bake for 10 minutes, or until starting to sizzle. Flip the zucchini. Scatter the scallions over the pan, pressing with a spatula to coat them with some of the oil and seasoning. Bake for 10 minutes, or until the scallions are wilting.

MAKES 4 SERVINGS

Per serving: 25 calories, 4 g carbohydrate, 1 g protein, 1 g fat, 0 g saturated fat, 0 mg cholesterol, 85 mg sodium, 1 g fiber

Carbohydrate Choices: 0

Dietary Exchanges: 1 vegetable

PARMESAN ROASTED ASPARAGUS

This unique and easy way to cook asparagus seals in all of the flavor and nutrients. Feature it in the springtime when local asparagus appears in the markets.

Preparation time: 4 minutes ● **Cooking time: 10 minutes**

1 pound asparagus, trimmed, cut into thirds

1 tablespoon (½ ounce) grated Parmesan cheese

2 teaspoons olive oil, preferably extra virgin

Pinch of salt

Ground black pepper

4 lemon wedges or white wine vinegar

1. Preheat the oven to 425°F. In a baking pan large enough to hold the asparagus in a single layer, combine the asparagus, cheese, oil, and salt. Toss to coat the asparagus evenly.

2. Bake for 8 to 10 minutes, or until the asparagus is tender (time will vary depending upon the thickness of the asparagus). Season to taste with pepper. Serve with lemon wedges or a splash of vinegar.

MAKES 4 SERVINGS

Per serving: 51 calories, 5 g carbohydrate, 3 g protein, 3 g fat, 1 g saturated fat, 1 mg cholesterol, 55 mg sodium, 3 g fiber

Carbohydrate Choices: 0

Dietary Exchanges: 1 vegetable, ½ fat

GINGERED SWEET POTATOES

This autumn vegetable side dish is perfect with roast pork, sautéed mushrooms, or sage-seasoned white beans.

Preparation time: 4 minutes ● **Cooking time: 12 minutes**

1¼ **pounds sweet potatoes, peeled, cut into small cubes**

2 **teaspoons Better Butter (page 323) or trans-fat free spread**

½ **teaspoon grated fresh ginger**

⅛ **teaspoon salt**

Minced chives or scallion greens (optional)

1. Place the potatoes in a microwaveable dish in a single layer (8" × 8" works well). Cover with plastic wrap, making a vent in one corner. Cook on high power, rotating occasionally, for about 8 minutes, or until very soft. Let stand for about 3 minutes.

2. Carefully remove the plastic by pulling it toward you so the steam rises away from you. With a potato masher, smash the potatoes. Add the Better Butter or spread, ginger, and salt. Stir with the masher to mix. Serve right away sprinkled with minced chives or scallion greens, if using.

MAKES 4 SERVINGS

Per serving: 136 calories, 28 g carbohydrate, 2 g protein, 2 g fat, 1 g saturated fat, 0 mg cholesterol, 127 mg sodium, 4 g fiber

Carbohydrate Choices: 2

Dietary Exchanges: 1½ starch, ½ fat

GREEN BEANS AND MUSTARD SEEDS

Tiny whole mustard seeds are popular in Indian seasoning mixes. They are a spunky sodium-free seasoning. Look for them in the spice section of the supermarket.

Preparation time: 4 minutes ● **Cooking time: 9 minutes**

1 pound green beans, broken into 2" lengths

2 teaspoons canola oil

1 teaspoon yellow mustard seeds

½ teaspoon minced garlic

⅛ teaspoon salt

1. Pour enough water into a large skillet to come ½" up the sides. Cover and bring to a boil over high heat. Add the beans. Cover and cook, tossing occasionally, for about 6 minutes or until bright green and crisp-tender. Reserve ¼ cup of the cooking water. Drain the beans and return to the pan.

2. Set the pan over medium-high heat. Add the oil, seeds, garlic, and salt. Toss to evenly coat the beans with the seasonings. Cook over medium heat, tossing frequently, for about 3 minutes, or until the beans start to brown. Add a few drops of the reserved cooking water and reduce the heat slightly if the pan bottom starts to brown too quickly.

MAKES 4 SERVINGS

Per serving: 54 calories, 7 g carbohydrate, 2 g protein, 3 g fat, 0 g saturated fat, 0 mg cholesterol, 73 mg sodium, 4 g fiber

Carbohydrate Choices: ½

Dietary Exchanges: 1 vegetable, ½ fat

HOT AND SPICY ASIAN EGGPLANT

Be sure to choose the small Asian or Italian eggplants for this dish. They're milder than large pear-shaped eggplants, so there's no need to peel them.

Preparation time: 5 minutes ● Cooking time: 45 minutes

¾ pound small Italian or Asian eggplant, cut into 1" cubes

¾ cup shredded carrots

½ cup canned tomato puree

2 teaspoons minced garlic

⅛ teaspoon salt

Pinch of red-pepper flakes

2 teaspoons toasted sesame oil

2 tablespoons chopped cilantro (optional)

1. Preheat the oven to 375°F. In a 13" × 9" nonstick baking pan, combine the eggplant, carrots, tomato puree, garlic, salt, and pepper flakes. Toss to mix well. Cover the pan tightly with aluminum foil.

2. Bake for about 45 minutes, stirring occasionally, or until the eggplant is very tender. Drizzle with the sesame oil. Toss. Serve, sprinkled with cilantro, if using.

MAKES 4 SERVINGS

Per serving: 68 calories, 10 g carbohydrate, 2 g protein, 3 g fat, 1 g saturated fat, 0 mg cholesterol, 141 mg sodium, 4 g fiber

Carbohydrate Choices: 1

Dietary Exchanges: 2 vegetable, ½ fat

NOTE: This dish actually improves in flavor if prepared in advance. Reheat, covered, for 2 or 3 minutes in a microwave on medium power, or until heated through.

PORTOBELLO MUSHROOM BARLEY

This robustly flavored imitation of Italian risotto is made more nutritious by replacing white rice with barley.

Preparation time: 8 minutes ● **Cooking time: 16 minutes**

2 teaspoons olive oil, preferably extra virgin

1 cup sliced baby portobello mushrooms, chopped

¼ cup sliced scallions

1 bay leaf

½ teaspoon minced fresh or crumbled dry rosemary

¼ teaspoon salt

⅛ teaspoon ground black pepper

½ cup instant barley

¾ cup chicken broth

2 teaspoons balsamic vinegar

1. Coat a wide shallow saucepan or skillet with vegetable spray. Set over medium-high heat for 1 minute. Add the oil and swirl to coat the pan. Heat for 1 minute. Add the mushrooms, scallions (reserve a few greens for garnish), bay leaf, rosemary, salt, and pepper. Stir. Cover and cook, stirring frequently, for 2 minutes, or until the mushrooms give off liquid.

2. Add the barley. Cook, stirring, for 2 minutes, or until the barley is coated with the seasonings. Add the broth and bring to a boil.

3. Cover and cook over medium-low heat for about 10 minutes, or until the barley is tender. Remove and let stand, covered, for a few minutes, or until all of the liquid is absorbed and the flavor develops.

4. Remove and discard the bay leaf. Stir in the vinegar. Serve, garnished with the reserved scallion greens.

MAKES 4 SERVINGS

Per serving: 115 calories, 19 g carbohydrate, 4 g protein, 3 g fat, 1 g saturated fat, 0 mg cholesterol, 177 mg sodium, 4 g fiber

Carbohydrate Choices: 1

Dietary Exchanges: 1 starch, ½ fat

NOTE: It's no more work to prepare a double batch of this dish (don't increase the salt) and set half aside to cool. Refrigerate in an airtight container for several days, or freeze in serving-size portions in resealable plastic freezer bags for up to 1 month. Reheat in the microwave for a side dish or as an addition to vegetable soup.

VEGETABLE FRIED RICE

When cooking rice as a side dish, make extra to refrigerate for fried rice later in the week. Substitute any chopped cooked vegetables for the peas and carrots.

Preparation time: 10 minutes ● **Cooking time: 5 minutes**

---

   1   egg
   2   tablespoons chicken broth or water
1½   teaspoons soy sauce
   1   teaspoon toasted sesame oil
   2   teaspoons canola oil
   ⅓   cup finely chopped onion
   ⅓   cup shredded carrots
   ⅓   cup frozen baby peas
1½   cups cold cooked brown rice

1. In a small bowl, combine the egg, broth or water, soy sauce, and sesame oil. Beat with a fork until smooth. Set aside.

2. Set a nonstick skillet over high heat for 1 minute. Add the canola oil and swirl to coat the pan bottom. Heat for 30 seconds. Add the onion, carrots, and peas. Toss. Reduce the heat to medium-high. Cook, tossing occasionally, for 1 minute, or until sizzling. Add the rice. Toss and cook for 1 minute, or until sizzling.

3. Reduce the heat to medium. Scrape the rice mixture to the sides of the pan. Pour the egg mixture into the well. Cook, stirring the egg mixture into the rice mixture, for 1 to 2 minutes, or until the eggs are cooked.

MAKES 4 SERVINGS

Per serving: 152 calories, 21 g carbohydrate, 5 g protein, 6 g fat, 1 g saturated fat, 53 mg cholesterol, 296 mg sodium, 2 g fiber

Carbohydrate Choices: 1½

Dietary Exchanges: 1 starch, ½ vegetable, 1 fat

FILL UP ON WHOLE FOODS

Peas, Please

A good source of fiber, loose-pack baby peas should be a freezer staple in every kitchen. Here is a podful of easy ways to please with delightful, sweet peas.

1. Toss some peas into tuna or chicken salad.

2. Add peas to pasta with red sauce.

3. Heat frozen peas with a dash of toasted sesame oil in a microwaveable bowl.

4. For a souper-fast lunch, add some precooked brown rice and peas to reduced-sodium chicken broth.

5. Make a cool salad by mixing ⅓ cup peas, some snipped scallion or chives, and a drizzle of balsamic vinegar. Toss.

STIR-FRIED CURLY KALE

If there were an Olympic event for healthful vegetables, kale would take the gold! It supplies ample amounts of vitamins A and C, folate, calcium, and iron.

Preparation time: 4 minutes ● **Cooking time: 8 minutes**

1 tablespoon extra virgin olive oil

2 teaspoons minced garlic

1 pound kale leaves, chopped or torn into small pieces

¼ teaspoon salt

Ground black pepper

Place the oil and garlic in a large skillet or large pot set over low heat. Cook for about 3 minutes, or until the garlic is softened. Do not brown. Increase the heat to high. Add half the kale to the pan; toss with tongs. Cover for about 1 minute, or until the leaves start to wilt. Add the remaining kale. Toss and cover for 1 minute. Uncover and cook, tossing, for about 2 minutes, or until the leaves are wilted, brightly colored, and glossy. Add the salt. Season with pepper to taste. Toss to combine.

MAKES 4 SERVINGS

Per serving: 90 calories, 12 g carbohydrate, 4 g protein, 5 g fat, 0.5 g saturated fat, 0 mg cholesterol, 190 mg sodium, 2 g fiber

Carbohydrate Choices: 1

Dietary Exchanges: 2½ vegetable, 1 fat

NOTES: Wash the kale in plenty of cold water. Trim off and discard any really tough stems. Chop or tear the leaves (with the tender stems) into small pieces. Drain in a colander. (It's not necessary to dry the kale before cooking.)

Prewashed trimmed kale is sold bagged in some supermarkets.

Collards, chard, mustard, or turnip greens may replace the kale.

BRAISED GERMAN RED CABBAGE

An ideal side dish for wintry meals, this cabbage pairs beautifully with roast pork loin and some hearty rye bread.

Preparation time: 5 minutes ● **Cooking time: 35 minutes**

---

2 teaspoons vegetable oil

½ cup chopped onion

4 cups shredded red cabbage
  (8 ounces)

1 can (15 ounces) sliced beets, rinsed,
  drained, cut into sticks

2 tablespoons red wine vinegar

1 tablespoon brown sugar

2 bay leaves

⅛ teaspoon salt

  Pinch of ground cloves or allspice

  Ground black pepper

8 teaspoons sour cream (optional)

1. Place the oil and onion in a large pot set over medium-low heat. Cook for about 3 minutes, or until the onion sizzles. Do not brown. Add the cabbage, beets, vinegar, sugar, bay leaves, salt, and cloves or allspice. Cook, stirring, for 2 minutes, or until sizzling. Reduce the heat to medium-low.

2. Cover and cook, stirring occasionally, for 30 minutes, or until the cabbage is very tender. Remove and discard the bay leaves. Season to taste with pepper. Serve with a teaspoon dollop of sour cream, if using.

MAKES 8 SERVINGS

Per serving: 34 calories, 6 g carbohydrate, 1 g protein, 1 g fat, 0 g saturated fat, 0 mg cholesterol, 113 mg sodium, 2 g fiber

Carbohydrate Choices: ½

Dietary Exchanges: 1 vegetable

CURRIED CAULIFLOWER

Cooking spices in a small amount of oil releases their aroma and flavor. To keep calories to a minimum, we're precooking the cauliflower in water and then stir-frying with some oil, garlic, and curry powder.

Preparation time: 4 minutes ● **Cooking time: 10 minutes**

1 **pound cauliflower florets, cut into walnut-size pieces**

2 **teaspoons olive oil**

1 **teaspoon minced garlic**

½ **teaspoon curry powder**

¼ **teaspoon salt**

1 **tablespoon finely chopped parsley (optional)**

Ground black pepper

1. Fill a large skillet with enough water to come ½" up the sides of the pan. Cover and bring to a boil over high heat. Add the cauliflower. Cover and cook, stirring once, over medium-high heat for about 3 minutes, or until tender but still crisp.

2. Tip the pan and spoon out most of the water into a measuring cup. Set aside. Return the pan to medium-high heat. Add the oil, garlic, curry powder, and salt. Cook over medium-high heat, tossing frequently and adding a tablespoon at a time of the reserved water. Scrape the bottom of the pan to release the flavorful browned bits. Cook for about 5 minutes, or until the cauliflower is golden brown. Sprinkle on the parsley, if using. Season to taste with pepper.

MAKES 4 SERVINGS

Per serving: 53 calories, 7 g carbohydrate, 2 g protein, 3 g fat, 1 g saturated fat, 0 mg cholesterol, 180 mg sodium, 3 g fiber

Carbohydrate Choices: ½

Dietary Exchanges: 1 vegetable, ½ fat

NOTES: A touch of fresh green sparks this dish. If you don't have parsley, toss in 1 tablespoon of minced scallion greens or 2 tablespoons of frozen baby peas. Toss with the cauliflower for about 1 minute, or until heated through.

For variety, you can replace the cauliflower with broccoli or broccoflower.

SNOW PEAS AND PEPPERS IN PEANUT SAUCE

For a satisfying yet light meal, start with egg drop soup, followed by this tasty vegetable dish and a serving of steamed brown rice.

Preparation time: 4 minutes ● **Cooking time: 6 minutes**

2 tablespoons chicken or vegetable broth

1 tablespoon natural peanut butter

1 teaspoon soy sauce

½ teaspoon minced garlic

½ teaspoon sugar

1 teaspoon canola oil

12 ounces Chinese snow peas

½ cup thinly sliced red bell pepper

1. In a small bowl, combine the broth, peanut butter, soy sauce, garlic, and sugar. Whisk to blend. Set aside.

2. Coat a skillet or wok with vegetable oil spray. Set over high heat for 1 minute. Add the oil and swirl around the pan to coat. Let stand for 30 seconds. Add the snow peas and pepper. Toss. Cover and cook for 2 minutes, or until the peas are bright green.

3. Reduce the heat to low. Add the reserved peanut butter mixture. Cook, tossing for 2 minutes, or until heated through.

MAKES 4 SERVINGS

Per serving: 81 calories, 9 g carbohydrate, 4 g protein, 4 g fat, 1 g saturated fat, 0 mg cholesterol, 68 mg sodium, 3 g fiber

Carbohydrate Choices: 1

Dietary Exchanges: ½ starch, ½ fat

NOTE: Sugar snap peas can replace the Chinese snow peas if desired. Orange or yellow bell pepper can replace the red bell pepper.

BAKED BEANS

Azuki beans are naturally sweet and are actually used in desserts in some Asian cuisines. By using azuki beans in this all-American recipe, we were able to reduce the typical amount of sweetening.

Preparation time: 5 minutes ● **Cooking time: 1 hour** ● **Standing time: 15 minutes**

---

4 cups cooked azuki beans or canned azuki beans, rinsed and drained

¼ cup finely chopped onion

2 slices (2 ounces) Canadian bacon, finely chopped

¾ cup canned tomato puree

2 tablespoons pure maple syrup

¾ teaspoon mustard powder

¼ teaspoon salt

¼ teaspoon ground black pepper

¼ teaspoon hot-pepper sauce

¼ teaspoon ground cloves or allspice

1. Preheat the oven to 325°F. Coat an 8" × 8" baking dish with vegetable oil spray. Add the beans, onion, bacon, tomato puree, syrup, mustard, salt, pepper, hot-pepper sauce, and cloves or allspice. Stir to combine.

2. Cover the dish tightly with aluminum foil. Bake for 1 hour. Turn off the oven and let the beans stand inside for about 15 minutes.

MAKES 8 SERVINGS

Per serving: 184 calories, 35 g carbohydrate, 11 g protein, 1 g fat, 0 g saturated fat, 4 mg cholesterol, 277 mg sodium, 9 g fiber

Carbohydrate Choices: 2

Dietary Exchanges: 2 starch, ½ vegetable

NOTE: The beans can also be cooked in a slow cooker on the low setting for 2 hours.

BROCCOLI WITH CHEDDAR CRUMBLES

Selecting the best-tasting aged Cheddar you can find is the flavor secret to this vegetable dish.

Preparation time: 5 minutes ● **Cooking time: 8 minutes**

---

1 **pound broccoli, cut into walnut-size pieces**

1 **tablespoon Better Butter (page 323) or trans-fat free spread**

2 **tablespoons dry whole grain bread crumbs**

⅛ **teaspoon salt**

2 **tablespoons shredded extra-sharp Cheddar cheese**

1. Bring ½" water to a boil in a nonstick skillet. Add the broccoli. Cover and cook, tossing occasionally, for 2 minutes, or until bright green and crisp-tender. Drain the broccoli. Set aside.

2. Wipe the skillet dry and place over high heat for 1 minute. Add the Better Butter or spread, bread crumbs, and salt. Stir to mix. Return the broccoli to the pan. Cook over medium heat, tossing for 3 minutes, or until the crumbs are toasted. Remove from the heat. Scatter on the cheese. Toss for about 1 minute, or until the cheese coats the broccoli and starts to melt.

MAKES 4 SERVINGS

Per serving: 88 calories, 10 g carbohydrate, 4 g protein, 4 g fat, 2 g saturated fat, 4 mg cholesterol, 180 mg sodium, 3 g fiber

Carbohydrate Choices: 1

Dietary Exchanges: 1½ vegetable, 1 fat

NOTE: Cauliflower can replace the broccoli if you like.

ROASTED ROOT VEGETABLES

Robust winter vegetables become oh-so-sweet when baked. If you ...
salad, they're hearty enough to make a meal.

Preparation time: 10 minutes ● **Cooking time: 45 minutes**

1 onion (8 ounces), cut into walnut-size chunks

1 sweet potato (8 ounces), cut into walnut-size chunks

1 turnip (6 ounces), cut into walnut-size chunks

1 russet potato (6 ounces), cut into walnut-size chunks

2 tablespoons olive oil, preferably extra virgin

2 teaspoons herbes des Provence

¼ teaspoon salt

1. Preheat the oven to 375°F. In a 13" × 9" baking dish, combine the onion, sweet potato, turnip, russet potato, oil, herbes de Provence, and salt. Toss to coat the vegetables with the seasoning.

2. Roast for about 45 minutes, stirring occasionally, or until golden and tender.

MAKES 8 SERVINGS

Per serving: 90 calories, 15 g carbohydrate, 2 g protein, 4 g fat, 0 g saturated fat, 0 mg cholesterol, 190 mg sodium, 2 g fiber

Carbohydrate Choices: 1

Dietary Exchanges: 1 starch, 1 vegetable, 1 fat

NOTE: Store any leftovers in an airtight plastic container. For a quick and satisfying roasted vegetable soup, reheat 1 serving of the vegetables with 1 cup of chicken or vegetable broth.

UNLEASH NUTRIENTS

Repeal Peeling

Don't peel fruits and vegetables unless you absolutely must for edibility. Scrub them really well under cold running water instead. You'll get extra nutrients and fiber—and it cuts preparation time.

BALSAMIC BELL PEPPERS WITH PINE NUTS

This dish is a good choice for a buffet because it tastes as good at room temperature as it does hot from the skillet. Any leftovers make a wonderful filling for a breakfast omelet.

Preparation time: 5 minutes ● **Cooking time: 6 minutes**

---

2 teaspoons olive oil, preferably extra virgin

1 pound orange or yellow bell peppers, cut into strips

⅛ teaspoon salt

2 teaspoons minced garlic

Balsamic vinegar

1 tablespoon pine nuts, toasted and chopped

Set a skillet over medium heat for 1 minute. Add the oil. Heat for 30 seconds. Add the peppers and salt. Toss to combine. Cover and cook, tossing occasionally, for about 3 minutes, or until the peppers are starting to soften. Add the garlic. Cook, tossing, for about 1 minute, or until the garlic is fragrant. Drizzle with vinegar to taste. Toss to heat through. Serve sprinkled with the nuts.

MAKES 4 SERVINGS

Per serving: 78 calories, 9 g carbohydrate, 2 g protein, 4 g fat, 1 g saturated fat, 0 mg cholesterol, 77 mg sodium, 1 g fiber

Carbohydrate Choices: 1

Dietary Exchanges: 1 vegetable, 1 fat

NOTE: To toast pine nuts, place in a cold skillet. Set over medium heat. Cook, stirring frequently, for about 4 minutes, or until golden. Watch the nuts carefully so they don't burn.

ORANGE-GLAZED FENNEL AND RED ONION

Once an oddity, the fresh vegetable Florence fennel—often mislabeled as anise—is now widely available in supermarkets. When it's skillet braised in a small amount of liquid, it makes a delightful pairing with grilled fish or seafood.

Preparation time: 10 minutes ● **Cooking time: 8 minutes**

1¼ **pounds bulb fennel**

½ **red onion (4 ounces)**

1 **tablespoon olive oil, preferably extra virgin**

2 **tablespoons orange juice**

⅛ **teaspoon salt**

½ **teaspoon grated orange peel**

1. Cut off the tall fennel stalks. Save some of the leafy greens for garnish. Discard the stalks. Chop about 1 tablespoon leaves and set aside. Quarter the bulbs. Cut out the core and discard. Cut the bulbs into ½"-thick slices. Halve the onion and cut into ½"-thick slices.

2. Coat a skillet with vegetable oil spray. Set over high heat for 1 minute. Add the oil and swirl to coat the pan bottom. Heat for 30 seconds. Add the sliced fennel, onion, juice, and salt. Toss. Reduce the heat to medium. Cover and cook for 7 to 8 minutes, or until glazed and brown. Add a few drops of water to the pan occasionally and reduce the heat slightly if the mixture is browning too fast. Add the peel and reserved leaves for garnish. Toss and serve.

MAKES 4 SERVINGS

Per serving: 91 calories, 14 g carbohydrate, 2 g protein, 4 g fat, 1 g saturated fat, 0 mg cholesterol, 147 mg sodium, 5 g fiber

Carbohydrate Choices: 1

Dietary Exchanges: 2 vegetable, 1 fat

SESAME SPINACH

This Japanese-style seasoning is also appetizing with cooked kale, mustard greens, or chard.

Preparation time: 4 minutes ● **Cooking time: 4 minutes**

1 teaspoon sesame seeds
2 teaspoons canola oil
½ teaspoon minced garlic
1 pound baby spinach leaves
2 tablespoons water
1½ teaspoons reduced-sodium soy sauce

Place the sesame seeds in a skillet. Cook over medium-high heat, stirring frequently, for about 2 minutes, or until golden. Remove to a bowl. Return the skillet to medium-low heat. Add the oil and garlic. Cook for 30 seconds, or until fragrant. Add the spinach, water, and soy sauce to the pan; toss with tongs. Cover for about 1 minute, or until the leaves wilt. Serve sprinkled with the sesame seeds.

MAKES 4 SERVINGS

Per serving: 74 calories, 12 g carbohydrate, 3 g protein, 3 g fat, 0 g saturated fat, 0 mg cholesterol, 256 mg sodium, 5 g fiber

Carbohydrate Choices: 1

Dietary Exchanges: 2 vegetable, ½ fat

SOUTHERN COLLARDS

Pair these flavorful greens with baked catfish or Baked Beans (page 229) for a taste of the South.

Preparation time: 5 minutes   ● Cooking time: 7 minutes

1 slice (1 ounce) Canadian bacon, finely chopped
¼ cup finely chopped onion
1 teaspoon canola oil
1 pound collard greens, chopped or torn into small pieces
¼ teaspoon salt
Pinch of ground red pepper
Wine or cider vinegar

In a large skillet, combine the bacon, onion, and oil. Set over low heat. Cook, stirring occasionally, for about 3 minutes, or until sizzling. Increase the heat to medium-high. Add the greens to the pan; toss with tongs. Cover and cook, tossing occasionally, for about 4 minutes, or until the leaves are brightly colored and glossy. Add the salt and pepper. Serve with vinegar to drizzle at the table.

MAKES 4 SERVINGS

Per serving: 54 calories, 8 g carbohydrate, 4 g protein, 1 g fat, 0 g saturated fat, 4 mg cholesterol, 313 mg sodium, 4 g fiber

Carbohydrate Choices: ½

Dietary Exchanges: 2 vegetable

NOTE: To prep the collard greens for cooking, wash them in a large amount of cold water. Drain the greens (some water clinging to the leaves is fine). Chop off and discard any browned bottom stems. Place a big bunch of the leaves on a work surface. Holding the bunch tightly in one hand, use a cleaver or chef's knife to slice crosswise into shreds. Continue until all of the leaves are sliced.

CHAPTER 9

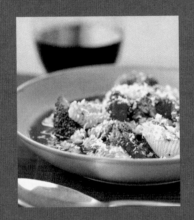

DINNERS

ORANGE-SOY SALMON WITH VEGETABLES

Salmon, a popular source of good-for-you omega-3 fats, is paired with vitamin-rich spinach and carrots and sweetened with citrus.

Preparation time: 5 minutes ● **Cooking time: 7 minutes**

Grated peel and juice of ½ orange

1½ tablespoons reduced-sodium soy sauce

1 tablespoon hoisin sauce

1 teaspoon grated fresh ginger

1 teaspoon toasted sesame oil

1 bag (6 ounces) baby spinach

5 teaspoons water, divided

4 skinless salmon fillets (about 5 ounces each), 1" thick

8 ounces sugar snap peas

1 cup matchstick-cut carrots

2 scallions, sliced

1. In a small bowl, combine the orange peel and juice, soy sauce, hoisin sauce, ginger, and sesame oil. Mix to blend and set aside. Place the spinach in a mound to cover ⅔ of a microwaveable dish. Drizzle and toss with 2 teaspoons of the water. Place the salmon fillets on top. On the other side of the dish, toss the snap peas, carrots, 1 tablespoon of the soy mixture, and the remaining 3 teaspoons water. Drizzle 2 tablespoons of the soy mixture over the salmon.

2. Cover with vented plastic wrap (keep wrap about 1" above food), and microwave on high power for 5 to 7 minutes, or until the salmon is slightly opaque in the center and the vegetables are tender. Drizzle the remaining soy mixture over the salmon and vegetables. Sprinkle with the scallions.

MAKES 4 SERVINGS

Per serving: 347 calories, 15 g carbohydrate, 40 g protein, 13 g fat, 2 g saturated fat, 100 mg cholesterol, 595 mg sodium, 4 g fiber

Carbohydrate Choices: 1

Dietary Exchanges: ½ starch, 1 vegetable, 5 meat, 2 fat

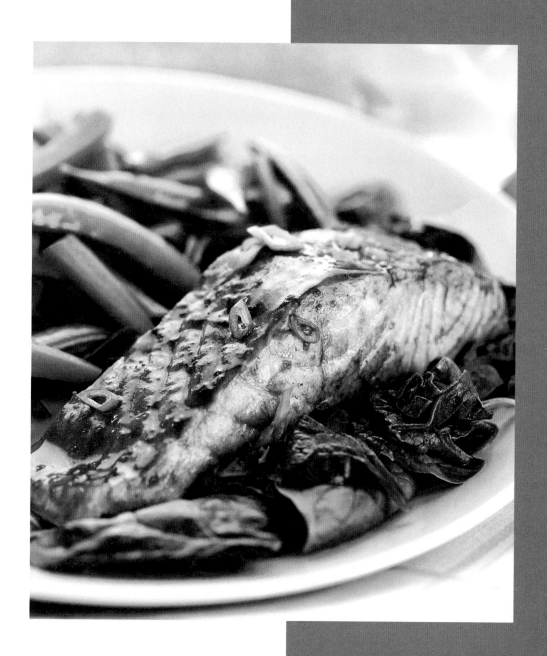

WILD PACIFIC SALMON WITH CREAMY AVOCADO SAUCE

If wild salmon isn't available, you can substitute farm-raised salmon for this elegant dinner.

Preparation time: 10 minutes ● Cooking time: 10–12 minutes

---

6 wild Pacific salmon fillets (6 ounces each), about 1" thick

½ large avocado, peeled, pitted, and quartered

¼ cup fat-free sour cream

1 tablespoon reduced-fat mayonnaise

1 teaspoon lemon juice

1 teaspoon minced garlic

¼ teaspoon hot-pepper sauce

¼ teaspoon Worcestershire sauce

¼ teaspoon salt

¼ teaspoon ground black pepper

1. Place the salmon fillets, skin side down, on an aluminum foil–lined baking sheet. Coat the fish with vegetable oil spray.

2. Preheat the broiler. Cook the salmon for 10 to 12 minutes, or until the fish is opaque.

3. While the fish is cooking, in the bowl of a food processor fitted with a metal blade, combine the avocado, sour cream, mayonnaise, lemon juice, garlic, hot-pepper sauce, Worcestershire sauce, salt, and pepper. Process, scraping down the bowl occasionally, until the mixture is smooth.

4. With a spatula, lift each salmon fillet away from the skin and set on dinner plates. Serve a dollop of the sauce with each salmon fillet.

MAKES 6 SERVINGS (1 SALMON FILLET AND 2 TABLESPOONS OF SAUCE)

Per serving: 290 calories, 4 g carbohydrate, 38 g protein, 13 g fat, 2.5 g saturated fat, 80 mg cholesterol, 215 mg sodium, 1 g fiber

Carbohydrate Choices: 0

Dietary Exchanges: 5 meat, 2 fat

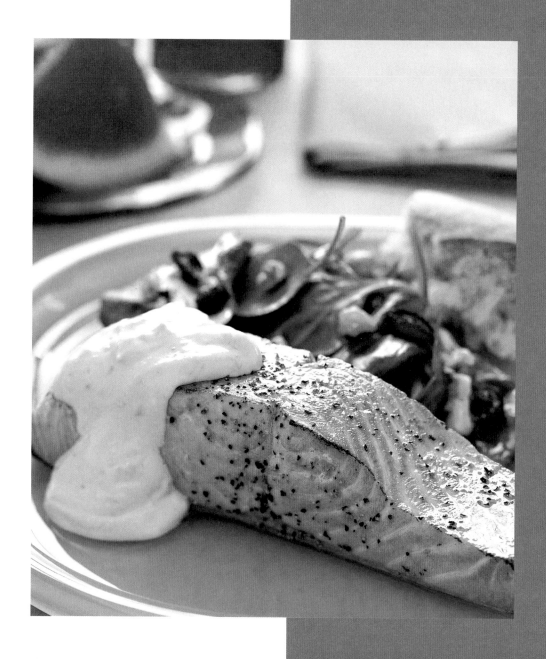

ASIAN-INSPIRED COD

Take your daily dose of ginger, fresh and preserved, in this sesame-flavored cod.

Preparation time: 10 minutes ● **Cooking time: 20 minutes**

---

1 piece (2") fresh ginger, cut into matchsticks

1 bunch scallions, cut into matchsticks

1 medium carrot, cut into matchsticks

1 tablespoon minced garlic

4 cod fillets (about 8 ounces each)

2 tablespoons chopped cilantro + sprigs for garnish

1½ tablespoons reduced-sodium soy sauce

2 tablespoons ginger preserves

¼ cup water

2 tablespoons toasted sesame oil

1. Preheat the oven to 400°F. Coat a 13" × 9" baking dish with vegetable oil spray. Add the ginger, scallions, carrot, and garlic to the dish. Toss to mix.

2. Place the fillets over the ginger-scallion mixture. Sprinkle with the chopped cilantro.

3. In a small bowl, combine the soy sauce, preserves, water, and oil. Pour the mixture over the fish.

4. Cover and seal the dish with aluminum foil. Bake for 20 minutes, or until the fish flakes. Garnish with cilantro sprigs, if desired.

MAKES 4 SERVINGS

Per serving: 310 calories, 12 g carbohydrate, 42 g protein, 10 g fat, 1.5 g saturated fat, 100 mg cholesterol, 338 mg sodium, 1 g fiber

Carbohydrate Choices: 1

Dietary Exchanges: ½ starch, 1 vegetable, 6 meat, 1½ fat

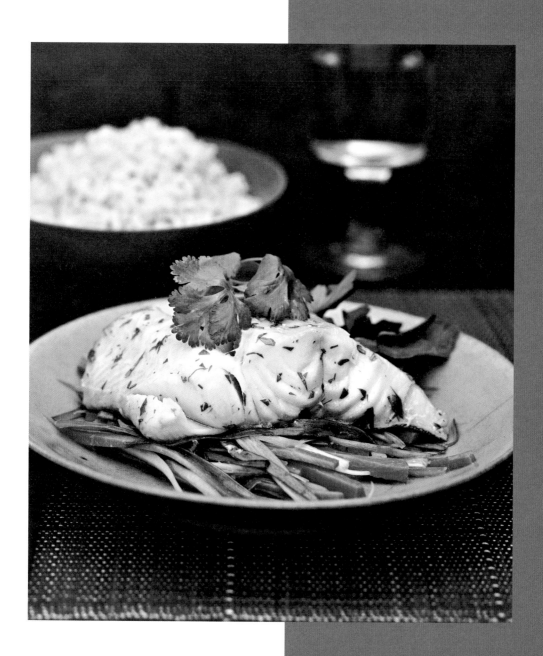

POACHED HALIBUT IN VEGETABLE BROTH

Be sure to sip every drop of the delicious and filling broth in this seafood dinner.
If you can't find sodium-free vegetable broth, replace half of regular vegetable
broth with water.

Preparation time: 25 minutes ● **Cooking time: 10 minutes**

4 halibut fillets (4 ounces each)

2 cups matchstick-cut snow peas

1 cup bean sprouts

2 red bell peppers, cut into matchsticks

1 red onion, cut into matchsticks

1 cup matchstick-cut carrots

¼ cup minced garlic (about 10 cloves)

1 tablespoon minced fresh ginger

1 teaspoon grated lemon peel

3 cups sodium-free vegetable broth

1 cup sherry (optional)

3 tablespoons chopped cilantro

1. In a large skillet with a lid, combine the fish, snow peas, bean sprouts, peppers, onion, carrots, garlic, ginger, lemon peel, broth, and sherry (if desired).

2. Cover and bring to a simmer over high heat. Reduce the heat to low. Cover and cook 6 minutes, or until the fish flakes easily. Sprinkle on the cilantro. Serve in pasta bowls with the broth.

MAKES 4 SERVINGS

Per serving: 214 calories, 19 g carbohydrate, 27 g protein, 3 g fat, 0.5 g saturated fat, 36 mg cholesterol, 360 mg sodium, 4 g fiber

Carbohydrate Choices: 1

Dietary Exchanges: 2½ vegetable, 3½ meat

LOOSEN UP/GET MOVING

The Path to Living Longer

Hit the walking trail to improve the quality and the quantity of your life! Researchers at the Centers for Disease Control and *Prevention* say walking—even just a little—can lower the risk of death for those with adult-onset diabetes. They studied 2,896 adults, average age around 59, who'd had diabetes for about 11 years. Those in the study group who walked as little as 2 hours per week had a 39 percent lower death rate from all causes and a 34 percent lower risk of death from heart disease. Those who walked 3 to 4 hours a week had the lowest overall death rates.

SALMON WITH WHITE BEAN AND CITRUS SALAD

This sophisticated main dish brings together some unlikely ingredients in perfect harmony. Tart-sweet grapefruit, orange, and lemon play counterpoint to earthy beans and richly flavored salmon.

Preparation time: 15 minutes ● **Cooking time: 15 minutes**

1 tablespoon olive oil

1 red onion, thinly sliced

1 can (15 ounces) cannellini beans, rinsed and drained

¼ cup chopped flat-leaf parsley

2 teaspoons grated lemon peel

¼ teaspoon salt, divided

¼ teaspoon ground black pepper, divided

1 pink grapefruit, peeled and cut into segments

1 navel orange, peeled and cut into segments

1 tablespoon lemon juice

4 center-cut salmon fillets (4 ounces each), with skin

1. In a medium skillet, heat the oil over medium heat. Add the onion and cook, stirring, for 5 minutes, or until softened. Stir in the beans, parsley, lemon peel, ⅛ teaspoon salt, and ⅛ teaspoon pepper. Cook, stirring, for 3 minutes, or until heated through. Stir in the grapefruit, orange, and lemon juice. Remove from the heat and set aside.

2. Season the salmon with the remaining ⅛ teaspoon salt and ⅛ teaspoon pepper. Heat a large nonstick skillet over medium-high heat. Place the salmon, skin side down, in the pan. Cook for 2 minutes. Turn the salmon and cook for about 2 minutes on each of the remaining sides, until the fish is browned and opaque.

3. Transfer the salmon to serving plates and spoon the salad on the side.

MAKES 4 SERVINGS

Per serving: 285 calories, 26 g carbohydrate, 27 g protein, 8 g fat, 1 g saturated fat, 59 mg cholesterol, 395 mg sodium, 6 g fiber

Carbohydrate Choices: 2

Dietary Exchanges: 1 starch, 1 fruit, 1 vegetable, 3 meat, 1 fat

THE GREENHOUSE CRAB CAKES

Crab cakes are indeed a special treat, but if you ever want to enjoy other seafood cakes, simply use scallops or any mild white-fleshed fish, such as tilapia, snapper, or catfish, in this dish.

Preparation time: 20 minutes ● **Cooking time: 10 minutes**

1	pound crabmeat
1	egg
1	cup finely chopped celery
1	tablespoon fat-free mayonnaise
1	tablespoon lemon juice
½	teaspoon ground white pepper
¼	teaspoon curry powder
⅛	teaspoon ground red pepper
⅛	teaspoon mustard powder
2	tablespoons chopped fresh chives
1–2	tablespoons unseasoned dry bread crumbs
3	drops hot-pepper sauce
8–16	slices sprouted wheat bread, cut into 3"–4" rounds and toasted (optional)

1. In a large bowl, combine the crabmeat, egg, celery, mayonnaise, lemon juice, white pepper, curry powder, red pepper, mustard powder, chives, bread crumbs, and hot-pepper sauce. Toss to mix. Form into 8 patties.

2. Heat the patties in a medium nonstick skillet over low heat until brown, 4 to 5 minutes per side. Serve warm alone, on 1 toast round, or between 2 rounds as a sandwich.

MAKES 8 CRAB CAKES

Per serving: (1 crab cake without bread): 67 calories, 2 g carbohydrate, 11 g protein, 2 g fat, 0.5 g saturated fat, 71 mg cholesterol, 212 mg sodium,1 g fiber

Per serving: (1 crab cake with 2 rounds of bread): 202 calories, 26 g carbohydrate, 16 g protein, 3.5 g fat, 1 g saturated fat, 71 mg cholesterol, 487 mg sodium, 3 g fiber

Carbohydrate Choices: 2

Dietary Exchanges: 2 starch, 1½ meat

NOTE: High-fiber, sprouted grain bread is available in the freezer section of most grocery and natural food stores. Multigrain bread can be used as an alternative.

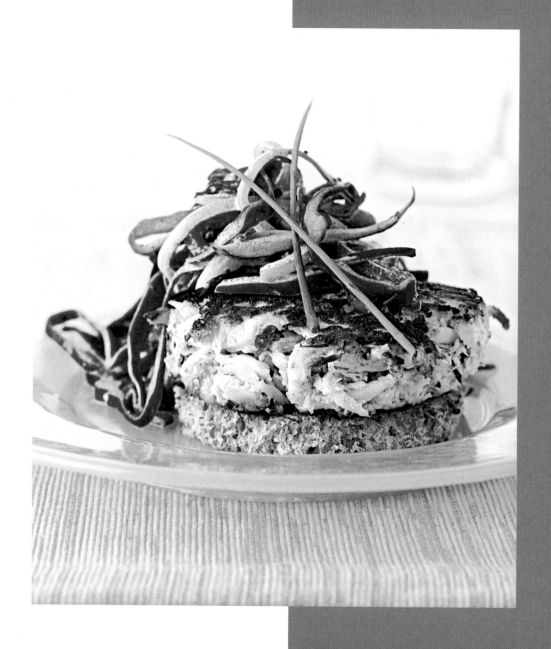

SEARED SHRIMP WITH GINGER STIR-FRIED VEGETABLES

Just because you're dining solo doesn't mean you can't enjoy great-tasting food, as this single-serving recipe proves.

Preparation time: 17 minutes ● **Cooking time: 13 minutes**

2 ounces peeled and deveined medium shrimp

Pinch of coarsely ground sea salt

Pinch of freshly ground black pepper

1 teaspoon canola oil

1 tablespoon lime juice

2 teaspoons crushed fresh ginger

1 teaspoon cornstarch

1 teaspoon minced garlic

1 teaspoon toasted sesame oil

1 cup broccoli florets

½ cup snow peas

½ cup matchstick-cut carrots

½ cup whole shiitake mushrooms

2 teaspoons low-sodium soy sauce

2 tablespoons water

1. Season the shrimp to taste with salt and pepper. Heat the canola oil in a large heavy skillet over high heat. The pan should be as hot as possible. Place the shrimp in the pan and sear for 45 to 60 seconds. Remove and set aside.

2. In a large bowl, blend the lime juice, ginger, cornstarch, garlic, and sesame oil until the cornstarch is dissolved. Mix in the broccoli, peas, carrots, and mushrooms, tossing to lightly coat. In the same pan used for the shrimp, cook the vegetables for 2 minutes, stirring constantly. Stir in the soy sauce and water. Cook for about 10 minutes, or until the vegetables are crisp-tender.

3. Place the vegetables on a plate and top with the shrimp.

MAKES 1 SERVING

Per serving: 270 calories, 24 g carbohydrate, 18 g protein, 11 g fat, 1.5 g saturated fat, 85 mg cholesterol, 520 mg sodium, 6 g fiber

Carbohydrate Choices: 1½

Dietary Exchanges: 2½ vegetable, 1½ meat, 2 fat

ROASTED CHILI-RUBBED SALMON

Try purchasing individually quick-frozen fish fillets sometimes. Often, they can be "fresher" than the fish displayed at the fish counter because they are frozen immediately after being caught.

Preparation time: 10 minutes ● **Cooking time: 20 minutes**

---

1 tablespoon olive oil

½ cup coarsely chopped red onion

2½ teaspoons chili powder, divided

1 bag (14 ounces) frozen corn kernels

1 cup frozen mixed bell pepper strips

¼ cup chopped cilantro + 4 sprigs for garnish

4 boneless, skinless salmon fillets (4 ounces each), about 1" thick

½ teaspoon salt

¼ teaspoon ground black pepper

1. Preheat the oven to 450°F.

2. Heat the oil over medium heat in a large ovenproof skillet or shallow stovetop-to-oven baking dish. Add the onion and cook, stirring, for 2 minutes.

3. Add 1½ teaspoons of the chili powder and stir to blend. Add the corn and bell pepper strips. Cook over medium heat, stirring, for about 3 minutes, or until the vegetables are no longer icy. Stir in the chopped cilantro. Spread the vegetables in an even layer.

4. Sprinkle the remaining 1 teaspoon chili powder evenly on the fish. Place, chili side up, on the vegetables. Sprinkle with the salt and pepper.

5. Place in the oven and roast for about 12 minutes, or until the fish is opaque. Serve each fillet on a bed of vegetables and garnish with a cilantro sprig.

MAKES 4 SERVINGS

Per serving: 350 calories, 26 g carbohydrate, 26 g protein, 17 g fat, 3 g saturated fat, 65 mg cholesterol, 380 mg sodium, 4 g fiber

Carbohydrate Choices: 2

Dietary Exchanges: 1 starch, 3 meat, ½ vegetable, 1½ fat

MEDITERRANEAN COD

Any mild-flavored white-fleshed fish, such as tilapia, turbot, or snapper, is fine for this dish. Shop for fish where the fillets are displayed on a bed of ice. They should look firm and glistening, never sunken or soggy.

Preparation time: 17 minutes ● **Cooking time: 9 minutes**

¼ cup sun-dried tomato pesto

1 pound cod fillets, cut into 4 portions

2 bunches fennel (¾ pound), trimmed, halved, and sliced very thin crosswise

2 tablespoons chopped fennel fronds

¼ cup halved pitted kalamata olives

1 cup whole fresh parsley leaves

1½ teaspoons lemon juice

1½ teaspoons olive oil

⅛ teaspoon salt

1. Preheat the oven to 400°F. Coat an oven-proof skillet with vegetable oil spray.

2. Spoon 1 tablespoon of the pesto on each fillet. Arrange in the prepared pan with space in between. Roast for 9 minutes, or until the fish flakes easily. Remove from the oven.

3. Meanwhile, in a large bowl, combine the sliced fennel and fronds, olives, parsley, lemon juice, oil, and salt. Toss to mix.

4. Divide the salad among 4 plates and top each with one roasted cod portion.

MAKES 4 SERVINGS

Per serving: 162 calories, 9 g carbohydrate, 22 g protein, 4 g fat, 1 g saturated fat, 50 mg cholesterol, 440 mg sodium, 3 g fiber

Carbohydrate Choices: 1

Dietary Exchanges: 1½ vegetable, 3 meat, ½ fat

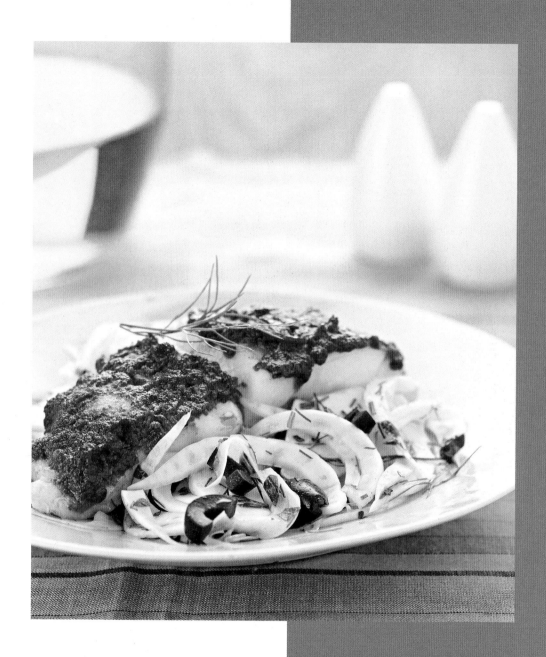

SCALLOP-ASPARAGUS LINGUINE

Scallops make this a special occasion dish. For a weekday alternative, replace the scallops with catfish, cut into scallop-size chunks.

Preparation time: 22 minutes ● **Cooking time: 11 minutes**

---

1 bunch asparagus, cut diagonally into 2" pieces

8 ounces spinach linguine

16 sea scallops (about 1 pound)

Ground black pepper

¼ teaspoon salt

2 teaspoons olive oil

2 tablespoons lemon juice

Strip lemon peel, ½" × 3", thinly sliced

¼ cup water

¼ cup chopped fresh basil + additional leaves for garnish

1. In a large pot, bring 3 quarts of water to a boil. Add the asparagus and cook for 1 minute, or until bright green and crisp-tender. Remove with tongs, rinse in cool water, and set aside.

2. In the same pot, cook the linguine for about 10 minutes, or until al dente.

3. Meanwhile, season the scallops with pepper to taste and ⅛ teaspoon salt. Heat a large skillet over medium-high heat. Add the oil to the pan. Add the scallops and cook for 5 minutes. Flip the scallops and cook for about 3 minutes, or until opaque. Remove and set aside.

4. In the same skillet, combine the lemon juice, lemon peel, ¼ cup of water, and the remaining ⅛ teaspoon of salt. Cook, stirring, for about 1 minute, or until slightly reduced.

5. Drain the pasta and toss with the asparagus, chopped basil, and lemon juice mixture. Serve in pasta bowls topped with the scallops and garnished with basil leaves.

MAKES 4 SERVINGS

Per serving: 340 calories, 49 g carbohydrate, 27 g protein, 5 g fat, 0 g saturated fat, 35 mg cholesterol, 350 mg sodium, 4 g fiber

Carbohydrate Choices: 3

Dietary Exchanges: 3 starch, ½ vegetable, 3 meat, ½ fat

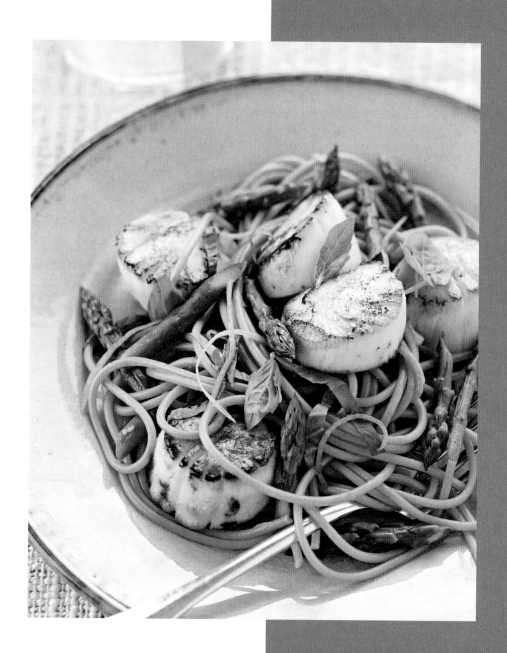

ROASTED CATFISH WITH CUMIN SWEET POTATOES

Anyone who (wrongly) believes that fish is difficult to cook will be won over by this recipe. There's nothing to do but season the fish and bake it!

Preparation time: 10 minutes ● **Cooking time: 1 hour**

1 pound sweet potatoes, peeled and sliced ¼" thick

½ teaspoon ground cumin

1 tablespoon canola oil

4 catfish fillets (5 ounces each)

1 teaspoon chili powder

½ cup diagonally sliced scallions

1 bag (10 ounces) frozen corn kernels, thawed

1 medium green bell pepper, chopped

2 tablespoons fresh lime juice

1 tablespoon chopped cilantro

1 teaspoon finely chopped jalapeño chile pepper, or more to taste

1. Preheat the oven to 400°F. In a 13" × 9" baking dish, combine the potatoes, cumin, and oil. Toss to coat. Spread in an even layer and roast for about 45 minutes, or until the potatoes are browned.

2. Remove the potatoes from the oven. Increase the temperature to 450°F. Use a wide spatula to gently turn the potato slices. Arrange the fish on top of the potatoes. Sprinkle with chili powder and scallions.

3. Return the fish and potatoes to the oven. Roast for 8 to 10 minutes per inch of thickness, or until the fish flakes easily.

4. Meanwhile, in a bowl, combine the corn, bell pepper, lime juice, cilantro, and jalapeño pepper.

5. With a wide spatula, lift a portion of potatoes and fish onto serving plates. Spoon the corn salad on top.

MAKES 4 SERVINGS

Per serving: 393 calories, 40 g carbohydrate, 26 g protein, 15 g fat, 3 g saturated fat, 67 mg cholesterol, 112 mg sodium, 6 g fiber

Carbohydrate Choices: 3

Dietary Exchanges: 2 starch, ½ vegetable, 3 meat, 1 fat

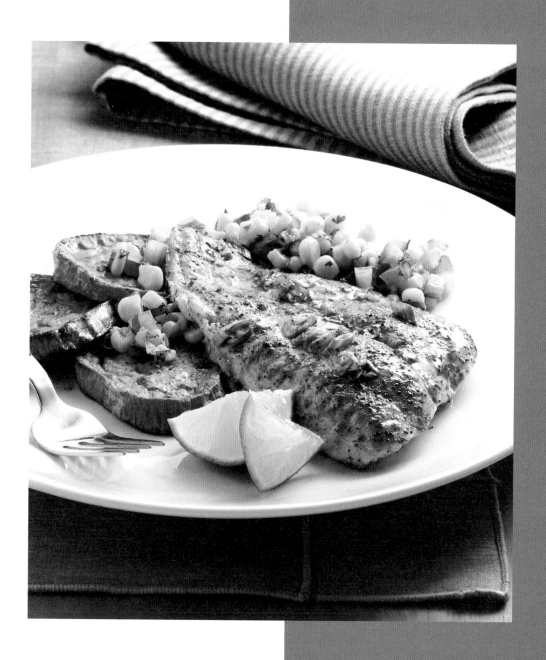

ROASTED FLOUNDER WITH ARTICHOKES

Whole wheat couscous takes just 10 minutes to prepare and goes beautifully with this Mediterranean-flavored fish.

Preparation time: 10 minutes ● **Cooking time: 47–50 minutes**

2 large red onions, cut into ¼" wedges

2 tablespoons olive oil, preferably extra virgin

1 package (10 ounces) frozen artichoke hearts, thawed (about 2 cups)

1 cup cherry or grape tomatoes

2 tablespoons chopped parsley

1 teaspoon grated orange peel

1 teaspoon minced garlic

4 skinless flounder fillets (5 ounces each)

1. Preheat the oven to 400°F. In a 13" × 9" baking dish, combine the onions and oil. Spread in an even layer.

2. Roast for about 35 minutes, or until the onions are golden. Remove from the oven. Stir in the artichokes and tomatoes.

3. In a small bowl, combine the parsley, orange peel, and garlic. Set aside.

4. Increase the oven temperature to 450°F. Push the vegetables to one side of the dish and add the fish. Spoon the vegetables over the fish. Sprinkle with the reserved parsley mixture.

5. Return the fish to the oven and roast for about 5 minutes (for thin fillets), 12 to 15 minutes (for thicker fillets), or until the fish flakes easily.

MAKES 4 SERVINGS

Per serving: 262 calories, 15 g carbohydrate, 30 g protein, 9 g fat, 1.5 g saturated fat, 68 mg cholesterol, 152 mg sodium, 4 g fiber

Carbohydrate Choices: 1

Dietary Exchanges: 3 vegetable, 4 meat, 1 fat

TANGERINE-SESAME NOODLES WITH SEARED SCALLOPS

Citrus has a special affinity for seafood. In addition to tangerines, clementines, navel oranges, or tangelos would work well in this dish.

Preparation time: 20 minutes ● **Cooking time: 20 minutes**

¼ cup fresh tangerine juice

3 tablespoons reduced-sodium soy sauce

3 tablespoons creamy natural peanut butter

2 tablespoons toasted sesame oil

2 teaspoons grated fresh ginger

2 teaspoons grated tangerine peel

¼ teaspoon ground red pepper, divided

1 cup snow peas

8 ounces whole wheat spaghetti

2 carrots, cut into matchsticks

16 sea scallops (1 pound), patted dry

Pinch of salt

1 tablespoon canola oil

3 scallions, cut into thin diagonal slices

1. In a large bowl, combine the juice, soy sauce, peanut butter, sesame oil, ginger, tangerine peel, and ⅛ teaspoon pepper. Set aside.

2. Bring a large pot of water to a boil. Add the peas and cook for 1 minute. Remove with a slotted spoon and plunge into a bowl of cold water (save the pot of hot water for the spaghetti). Drain the peas and set aside.

3. Bring the reserved water back to boiling. Cook the spaghetti according to the package directions, omitting the salt. Drain and transfer to the bowl with the peanut butter mixture. Add the peas and carrots. Toss to mix. Set aside.

4. Season the scallops with salt and the remaining ⅛ teaspoon pepper. In a large skillet, heat the canola oil over high heat. Cook the scallops in two batches, without touching each other, 3 to 4 minutes on each side, or until golden brown and opaque in the center.

5. Arrange the pasta on serving plates. Top with the scallops and sprinkle with the scallions.

MAKES 4 SERVINGS

Per serving: 457 calories, 55 g carbohydrate, 23 g protein, 18 g fat, 2 g saturated fat, 20 mg cholesterol, 474 mg sodium, 10 g fiber

Carbohydrate Choices: 4

Dietary Exchanges: 3 starch, 1 vegetable, 2 meat, 3 fat

WHOLE WHEAT PENNE WITH SHRIMP AND BROCCOLI RABE

Broccoli rabe, also known as rape and rapini, is a pleasingly bitter leafy green vegetable with tiny broccoli-like florets. Very popular in the Italian kitchen, it's related to both the cabbage and turnip families.

Preparation time: 7 minutes ● **Cooking time: 18 minutes**

---

1 bunch (about 1 pound) broccoli rabe or broccolini, cut into 3" lengths

8 ounces whole wheat penne

4 tablespoons olive oil, divided

1 pound medium raw shrimp, peeled and deveined

2 teaspoons minced garlic

¼–½ teaspoon red-pepper flakes

⅓ cup chicken or vegetable broth

½ cup chopped fresh basil

⅓ cup (about 1¾ ounces) grated Parmesan cheese

1. Bring 4 quarts of water to a boil in a large pot over high heat. Add the broccoli rabe or broccolini and cook for about 1½ minutes, or until crisp-tender. Remove with a slotted spoon or tongs and plunge into a bowl of cold water. Drain and set aside.

2. Return the pot of water to boiling. Add the penne and cook according to the package directions, omitting the salt.

3. Meanwhile, heat 2 tablespoons oil over medium heat in a large heavy pan. Place the shrimp in the pan in a single layer. Cook for about 2 minutes, stirring once or twice, until the shrimp are opaque. With a slotted spoon or tongs, transfer the shrimp to a medium bowl and set aside.

4. Add the remaining 2 tablespoons oil to the pan and cook the garlic over medium heat for 30 seconds, until fragrant. Add ¼ teaspoon red-pepper flakes and the reserved broccoli rabe or broccolini. Cook for about 2 minutes, or until tender. Add the shrimp, broth, and basil. Cook for about 1 minute just to heat.

5. Drain the pasta and transfer to a large serving bowl. Add the cheese and toss. Add the shrimp mixture and toss. Serve immediately.

MAKES 4 SERVINGS

Per serving: 512 calories, 50 g carbohydrate, 34 g protein, 19 g fat, 3.6 g saturated fat, 157 mg cholesterol, 299 mg sodium, 5 g fiber

Carbohydrate Choices: 3

Dietary Exchanges: 3 starch, 1½ vegetable, 3 meat, 3 fat

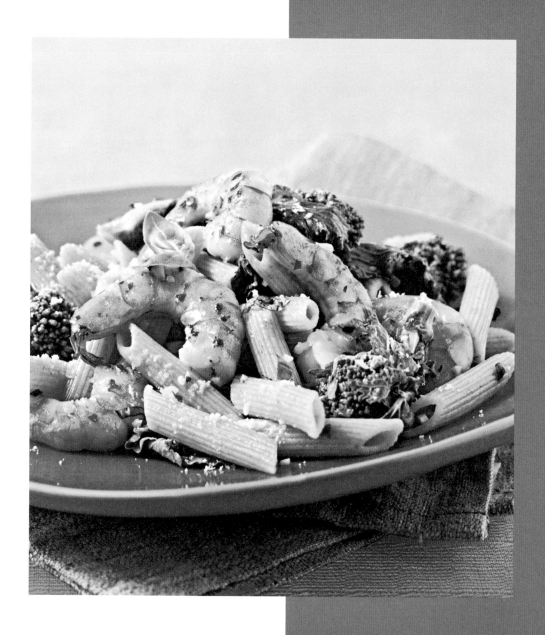

GREEK LEMON CHICKEN

This dish offers the best of the Mediterranean diet: lean protein, lots of vegetables, garlic, and heart-healthy olive oil.

Preparation time: 12 minutes ● **Cooking time: 45 minutes**

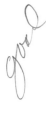

2 tablespoons olive oil, preferably extra virgin

Grated peel and juice of 1 lemon

1 tablespoon minced garlic

1 teaspoon dried oregano

¼ teaspoon salt

¾ teaspoon ground black pepper

¾ teaspoon paprika

4 each skinless, fat-trimmed chicken legs and thighs (about 1½ pounds total)

1 medium red bell pepper, cut into 8 wedges

1 medium orange bell pepper, cut into 8 wedges

2 medium Yukon gold potatoes, each cut into 8 wedges

1 medium red onion, cut into 8 wedges

8 pitted kalamata olives, each quartered lengthwise

Chopped fresh mint or parsley, grated lemon peel, and lemon wedges (optional)

1. Preheat the oven to 400°F. Coat a 17" × 12" rimmed baking pan with vegetable oil spray. Add the oil, lemon peel and lemon juice, garlic, oregano, salt, black pepper, and paprika.

2. Place the chicken on one side of the pan and the bell peppers, potatoes, and onion on the other. Toss to coat with seasonings.

3. Roast for 20 minutes. Turn the chicken and stir the vegetables. Roast for 20 to 25 minutes, or until the chicken is cooked through and the vegetables are lightly browned and tender. Sprinkle with the olives. Garnish with the mint or parsley, grated lemon peel, and lemon wedges, if using.

MAKES 4 SERVINGS

Per serving: 307 calories, 25 g carbohydrate, 22 g protein, 13 g fat, 2 g saturated fat, 80 mg cholesterol, 530 mg sodium, 4 g fiber

Carbohydrate Choices: 2

Dietary Exchanges: 1 starch, 1½ vegetable, 2½ meat, 2½ fat

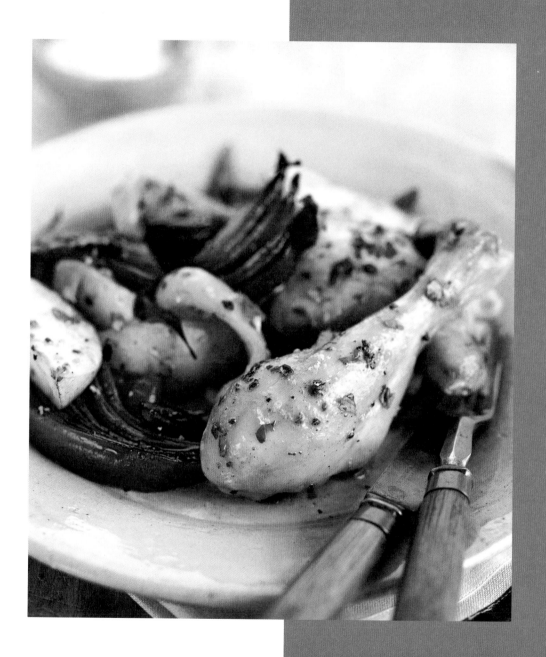

SEARED HERBED CHICKEN BREAST

The chicken breast is the little black dress of main dishes. Adapt this quick and easy poultry by substituting whatever herb or spice blend you prefer.

Preparation time: 5 minutes ● **Cooking time: 15 minutes**

4 **boneless, skinless chicken breasts (about 1½ pounds)**

2 **teaspoons minced garlic**

2 **tablespoons herbes de Provence**

¼ **teaspoon salt**

2 **tablespoons + 2 teaspoons olive oil, preferably extra virgin**

1. Preheat the oven to 475°F. Make several deep, diagonal cuts into the smoother, rounder side of each chicken breast. In a small bowl, combine the garlic, herbes de Provence, salt, and 2 tablespoons of the oil. Brush mixture on chicken.

2. Place an ovenproof skillet over high heat. Pour in the remaining 2 teaspoons oil and add the chicken, cut side down. Cover and cook for 5 minutes. Uncover, flip chicken, and slide skillet into preheated oven. Cook for 10 minutes, or until no longer pink and the juices run clear. Cut chicken diagonally into slices or serve whole.

MAKES 4 SERVINGS

Per serving: 274 calories, 1 g carbohydrate, 39 g protein, 11 g fat, 2 g saturated fat, 98 mg cholesterol, 257 mg sodium, 0 g fiber

Carbohydrate Choices: 0

Dietary Exchanges: 6 meat, 2 fat

SZECHUAN CHICKEN

Cook some instant brown rice while preparing the stir-fry to have a complete meal. Chilled pineapple drizzled with 1 teaspoon each of sour cream and brown sugar makes a delightful dessert.

Preparation time: 10 minutes ● **Cooking time: 6 minutes**

1 teaspoon minced garlic

1 teaspoon grated fresh ginger

½ teaspoon salt-free lemon-pepper seasoning

½ teaspoon crushed fennel seeds

Pinch of ground cloves

1 pound chicken tenders, cut into ½"-thick crosswise slices

1 tablespoon canola oil

12 ounces bok choy, cut into ½"-thick crosswise slices

¼ cup chicken broth

1 tablespoon reduced-sodium soy sauce

Red-pepper flakes (optional)

1. In a mixing bowl, combine the garlic, ginger, lemon-pepper seasoning, fennel seeds, and cloves. Add the chicken. With your hands or a fork, toss well to coat all the pieces with seasoning.

2. Set a wok or large skillet over high heat until very hot. Add the oil and swirl to coat the pan. Place the chicken pieces in the pan so they are separated. Cook for 1 minute, or until browned on the bottom. Turn and cook for 1 minute, until browned. Reduce the heat to medium-high. Add the bok choy. Cook, tossing, for about 2 minutes, or until the bok choy leaves are wilting. Add the broth and soy sauce. Bring almost to a boil. Reduce the heat and simmer for 2 minutes, or until the chicken is no longer pink and the juices run clear. Serve, garnished with red-pepper flakes, if desired.

MAKES 4 SERVINGS

Per serving: 156 calories, 3 g carbohydrate, 28 g protein, 4 g fat, 0.5 g saturated fat, 67 mg cholesterol, 263 mg sodium, 1 g fiber

Carbohydrate Choices: 0

Dietary Exchanges: ½ vegetable, 3 meat, 1 fat

STIR-FRIED CHICKEN WITH ASPARAGUS

If asparagus isn't in season, try green beans in this quick dish. Serve with steamed brown rice or whole wheat couscous.

Preparation time: 5 minutes ● **Cooking time: 5 minutes**

2 teaspoons reduced-sodium soy sauce

1 teaspoon honey

2 teaspoons toasted sesame oil

1 large bunch asparagus (about 1¾ pounds), trimmed and cut diagonally into 1" pieces

1 teaspoon minced garlic

2½ cups sliced cooked chicken breasts

1 teaspoon sesame seeds (optional)

In a small bowl, combine the soy sauce and honey. Set aside. Heat the oil in a large skillet or wok over medium-high heat. Add the asparagus and garlic. Cook for 4 minutes, stirring frequently. Toss in the chicken and soy sauce–honey mixture. Heat thoroughly. Sprinkle with sesame seeds, if desired.

MAKES 4 SERVINGS

Per serving: 209 calories, 8 g carbohydrate, 31 g protein, 6 g fat, 1 g saturated fat, 74 mg cholesterol, 170 mg sodium, 4 g fiber

Carbohydrate Choices: ½

Dietary Exchanges: 1½ vegetable, 4 meat, 1 fat

LET YOURSELF GO/STRESS LESS

Massage is a powerful tool for releasing the physical and mental symptoms of stress. It ranks behind relaxation techniques and chiropractic as the third most popular form of alternative therapy in the country. Scientists believe that the physical sensations experienced during massage trigger a natural relaxation response in the body. For more information about the different styles of massage or the name of a professional massage therapist near you, consult the American Massage Therapy Association, which represents more than 55,000 massage therapists in 27 countries. Visit www.amtamassage.org or phone 877-905-2700.

LIME-MARINATED CHICKEN WITH SALSA

Never eat dry chicken breasts again! If you've been overcooking chicken because you're not certain when it's done, use an instant-read digital thermometer to gauge the internal temperature. Your poultry will be moist every time.

Preparation time: 20 minutes ● Marinating time: 1 hour ● Cooking time: 13–15 minutes

- 4 boneless, skinless chicken breasts (about 1½ pounds)
- 3 tablespoons lime juice + 4 lime wedges for garnish
- 2 tablespoons olive oil
- 1¼ teaspoons ground cumin
- ¼ teaspoon salt
- 3 medium tomatoes, chopped
- ½ avocado, peeled, pitted, and chopped
- ½ cup chopped sweet onion, such as Vidalia
- ½ cup chopped cilantro + 4 sprigs for garnish
- 1 small jalapeño chile pepper, seeded and finely chopped (wear plastic gloves when handling)
- Salt

1. Put the chicken into a large resealable plastic bag.

2. In a small bowl, whisk the lime juice, oil, cumin, and ¼ teaspoon salt. Transfer 2 tablespoons of lime marinade to a medium glass bowl for the salsa, and cover with plastic wrap. Pour the remaining marinade over the chicken and squeeze the bag to coat. Let the chicken marinate in the refrigerator for at least 1 hour.

3. Coat a grill rack or broiler pan with vegetable oil spray. Preheat the grill (to medium-high) or broiler. Grill or broil the chicken for about 6 minutes on each side, or until a thermometer inserted into the thickest portion registers 160°F and the juices run clear.

4. Meanwhile, add the tomatoes, avocado, onion, cilantro, and chile pepper to the bowl with the reserved marinade. Gently toss to mix, and season to taste with salt.

5. To serve, place the chicken onto 4 plates and top each with ¾ cup salsa. Garnish with lime wedges and cilantro sprigs.

MAKES 4 SERVINGS

Per serving: 290 calories, 9 g carbohydrate, 35 g protein, 13 g fat, 2 g saturated fat, 80 mg cholesterol, 250 mg sodium, 4 g fiber

Carbohydrate Choices: 1

Dietary Exchanges: 1 vegetable, 5 meat, 2 fat

SPICE-RUBBED CHICKEN TORTILLAS WITH MANGO SALSA

Mangoes are a luscious tropical fruit that's bursting with vitamin A. Ripe peaches or nectarines can also be used in this dish.

Preparation time: 25 minutes ● **Cooking time: 22 minutes**

1½ tablespoons brown sugar

2 teaspoons ground cumin

1 teaspoon ground ginger

½ teaspoon salt

½ teaspoon ground red pepper

4 boneless, skinless chicken breasts (4 ounces each)

1 cup diced mango

1 jalapeño chile pepper, minced

2 tablespoons minced red onion

1 tablespoon lime juice

2 teaspoons olive oil

2 red bell peppers, thinly sliced

1 large red onion, halved and thinly sliced

¼ cup coarsely chopped cilantro + additional for garnish

4 whole wheat tortillas (10" diameter)

1. Preheat the broiler. Line a baking sheet with aluminum foil.

2. In a small bowl, combine the sugar, cumin, ginger, salt, and ground red pepper. Coat both sides of the chicken with the spice rub. Set aside.

3. In another small bowl, combine the mango, chile pepper, minced onion, and lime juice. Set aside.

4. Coat a large skillet with vegetable oil spray. Add the oil. Warm over medium heat. Add the bell peppers and sliced onion. Cook, stirring occasionally, for about 10 minutes, or until the vegetables are soft and lightly browned. Stir in the chopped cilantro. Turn off the heat. Cover the skillet to keep the vegetables warm.

5. Broil the chicken for about 6 minutes on each side, or until a thermometer inserted into the thickest portion registers 160°F and the juices run clear. Let the chicken cool slightly before cutting into ½"-thick slices.

6. Heat the tortillas by placing each one in a large dry skillet over medium heat for 30 seconds on each side, or until heated through.

7. To serve, spoon a portion of vegetables down the center of each tortilla. Arrange the chicken over the vegetables, and roll up. Spoon mango salsa over each tortilla. Garnish with cilantro.

MAKES 4 SERVINGS

Per serving: 380 calories, 45 g carbohydrate, 32 g protein, 7 g fat, 1 g saturated fat, 65 mg cholesterol, 490 mg sodium, 6 g fiber

Carbohydrate Choices: 3

Dietary Exchanges: 2 starch, ½ fruit, 2 vegetable, 4 meat, 1 fat

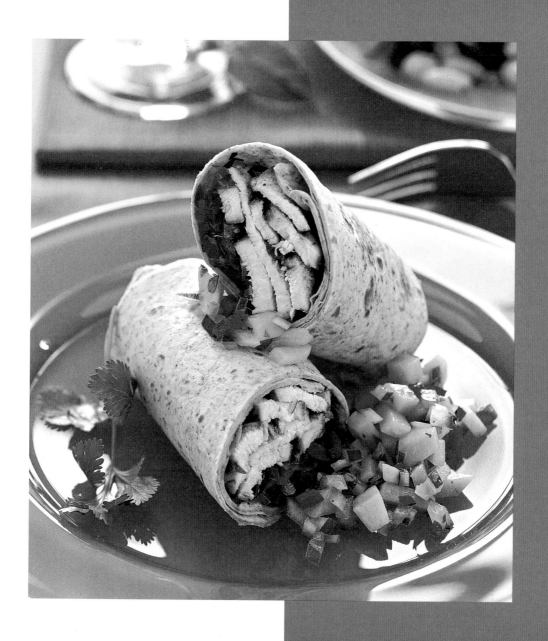

EASY CHICKEN FINGERS
WITH SWEET BEAN DIPPING SAUCE

If crunch is what you crave, try these oven-baked crispy chicken fingers. The same breading works beautifully with boneless, skinless fish fillets.

Preparation time: 25 minutes ● **Cooking time: 18–20 minutes**

1 cup honey crunch toasted wheat germ

¼ cup whole wheat flour

¼ teaspoon paprika

⅛ teaspoon ground black pepper

1 large egg

1 tablespoon fat-free milk

1¼ pounds boneless, skinless chicken tenders

Assorted raw vegetables

Sweet Bean Dipping Sauce (page 269)

1. Preheat the oven to 425°F. Coat a baking sheet with vegetable oil spray.

2. In a large resealable plastic bag, combine the wheat germ, flour, paprika, and pepper.

3. In a medium bowl, whisk the egg and milk. In batches, dip the chicken tenders into the egg-milk mixture. Place into the bag with the wheat germ mixture. Seal the bag and toss until the chicken tenders are evenly coated.

4. Place the chicken tenders on the reserved pan. Bake for 18 to 20 minutes, or until no longer pink and the juices run clear.

5. Divide the chicken fingers among 6 plates and serve with vegetables and dipping sauce.

MAKES 6 SERVINGS

Per serving: 306 calories, 17 g carbohydrate, 51 g protein, 4 g fat, 1 g saturated fat, 146 mg cholesterol, 117 mg sodium, 3 g fiber

Carbohydrate Choices: 1

Dietary Exchanges: 1 starch, 6 meat

Sweet Bean Dipping Sauce

This sauce can be paired with baked fish, too.

Preparation time: 12 minutes ● **Cooking time: 10 minutes**

1 tablespoon olive oil

1 small onion, chopped

1 teaspoon minced garlic

1 can (19 ounces) cannellini beans, rinsed and drained

¾ cup unsweetened applesauce

¼ teaspoon salt

1. Heat the oil in a medium skillet over medium heat. Add the onion and cook for 5 minutes, or until soft and translucent. Add the garlic and cook for 1 minute. Add the beans and applesauce. Cook for 4 minutes. Remove from heat. Stir in the salt.

2. Transfer the mixture to a blender or food processor fitted with a metal blade. Process until the mixture is smooth.

MAKES 6 SERVINGS (¼ CUP PER SERVING)

Per serving: 96 calories, 15 g carbohydrate, 3 g protein, 3 g fat, 0 g saturated fat, 0 mg cholesterol, 247 mg sodium, 3 g fiber

Carbohydrate Choices: 1

Dietary Exchanges: ½ starch, ½ fat

CHICKEN CACCIATORE

Come home to a trattoria-style meal with this slow-cooker version of the popular Italian ragout.

Preparation time: 8 minutes ● **Cooking time: 7–9 hours**

2 cans (14½ ounces each) no-sodium-added diced tomatoes

8 ounces shiitake mushrooms, stemmed and sliced ½" thick (3 cups)

2 large carrots, halved lengthwise, sliced ¼" thick (1 cup)

⅓ cup dry white wine

1 tablespoon chopped fresh thyme leaves or ½ teaspoon dried

1 clove garlic, minced

1 teaspoon dried basil

¼ teaspoon fennel seeds

¼ teaspoon red-pepper flakes

4 each skinless chicken drumsticks and thighs (about 2 pounds)

2 small yellow summer squash, sliced into ¾"-thick rounds

Thin strips basil leaves (optional)

1. In a 4-quart or larger slow cooker, combine the tomatoes (with juice), mushrooms, carrots, wine, thyme, garlic, basil, fennel seeds, and red-pepper flakes. Add the chicken and toss to coat. Place the squash on top.

2. Cover and cook on low setting for 7 to 9 hours, or until the chicken and vegetables are tender. Serve with sauce. Garnish with basil, if desired.

MAKES 4 SERVINGS

Per serving: 270 calories, 20 g carbohydrate, 30 g protein, 5 g fat, 1.5 g saturated fat, 105 mg cholesterol, 310 mg sodium, 6 g fiber

Carbohydrate Choices: 1

Dietary Exchanges: 3 vegetable, 4 meat

TURKEY TACOS WITH AVOCADO-CORN SALSA

Even non–vegetable lovers will go for veggies served inside terrific tacos.

Preparation time: 10 minutes ● Cooking time: 7 minutes

1 firm, ripe avocado, peeled, pitted, and chopped

1 cup canned sweet corn kernels, rinsed and drained

1 cup cherry tomatoes, halved

1 tablespoon lime juice

1 package (12) corn taco shells

12 ounces cooked boneless, skinless turkey breast, sliced into thin strips

¾ cup water

1 package (1¼ ounces) reduced-sodium taco seasoning mix

1. In a medium bowl, mix the avocado, corn, tomatoes, and lime juice. Set aside.

2. Warm the shells in the oven according to the package directions.

3. In a medium skillet, combine the turkey, water, and seasoning. Bring to a boil, reduce heat, and simmer 5 minutes, stirring occasionally.

4. Spoon the turkey mixture into the shells. Top with the salsa.

MAKES 6 SERVINGS (2 TACOS PER SERVING)

Per serving: 284 calories, 26 g carbohydrate, 20 g protein, 11 g fat, 2.5 g saturated fat, 39 mg cholesterol, 465 mg sodium, 4 g fiber

Carbohydrate Choices: 2

Dietary Exchanges: 1 starch, 2½ meat, 1½ fat

GINGER-GLAZED CHICKEN

A marinade infused with spices gives chicken a piquant kick that wakes up your circulation.

Preparation time: 10 minutes ● **Marinating time: 30 minutes** ● **Cooking time: 15 minutes**

⅓ cup orange juice

1 tablespoon grated orange peel

3 tablespoons honey

1 shallot, peeled and finely chopped

1 tablespoon minced garlic

1 tablespoon grated fresh ginger

4 boneless, skinless chicken breasts (about 1½ pounds)

Orange slices (optional, for garnish)

1. In a shallow bowl or pie plate, combine the orange juice, orange peel, honey, shallot, garlic, and ginger. Add the chicken and toss to coat. Cover and marinate, turning frequently, for at least 30 minutes.

2. Preheat the broiler and coat the broiler pan with vegetable oil spray. Remove the chicken from the marinade and place on pan. Reserve the marinade. Broil the chicken for 12 minutes, turning once, or until a thermometer inserted into the chicken reads 160°F and the juices run clear.

3. Meanwhile, bring the marinade to a boil in a small saucepan. Reduce the heat and simmer for 5 minutes, or until the mixture is slightly thickened.

4. Place the chicken on 4 plates and top with marinade. Garnish with orange slices, if desired.

MAKES 4 SERVINGS

Per serving: 250 calories, 17 g carbohydrate, 40 g protein, 2 g fat, 0.5 g saturated fat, 100 mg cholesterol, 110 mg sodium, 0 g fiber

Carbohydrate Choices: 1

Dietary Exchanges: 1 starch, 6 meat

NOTE: The chicken may be prepared ahead and marinated in the refrigerator overnight.

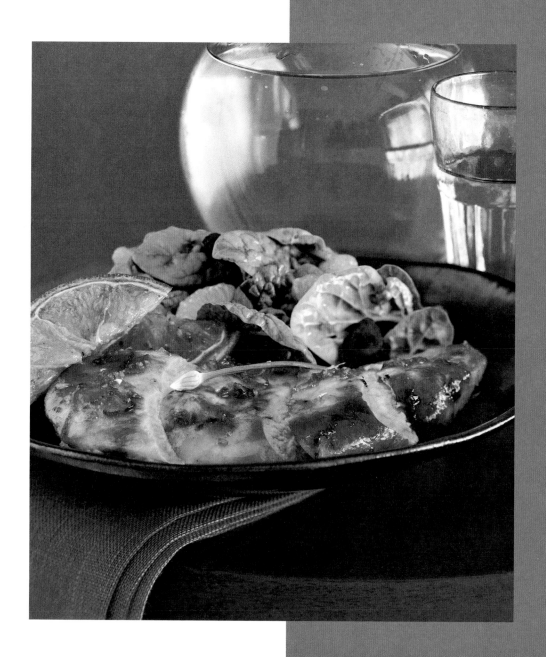

BROILED CORNISH HENS WITH LEMON, ORANGE, AND BASIL

Fragrant lemon and orange peel slipped beneath the skin infuse the meat with their flavor.

Preparation time: 15 minutes ● **Standing time: 15 minutes** ● **Cooking time: 20 minutes**

2 Cornish hens (about 1½ pounds each)
1 tablespoon finely grated lemon peel
2 teaspoons finely grated orange peel
1 teaspoon + 2 tablespoons olive oil, preferably extra virgin
½ teaspoon salt, divided
¼ teaspoon ground black pepper, divided
8–12 fresh basil leaves
8 cups mixed baby greens
2 tablespoons fresh orange juice
Orange segments (optional, for garnish)

1. With kitchen shears, remove the backbones of the hens. Halve the hens by cutting through the breastbone. Trim fat. Discard wing tips.

2. In a small bowl, combine the lemon and orange peels, 1 teaspoon oil, ¼ teaspoon salt, and ⅛ teaspoon pepper. Using fingers, separate the skin from the flesh of the hens and carefully stuff the peel mixture under the skin, spreading over the breast and thigh. Arrange 2 or 3 basil leaves under the skin and over the peel mixture in each half. Let stand for 15 minutes at room temperature.

3. Preheat the broiler. Coat the broiler pan with vegetable oil spray. Brush both sides of the hens with 1 tablespoon of the remaining oil and place skin side down on the pan. Broil for 10 minutes, 5" to 6" from the heat. Turn and broil for 8 to 10 minutes, or until the skin is browned and a thermometer inserted in a thigh registers 170°F and the juices run clear.

4. Toss the greens with the remaining 1 tablespoon of oil, ¼ teaspoon salt, and ⅛ teaspoon pepper. Add the juice and toss. Arrange the greens on serving plates, top with the hens, and garnish with orange segments, if desired.

MAKES 4 SERVINGS

Per serving: 430 calories, 5 g carbohydrate, 31 g protein, 32 g fat, 8 g saturated fat, 170 mg cholesterol, 422 mg sodium, 3 g fiber

Carbohydrate Choices: 0

Dietary Exchanges: 1 vegetable, 8 meat, 2½ fat

NOTE: Remove the skin before eating to lower fat content.

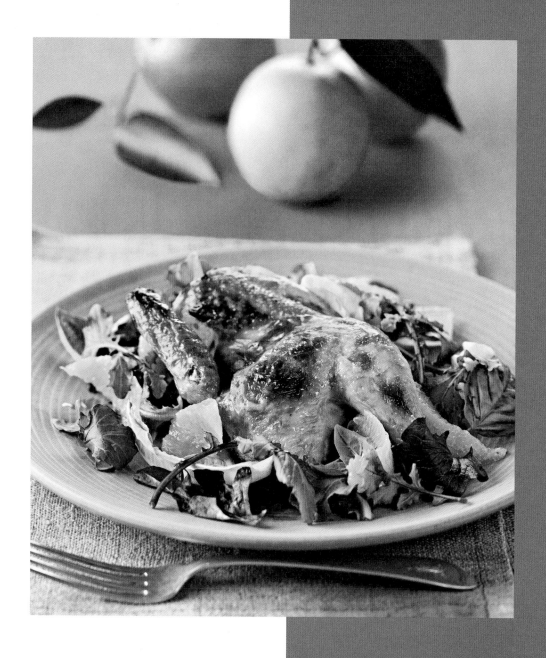

BLUE TORTILLA CHICKEN WITH CORN SALAD

The basic technique for "oven-frying" the chicken in this recipe is a versatile one. You can replace the corn chips with dry all-bran cereal or 100 percent whole grain crackers. Any salt-free herb or spice blend can stand in for the chili powder. Experiment to find your favorite combos.

Preparation time: 12 minutes ● Cooking time: 15 minutes ● Standing time: 5 minutes

4 boneless, skinless chicken breasts (4 ounces each)

1 egg white, beaten slightly

¾ cup no-salt-added blue corn chips, crushed

1 tablespoon chili powder

¼ teaspoon salt, divided

2 cups fresh corn kernels or frozen corn kernels, thawed

2 poblano chile or Cubanelle peppers, seeded and diced, or ½ green bell pepper, seeded and diced (wear plastic gloves when handling)

1 jalapeño chile pepper, seeded and diced (optional) (wear plastic gloves when handling)

¼ cup finely chopped cilantro

1 tablespoon + 2 teaspoons lime juice

1 lime, cut into wedges (optional, for garnish)

1. Preheat the oven to 400°F.

2. Coat a medium ovenproof skillet with vegetable oil spray. Dip the chicken into the egg white. Combine the chips with the chili powder, press mixture into chicken, and arrange in skillet, leaving space between each piece. Lightly coat the chicken with vegetable oil spray and sprinkle with ⅛ teaspoon salt. Place the pan in the oven and bake for about 15 minutes, or until a thermometer inserted in the thickest portion registers 160°F and the juices run clear.

3. Meanwhile, in a bowl, combine the corn; poblano, Cubanelle, or green bell pepper; jalapeño chile pepper (if using); cilantro; lime juice; and the remaining ⅛ teaspoon salt. Stir to mix. Set aside.

4. Remove the chicken and allow to rest for 4 minutes. Slice each piece crosswise into 5 pieces. Serve with the corn salad. Garnish with lime wedges, if desired

MAKES 4 SERVINGS

Per serving: 330 calories, 35 g carbohydrate, 31 g protein, 9 g fat, 1 g saturated fat, 65 mg cholesterol, 290 mg sodium, 4 g fiber

Carbohydrate Choices: 2

Dietary Exchanges: 1 starch, 4 meat

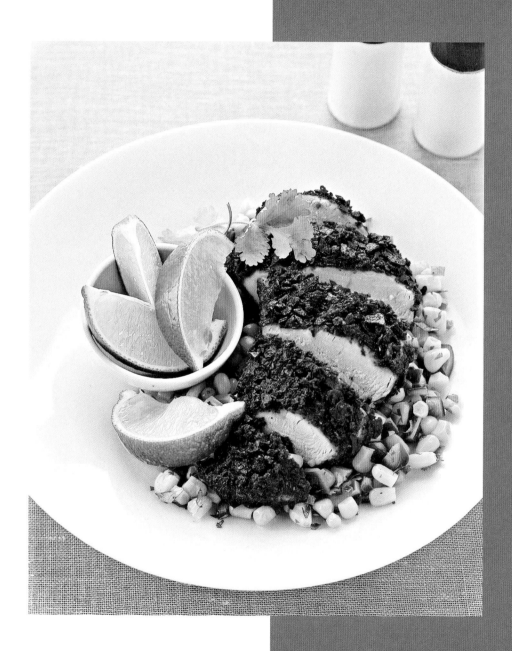

LIME CHICKEN WITH LENTILS AND DRIED FRUIT

Any dish becomes more dramatic when its flavors are enhanced with citrus juice and peel.

Preparation time: 15 minutes ● **Cooking time: 1 hour 20 minutes**

---

   4 **bone-in chicken thighs (about 1¼ pounds)**

 ¼ **teaspoon salt, divided**

 ⅛ **teaspoon ground allspice, divided**

 ⅛ **teaspoon ground red pepper, divided**

   1 **tablespoon olive oil**

 ¾ **cup small green and brown lentils, and a few red lentils, picked over and rinsed**

   3 **scallions, cut into 1" diagonal pieces**

   4 **large dried peaches or apricots (4 ounces), cut into thin strips**

 ½ **cup dried sour cherries or cranberries**

   2 **teaspoons finely chopped crystallized ginger**

   6 **tablespoons chopped cilantro, divided**

1½ **cups chicken broth**

   4 **teaspoons finely grated lime peel**

   1 **tablespoon fresh lime juice**
   Lime wedges (optional, for garnish)

1. Preheat the oven to 350°F. Season the chicken with ⅛ teaspoon salt, ¹⁄₁₆ teaspoon allspice, and ¹⁄₁₆ teaspoon pepper. In an oven-proof Dutch oven, heat the oil over medium-high heat. Cook the chicken for about 5 minutes on each side, or until browned. Transfer to a plate.

2. To the Dutch oven, add the lentils, scallions, peaches or apricots, cherries or cranberries, ginger, 3 tablespoons cilantro, and the remaining ⅛ teaspoon salt, ¹⁄₁₆ teaspoon allspice, and ¹⁄₁₆ teaspoon pepper. Cook, stirring, for 2 minutes. Add the broth. Return the chicken to the pot and submerge. Bring to a boil over high heat.

3. Remove from the heat, cover, and bake for 35 minutes. Uncover and bake for 30 minutes, or until the lentils are cooked through. Remove the chicken skins. Stir the lime peel and juice into the lentil mixture.

4. Arrange the lentils on serving plates. Top with the chicken, and sprinkle with the remaining 3 tablespoons cilantro. Garnish with lime wedges, if desired.

MAKES 4 SERVINGS

Per serving: 343 calories, 47 g carbohydrate, 26 g protein, 7 g fat, 2 g saturated fat, 59 mg cholesterol, 253 mg sodium, 14 g fiber

Carbohydrate Choices: 3

Dietary Exchanges: 1½ starch, 1½ fruit, 2½ meat, 1 fat

NOTE: This dish may be prepared with all green or brown lentils, if desired.

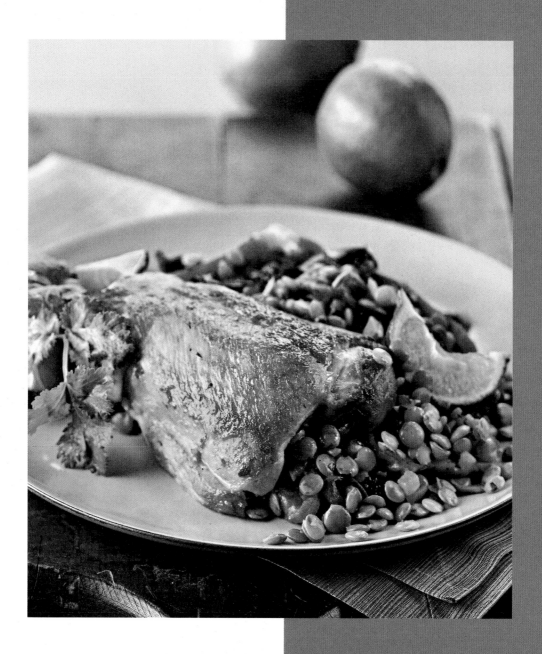

SPINACH-STUFFED CHICKEN ROULADE

Other greens such as arugula, chard, and baby kale can take the place of spinach in this dish.

Preparation time: 10 minutes ● **Cooking time: 30 minutes**

2 cups (2 ounces) baby spinach

¼ cup finely chopped onion

2 teaspoons olive oil, divided

1 teaspoon minced garlic

⅓ teaspoon red-pepper flakes

1 tablespoon water

¼ cup (1 ounce) grated Parmesan cheese

2 tablespoons chopped dry-packed sun-dried tomatoes

4 chicken cutlets (about 4 ounces each) or 4 chicken breast halves, trimmed and pounded thin into cutlets

½ cup chicken broth or dry white wine

1. Place the spinach in a large nonstick skillet with the washing water clinging to the leaves or a tablespoon or two of water if dried. Cover and cook for 2 minutes, tossing occasionally, or until wilted. Drain and press firmly with the back of a spoon or squeeze to remove excess moisture. There should be ½ cup spinach. Wipe out the skillet.

2. Meanwhile, in a medium nonstick skillet, combine the onion, 1 teaspoon oil, garlic, red-pepper flakes, and 1 tablespoon water. Turn the heat to medium. Cook for about 2 minutes, or until the onion sizzles. Reduce the heat to low. Cover and cook, stirring once, for about 3 minutes, or until softened. In a small

bowl, combine the onion mixture, cheese, and spinach. Stir to mix. Set aside.

3. Sprinkle the tomatoes evenly on the smooth side of the cutlets.

4. Divide the spinach mixture among the cutlets. Spread to the edges of 3 sides, leaving about 1" at the narrow tip free of spinach mixture. Loosely roll up the chicken, ending with the narrow tip, and secure with wooden picks.

5. Add the remaining 1 teaspoon oil to the large skillet and set over medium heat. Place the chicken in the pan. Cook, turning, for about 10 minutes, or until golden brown on all sides. Add the broth or wine, cover, and cook over low heat for about 7 minutes. Uncover and transfer chicken to a serving platter. Cover with foil to keep warm.

6. Boil the skillet juices for about 5 minutes, or until reduced to a glaze. Diagonally slice the chicken into 1"-thick pieces. Drizzle with pan juices and serve.

MAKES 4 SERVINGS

Per serving: 194 calories, 4 g carbohydrate, 27 g protein, 7 g fat, 2 g saturated fat, 70 mg cholesterol, 305 mg sodium, 2 g fiber

Carbohydrate Choices: 0

Dietary Exchanges: ½ vegetable, 3½ meat, 1 fat

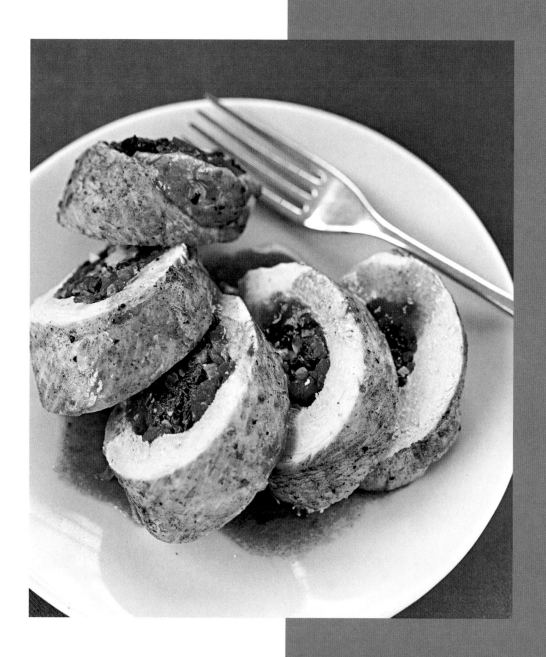

SAGE TURKEY CUTLETS WITH SQUASH

Sage, the predominant herb in poultry seasoning, is a natural complement to turkey. Paired with velvety butternut squash, this combination is a perfect autumn meal.

Preparation time: 5 minutes ● **Cooking time: 15 minutes**

  2 **pounds peeled, precut butternut squash, chopped into ¾" chunks**
  4 **thin turkey cutlets (4–6 ounces each), each cut into 2 pieces**
  ½ **teaspoon salt, divided**
     Ground black pepper
  8 **whole fresh sage leaves**
  3 **teaspoons olive oil, preferably extra virgin, divided**
  ¼ **cup balsamic vinegar**

1. Place the squash on a microwaveable plate. Cover with waxed paper. Cook on high power, rotating several times, for about 8 minutes, or until very tender when pierced with a fork.

2. Meanwhile, season the cutlets with ¼ teaspoon of the salt and pepper to taste. Press a sage leaf into the center of each.

3. Heat 1½ teaspoons of oil in a skillet set over medium-high heat. Place 4 cutlets in the skillet, leaf side down. Cook for about 1½ minutes, or until the edges whiten. Flip and cook through. Remove to a plate and set aside. Add the remaining 1½ teaspoons of oil to the skillet set over medium-high heat. Repeat cooking the remaining cutlets.

4. Pour the vinegar into the skillet. Cook for about 2 minutes, or until reduced by half. With a fork, mash the reserved squash. Season with the remaining ¼ teaspoon of salt and pepper to taste. Divide the squash among 4 plates and top with 2 cutlet pieces and a drizzle of balsamic sauce.

MAKES 4 SERVINGS

Per serving: 264 calories, 29 g carbohydrate, 30 g protein, 5 g fat, 0.5 g saturated fat, 45 mg cholesterol, 410 mg sodium, 5 g fiber

Carbohydrate Choices: 2

Dietary Exchanges: 4 vegetable, 3½ meat, 1 fat

NOTE: Butternut and other hard-shell squashes are easier to peel if cooked briefly in the microwave. Pierce several times with a sharp knife. Microwave on high power for about 4 minutes, rotating every minute. Let stand for 5 minutes before peeling.

TURKEY STUFFED WITH MUSHROOMS AND SPINACH

The mild flavor of turkey makes it companionable with many flavorings. In this preparation, earthy mushrooms and spinach add depth of flavor.

Preparation time: 15 minutes ● **Roasting time: 45 minutes** ● **Standing time: 15 minutes**

1 turkey London broil (about 1½ pounds)

2 teaspoons olive oil + additional for misting

1 cup sliced brown or white mushrooms, chopped

1 cup (1 ounce) baby spinach leaves

½ cup sliced scallions

¼ teaspoon poultry seasoning

⅛ teaspoon salt

Ground black pepper

2 tablespoons (½ ounce) shredded Swiss cheese

½ cup water

1. Preheat the oven to 350°F. Set the turkey on a work surface. With a sharp knife, cut through the middle to create a pocket. Set aside.

2. In an ovenproof skillet, warm 2 teaspoons oil over medium heat. Add the mushrooms, spinach, scallions, poultry seasoning, salt, and pepper to taste. Cook, stirring, for about 3 minutes, or until the spinach wilts. Spoon the mixture into the pocket in the turkey. Cover the stuffing with the cheese. Press the open edge down to seal. Fasten with toothpicks, if desired.

3. Add the water to the skillet. Cook over medium heat, scraping with a spatula to release the browned bits on the pan bottom. Bring to a boil. Turn off the heat. Place the turkey in the skillet. Mist lightly with olive oil.

4. Roast for about 45 minutes, or until an instant-read thermometer inserted in the center registers 165°F. Remove to a cutting board. Let stand for 15 minutes, until the internal temperature rises to 170°F. Slice the turkey. Reheat the juices in the skillet to drizzle over the turkey.

MAKES 6 SERVINGS

Per serving: 150 calories, 2 g carbohydrate, 29 g protein, 4 g fat, 0.5 g saturated fat, 47 mg cholesterol, 125 mg sodium, 6 g fiber

Carbohydrate Choices: 0

Dietary Exchanges: 3½ meat, ½ fat

GREEK MEATBALLS

This one-dish meal can be prepared through Step 2 and refrigerated for up to 24 hours before baking.

Preparation time: 10 minutes ● **Cooking time: 25 minutes**

2 cups cooked brown rice, cooled

¾ teaspoon dried oregano

4 tablespoons (1 ounce) reduced-fat crumbled feta cheese, divided

1 pound 95 percent lean ground beef

2 medium zucchini (1 pound total), cut into thin slices

1 cup bottled marinara sauce

1. Preheat the oven to 450°F. Coat a 13" × 9" baking dish with vegetable oil spray. In a large bowl, combine the rice, oregano, and 2 tablespoons of the cheese. Stir in the beef until combined.

2. Scatter the zucchini into the reserved baking dish in a single layer. Using a small ice cream scoop, shape the meat mixture into sixteen 1½" balls. Place the meatballs on top of the zucchini. Drizzle with the marinara sauce. Cover with aluminum foil.

3. Bake for about 22 minutes, or until the meatballs are no longer pink.

4. Uncover and top with the remaining 2 tablespoons of cheese. Let sit in the oven for about 1 minute, or until the cheese melts slightly.

MAKES 4 SERVINGS

Per serving: 333 calories, 32 g carbohydrate, 31 g protein, 9 g fat, 4 g saturated fat, 72 mg cholesterol, 433 mg sodium, 4 g fiber

Carbohydrate Choices: 2

Dietary Exchanges: 2 starch, 1 vegetable, 3½ meat, 1 fat

KIDNEY BEANS AND BEEF CHILI

Like most stews, this chili tastes better if you prepare it several days before serving. Or cool the finished stew and freeze it in single-serve portions for "instant" lunches and dinners.

Preparation time: 10 minutes ● **Cooking time: 40 minutes**

6 ounces lean beef top round, cut into chunks

½ cup chopped onion

½ cup chopped green bell pepper

1 tablespoon olive or canola oil

1 tablespoon minced garlic

1½ teaspoons chili powder

1 teaspoon ground cumin

½ teaspoon ground black pepper

¼ teaspoon salt

1¾ cups cooked red kidney beans (page 312) or 1 can (15 ounces) red kidney beans, rinsed and drained

1 cup crushed tomatoes

1 cup chicken broth

4 teaspoons sour cream

4 teaspoons grated extra-sharp Cheddar cheese

1 jalapeño chile pepper, minced (optional) (wear plastic gloves when handling)

Fresh cilantro leaves (optional)

1. In the bowl of a food processor fitted with a metal blade, pulse the beef for about 1 minute, or until coarsely ground. Set aside.

2. In a large pot, combine the onion, bell pepper, oil, garlic, chili powder, cumin, black pepper, and salt. Cook over medium heat, stirring occasionally, for 5 minutes, or until softened. Crumble the beef into the pot. Increase the heat to medium-high and cook, stirring, for 2 minutes, or until the beef is no longer pink. Stir in the beans, tomatoes, and broth. Reduce the heat to medium-low.

3. Cook, stirring occasionally, for about 30 minutes, or until the flavors are well blended.

4. Serve in shallow bowls. Dollop on the sour cream and sprinkle on the cheese. Garnish with chile pepper and cilantro, if using.

MAKES 4 SERVINGS

Per serving: 260 calories, 26 g carbohydrate, 19 g protein, 9 g fat, 3 g saturated fat, 20 mg cholesterol, 370 mg sodium, 9 g fiber

Carbohydrate Choices: 2

Dietary Exchanges: 1 starch, 1½ vegetable, 1½ meat, 1½ fat

MEXICAN STUFFED PEPPERS

If you love homestyle dishes but don't have the time to tend them, this slow-cooker dish is for you.

Preparation time: 15 minutes ● **Cooking time: 6–8 hours**

---

  2 cans (14½ ounces each) no-salt-added diced tomatoes
  1 tablespoon red wine vinegar
  1 teaspoon ground cumin
  ¼ teaspoon ground cinnamon
  ½ teaspoon salt
  4½ large bell peppers (preferably yellow and orange)
  8 ounces 95 percent lean ground beef
  ½ cup converted brown rice
  ⅓ cup finely chopped onion
  ¼ cup raisins
    Chopped parsley (for garnish)

1. In a medium bowl, combine the tomatoes (with juice), vinegar, cumin, cinnamon, and salt. Stir to mix. Pour 1⅓ cups of the sauce mixture into a 4-quart or larger slow cooker.

2. Finely chop the half bell pepper. Slice off the top ½" of the remaining peppers. Seed the peppers and reserve the tops.

3. In a large bowl, using your hands, combine the beef, rice, onion, raisins, chopped pepper, and the remaining sauce mixture. Spoon the mixture into the peppers and replace the tops. Place into the slow cooker.

4. Cover and cook on low for 6 to 8 hours, or until the peppers are tender and the meat is no longer pink. Serve topped with the cooking sauce. Garnish with parsley, if desired.

MAKES 4 SERVINGS

Per serving: 240 calories, 39 g carbohydrate, 16 g protein, 4 g fat, 1 g saturated fat, 30 mg cholesterol, 410 mg sodium, 6 g fiber

Carbohydrate Choices: 2½

Dietary Exchanges: ½ fruit, 2½ vegetable, 1½ meat

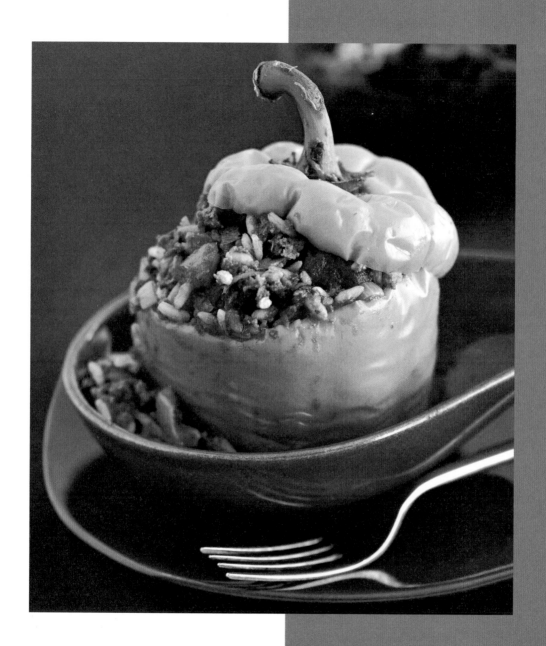

DIJON PEPPER STEAK

Serve mesclun—mixed baby greens—tossed with equal parts of extra virgin olive oil and red wine vinegar alongside this French-bistro inspired classic.

Preparation time: 5 minutes ● **Cooking time: 12 minutes**

2 tablespoons cracked or coarsely ground mixed peppercorns

¼ teaspoon salt

4 center-cut filet mignon steaks (6 ounces each), about 1¼" thick

1 teaspoon canola oil

¼ cup beef broth

3 tablespoons red wine or 2 tablespoons balsamic vinegar

2 teaspoons Dijon mustard

1. Sprinkle the peppercorns and salt on both sides of the steaks and press in.

2. Coat a large heavy skillet with vegetable oil spray. Place over high heat for 1 minute. Add the oil. When the oil is hot, reduce the heat to medium-high and place the steaks in the pan. Cook for 5 minutes per side, or until a thermometer inserted sideways in the center registers 145°F for medium-rare; 6 minutes for medium (160°F); or 7 minutes for well done (165°F).

3. Remove the steaks to a large plate. Set aside. Add the broth and wine or vinegar to the skillet. Simmer for 30 seconds. Stir in the mustard. Spoon the sauce over the steaks.

MAKES 4 SERVINGS

Per serving: 300 calories, 1 g carbohydrate, 36 g protein, 15 g fat, 5 g saturated fat, 105 mg cholesterol, 414 mg sodium, 0 g fiber

Carbohydrate Choices: 0

Dietary Exchanges: 5 meat, 2 fat

NOW YOU KNOW!

Eating fattier meats once in a while is okay as long as your total saturated fat intake for the day is within reason. Plus, because these fattier meats have more calories, you have to cut calories from somewhere else during the day if weight loss is a goal. It's all about balance. So if you crave beef chuck pot roast instead of grilled flank steak, you can eat a 3-ounce portion of the chuck instead of a 6-ounce portion of the flank.

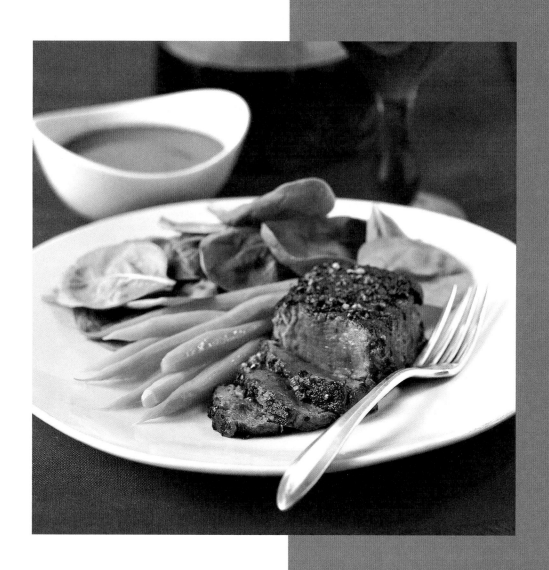

STEAK BURGERS

When you do indulge in a hamburger, choose lean ground beef and top with vitamin- and nutrient-rich veggies.

Preparation time: 10 minutes ● **Cooking time: 8 minutes**

1½ **pounds 95 percent lean ground beef**
    Ground black pepper
 6 **100 percent whole grain hamburger buns, sliced**
 6 **slices (½ ounce each) reduced-fat Swiss cheese**
 6 **red or green leaf lettuce leaves**
 6 **tomato slices**
 6 **thin red onion slices**
 6 **tablespoons chopped parsley**
 ¼ **cup steak sauce**

1. Preheat an indoor or outdoor grill to the highest heat setting.

2. Divide the meat and shape into six patties slightly larger in diameter than the buns (try not to overhandle or the meat will toughen). Season with plenty of pepper. Place on grill. Cook for 2 to 4 minutes per side, or until a thermometer inserted sideways registers 160°F and the meat is no longer pink.

3. Meanwhile, place the buns on the grill for about 1 minute, or until toasted. Add 1 slice cheese to each patty to melt just before the burgers are done.

4. Assemble the burgers by placing a lettuce leaf on the bottom of each bun followed by tomato, burger, and onion. Sprinkle with the parsley. Add 2 teaspoons of sauce to each burger. Cover with the bun top.

MAKES 6

Per serving: 321 calories, 25 g carbohydrate, 33 g protein, 10 g fat, 4 g saturated fat, 70 mg cholesterol, 441 mg sodium, 4 g fiber

Carbohydrate Choices: 2

Dietary Exchanges: 1½ starch, ½ vegetable, 4 meat, 1 fat

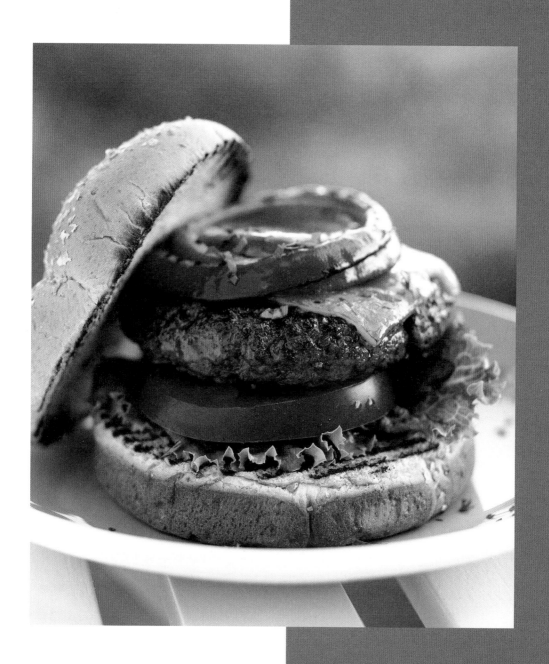

CHINESE BEEF AND RICE

This weeknight meal takes advantage of frozen ingredients to get dinner on the table quickly.

Preparation time: 10 minutes ● **Cooking time: 10 minutes**

1 ¾"-thick sirloin or top round steak (8 ounces), thinly sliced

2 tablespoons reduced-sodium soy sauce, divided

2 teaspoons canola oil

1 bag (14 ounces) frozen stir-fry or Asian vegetable mix

1 pouch (10 ounces) frozen brown rice

1 tablespoon finely chopped fresh ginger

2 teaspoons minced garlic

½ cup diagonally sliced scallions

¼ cup coarsely chopped dry-roasted peanuts

1. In a bowl, toss the meat with 1 tablespoon of the soy sauce.

2. Set a wok or large skillet over high heat for 1 minute. Add the oil. Place the meat in a single layer in the pan. Cook, without stirring, for about 1 minute, or until browned on the bottom. Stir. Cook 1 minute, stirring once or twice, until all pink is gone. With a slotted spoon or tongs, transfer the meat to a dish and set aside.

3. Add the vegetables to the pan. Stir-fry over medium heat about 5 minutes, or until the vegetables are tender.

4. Meanwhile, cook the rice per package directions.

5. Add the ginger and garlic to the pan. Stir-fry for 30 seconds. Add the reserved meat, rice, scallions, peanuts, and the remaining 1 tablespoon soy sauce. Stir-fry until heated through.

MAKES 4 SERVINGS

Per serving: 270 calories, 28 g carbohydrate, 19 g protein, 11 g fat, 2 g saturated fat, 35 mg cholesterol, 356 mg sodium, 5 g fiber

Carbohydrate Choices: 2

Dietary Exchanges: 1 starch, 1½ vegetable, 2 meat, 1 fat

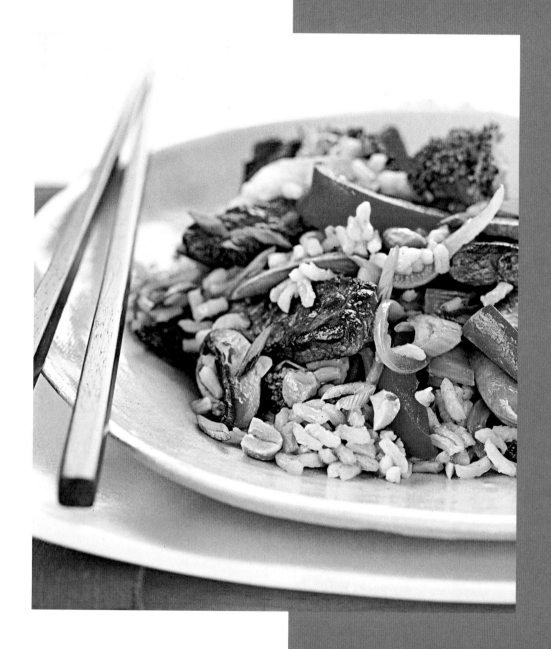

CINNAMON-RUBBED PORK LOIN
WITH ROASTED APPLES AND ONIONS

Spice-rubbed pork with maple-flavored apple puree can heat up the coldest day. Some studies have even identified a substance in cinnamon that helps control blood glucose levels.

Preparation time: 20 minutes ● **Roasting time: 50 minutes** ● **Standing time: 10 minutes**

---

2 teaspoons grated lemon peel

1 teaspoon ground cinnamon

½ teaspoon ground ginger

⅛ teaspoon ground allspice

⅛ teaspoon ground nutmeg

1 tablespoon olive oil

1 center-cut pork loin (1½ pounds)

Salt

Ground black pepper

3 apples, cut into wedges

3 medium onions, cut into wedges

¼ cup fresh lemon juice

½ cup apple juice

¼ cup maple syrup

1. Preheat the oven to 375°F. Coat a large roasting pan with vegetable oil spray. In a small bowl, combine the lemon peel, cinnamon, ginger, *[handwritten: decrease onion to 1 large — great flavor]* small bowl, spice mixtur pepper to ta oil mixture. S

2. In a large l wedges and ё lemon juice a   ...pice mixture. Place in the reserved pan with the pork and ½ cup water.

3. Roast, tossing the apple mixture once, for about 50 minutes, or until a thermometer inserted into the thickest portion registers 155°F and the juices run clear. Remove from the oven and allow to stand for 10 minutes.

4. Meanwhile, in a medium saucepan, bring the apple juice and maple syrup to a boil. Reduce the heat and simmer 1 to 2 minutes, until slightly thickened. Remove from heat.

5. In a food processor fitted with a metal blade, puree two-thirds of the apple mixture with the pan drippings until smooth. Add to the juice mixture. Season to taste with salt and pepper, if desired. Cook on medium-low heat until warm.

6. Cut the pork into thin slices. Garnish with the remaining raw apple wedges and remaining cooked onions. Serve with the sauce on the side.

MAKES 4 SERVINGS

Per serving: 440 calories, 44 g carbohydrate, 40 g protein, 12 g fat, 3.5 g saturated fat, 100 mg cholesterol, 440 mg sodium, 5 g fiber

Carbohydrate Choices: 3

Dietary Exchanges: 1 starch, 1 fruit, 2 vegetable, 5 meat, 2 fat

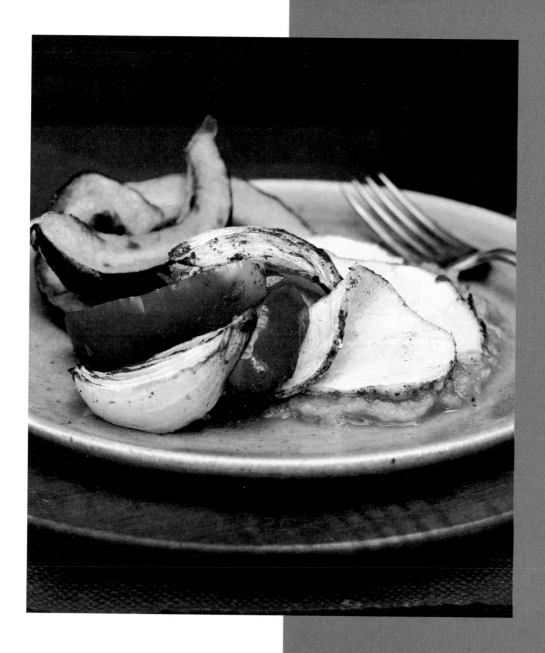

FIVE-SPICE PORK MEDALLIONS

Tenderloin contains the least fat of any cut of pork. It's boneless and quick to cook. What's not to like?

Preparation time: 4 minutes ● **Cooking time: 16 minutes** ● **Standing time: 5 minutes**

1 **pound pork tenderloin, trimmed of all visible fat**

2 **teaspoons five-spice powder**

¼ **teaspoon + pinch of salt**

4 **teaspoons Better Butter (page 323) or trans-fat free spread**

3 **large Granny Smith apples, cored and sliced in ½" wedges**

½ **cup dried cranberries**

½ **cup water**

1. Cut the tenderloin in half to create two equal pieces. Rub the spice powder and ¼ teaspoon salt over all sides of each piece.

2. In a small skillet, melt 2 teaspoons of the butter or spread over medium-high heat. Add the meat and cook, turning as needed, for about 4 minutes, or until browned on all sides. Cover and continue to cook, turning occasionally, for about 12 minutes, or until a thermometer inserted in the center reaches 155°F and the juices run clear. Remove and let stand for 5 minutes. Cut each piece into 6 medallions.

3. Meanwhile, in a heavy skillet set over medium-high heat, combine the apples, cranberries, remaining 2 teaspoons butter or spread, water, and the remaining pinch of salt. Cook, shaking the pan occasionally, until the liquid has almost evaporated and the apples soften. Serve with the pork medallions.

MAKES 4 SERVINGS

Per serving: 248 calories, 26 g carbohydrate, 25 g protein, 7 g fat, 2 g saturated fat, 80 mg cholesterol, 234 mg sodium, 3 g fiber

Carbohydrate Choices: 2

Dietary Exchanges: 1½ fruit, 3½ meat, 1 fat

NOTE: Five-spice powder is a Chinese seasoning mixture comprised of cinnamon, cloves, fennel seed, star anise, and Szechuan peppercorns. Look for it in the spice section of the supermarket.

SAUSAGE AND BROCCOLI RABE PASTA

Fusilli is a corkscrew-shaped dried pasta that has nooks and crannies to catch the savory sauce.

Preparation time: 5 minutes ● **Cooking time: 15 minutes**

1 pound broccoli rabe, 2" trimmed from ends, cut into 2" segments

8 ounces whole wheat fusilli pasta

1 tablespoon olive oil

6 ounces chicken sausage, cut into ½" slices

4 dry-packed sun-dried tomatoes, roughly chopped

3 cloves garlic, minced or put through garlic press

1. Bring a large pot of water to a boil. Add the broccoli rabe and blanch for 2 minutes. Remove from the pot and plunge into a bowl of cold water (save the pot of hot water for the pasta). Drain and set aside.

2. Add the pasta to the boiling water. Stir and cook for 10 minutes, or until al dente.

3. Meanwhile, heat the oil in a large skillet over medium-high heat. Add the sausage and cook, turning occasionally, for 5 minutes, or until browned. Add the tomatoes, garlic, and broccoli rabe to the pan. Cook for 2 minutes, or until the sausage is no longer pink.

4. Drain the pasta, reserving 2 tablespoons of the cooking water. Add the pasta and reserved water to the skillet. Toss with the sausage mixture.

MAKES 4 SERVINGS

Per serving: 370 calories, 50 g carbohydrate, 21 g protein, 9 g fat, 1.5 g saturated fat, 35 mg cholesterol, 300 mg sodium, 5 g fiber

Carbohydrate Choices: 3

Dietary Exchanges: 1 starch, 1½ vegetable, 1 meat, 1 fat

NOTE: Other shapes of dried pasta, such as rotini, butterflies, penne, or shells, can replace the fusilli.

CRANBERRY-APRICOT PORK ROAST

With the spices and citrus redolent of the winter celebrations, this roast is auspicious enough to grace a holiday table.

Preparation time: 10 minutes ● **Cooking time: 7–9 hours**

1 cup chopped cranberries

¼ cup quartered dried apricots

½ teaspoon grated orange peel

¼ cup orange juice

⅓ cup chopped shallot or onion

2 teaspoons cider vinegar

1 teaspoon dry mustard

1 teaspoon salt

1 teaspoon grated fresh ginger

2 pounds boneless pork loin roast

Snipped chives or scallion greens (optional)

1. In a 4-quart or larger slow cooker, combine the cranberries, apricots, orange peel and juice, shallot or onion, vinegar, mustard, salt, and ginger. Add the meat and spoon some of the cranberry mixture on top.

2. Cover and cook on the low setting for 7 to 9 hours, or until the pork is fork-tender.

3. Remove the pork to a cutting board. Spoon off any fat from the top of the cranberry mixture in the slow cooker. Cut the pork into 6 slices. Serve topped with the sauce. Garnish with chives or scallion greens, if desired.

MAKES 8 SERVINGS

Per serving: 250 calories, 7 g carbohydrate, 24 g protein, 13 g fat, 4.5 g saturated fat, 65 mg cholesterol, 340 mg sodium, 0 g fiber

Carbohydrate Choices: ½

Dietary Exchanges: ½ fruit, 3½ meat, 1 fat

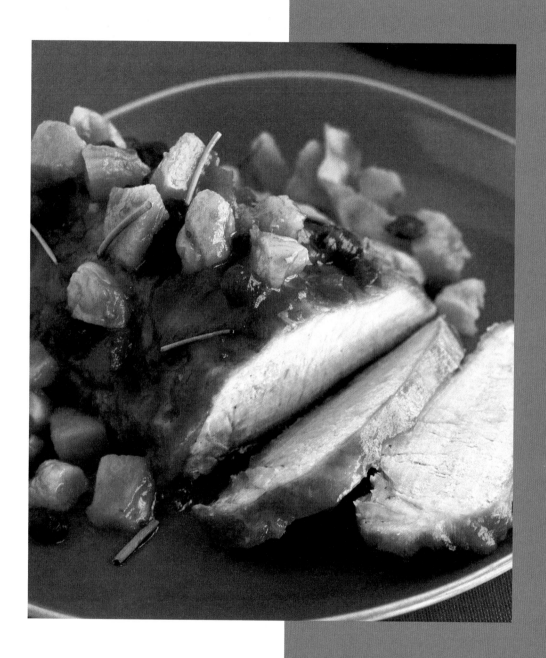

ITALIAN PORK CHOPS

Parmesan Roasted Asparagus (page 219) complements this main dish.

Preparation time: 5 minutes ● Cooking time: 18 minutes ● Standing time: 3 minutes

3 teaspoons olive oil, divided

4 boneless pork chops or cutlets (about 5 ounces each)

1 cup (4 ounces) bell pepper strips, any color

1 cup (4 ounces) sliced red onion

¾ teaspoon dried oregano

⅛ teaspoon salt

½ cup canned diced tomatoes
   Red-pepper flakes

4 lemon wedges (optional)

1. Coat a large heavy skillet with vegetable oil spray. Place over high heat for 1 minute. Add 1 teaspoon of the oil. Heat for 30 seconds. Place the chops or cutlets in the pan. Cook for 2 minutes on each side, or until browned. Remove to a plate and set aside.

2. Add the remaining 2 teaspoons of oil to the pan. Reduce the heat to medium. Add the pepper, onion, oregano, and salt. Toss. Cover the pan. Cook, tossing occasionally, for 4 minutes, or until softened.

3. Add the tomatoes (with juice). Stir to mix. Nestle the reserved chops under the vegetables. Cover and simmer over medium-low heat for about 6 minutes, or until a thermometer inserted sideways in the center of a chop registers 160°F and the juices run clear. Uncover and let stand for 3 minutes. Serve with red-pepper flakes and lemon, if desired.

MAKES 4 SERVINGS

Per serving: 255 calories, 5 g carbohydrate, 31 g protein, 12 g fat, 3.5 g saturated fat, 89 mg cholesterol, 219 mg sodium, 1 g fiber

Carbohydrate Choices: 0

Dietary Exchanges: 1 vegetable, 4 meat, 2 fat

BROCCOLI AND TOFU STIR-FRY WITH TOASTED ALMONDS

Turn to tofu—pressed cooked soybeans—if you would like to cut the amount of saturated fat you eat from animal protein. Tofu tastes pleasant and mild, making it a good base ingredient to absorb vivid flavorings.

Draining time: 30 minutes ● **Preparation time: 30 minutes** ● **Cooking time: 12 minutes**

---

1 package (16 ounces) firm tofu

4 cups broccoli florets

3 teaspoons toasted sesame oil, divided

1 bunch scallions, thinly sliced

1 tablespoon minced garlic

1 small jalapeño chile pepper, halved, seeded, and finely chopped (wear plastic gloves when handling)

3½ teaspoons soy sauce

2 tablespoons sliced almonds, lightly toasted

2 cups hot cooked brown rice

1. Place the tofu on a plate, and top with a cutting board. Place several cans of food on the board to weight it down. Let the tofu rest for 30 minutes while water is squeezed out. Cut the tofu into small cubes.

2. While the tofu drains, lightly steam the broccoli for about 5 minutes, or until crisp-tender. Set aside.

3. Coat a wok or large skillet with vegetable oil spray. Set over high heat for 1 minute. Add 2 teaspoons of oil. When hot, add the tofu and cook for about 5 minutes, stirring constantly, until browned. Transfer to a shallow bowl.

4. Add the remaining 1 teaspoon of oil to the wok, followed by the scallions, garlic, pepper, and broccoli. Stir-fry over medium-high heat for 2 minutes. Stir in the soy sauce, almonds, and tofu. Gently toss to combine. Serve each portion with ½ cup of brown rice.

MAKES 4 SERVINGS

Per serving: 307 calories, 32 g carbohydrate, 19 g protein, 13 g fat, 2 g saturated fat, 0 mg cholesterol, 184 mg sodium, 6 g fiber

Carbohydrate Choices: 2

Dietary Exchanges: 1½ starch, 1½ vegetable, 2 meat, 2 fat

MAGIC LASAGNA

There's no mystery about why this baked pasta dish is quicker to prepare. It starts with no-boil noodles to cut cooking time.

Preparation time: 25 minutes ● **Cooking time: 30 minutes** ● **Standing time: 10 minutes**

1 cup part-skim ricotta cheese

1 cup 1% cottage cheese

2 cups (8 ounces) shredded reduced-fat mozzarella cheese, divided

2 medium eggs

2 cups shredded carrots

1 package (10 ounces) frozen chopped broccoli, thawed and well drained

1 package (9 ounces) no-boil lasagna noodles

3 cups fat-free chunky garden-style pasta sauce

1. Preheat the oven to 400°F. Coat a 13" × 9" baking dish with vegetable oil spray.

2. In a large bowl, combine the ricotta, cottage cheese, 1 cup mozzarella, eggs, carrots, and broccoli.

3. Place 3 noodles in the reserved dish. Spread one-third of the cheese mixture evenly over the noodles. Drizzle on 1 cup of the sauce. Repeat the process two more times. Sprinkle with the remaining 1 cup mozzarella.

4. Bake for 30 minutes, or until bubbling. Allow to stand 10 minutes before serving.

MAKES 8 SERVINGS

Per serving: 320 calories, 36 g carbohydrate, 23 g protein, 9 g fat, 4.5 g saturated fat, 102 mg cholesterol, 541 mg sodium, 3 g fiber

Carbohydrate Choices: 2

Dietary Exchanges: 2½ vegetable, 1½ meat, ½ fat

UNLEASH NUTRIENTS

Dynamic Duo

Calcium plus vitamin D offers powerful protection against diabetes, according to a 20-year study of 83,779 women by scientists at Tufts–New England Medical Center in Boston. Those who got the highest levels of the combo—more than 1,200 milligrams of calcium and more than 800 IU of vitamin D—had a 33 percent lower risk of type 2 diabetes than women who got the least. The nutrients also worked alone, though not as well. Aim for three servings of low-fat dairy a day, and include foods that are good sources of vitamin D, such as fortified milk, whole eggs, cheese, and salmon. Consult your physician or dietitian about supplements if needed.

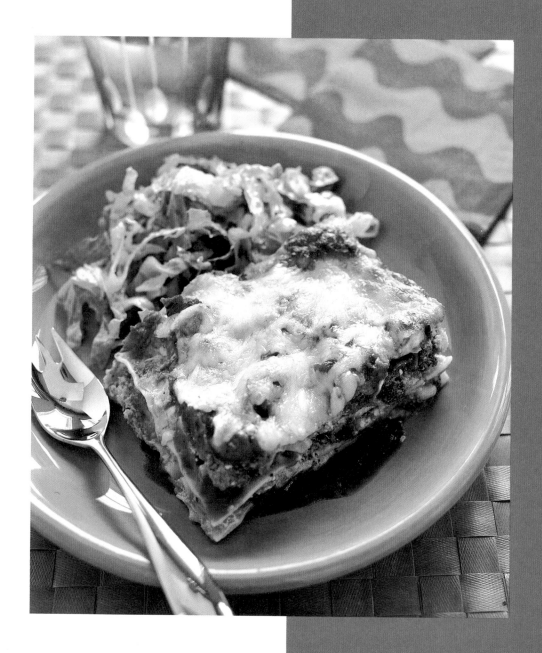

ITALIAN POTATO DUMPLING CASSEROLE

Gnocchi—tender dumpling morsels—are Italian comfort food.

Preparation time: 20 minutes ● **Baking time: 40 minutes** ● **Standing time: 15 minutes**

¾ cup part-skim ricotta cheese

¼ cup fresh basil, thinly sliced

½ cup (2 ounces) grated reduced-fat mozzarella, divided

2 tablespoons (½ ounce) grated Parmesan cheese

1 egg, lightly beaten

3 cups Basic Tomato Sauce (page 306)

1 package (16 ounces) potato gnocchi

2 cups spinach leaves, thinly sliced

1. Preheat the oven to 400°F. Lightly coat a 1½-quart casserole or gratin dish with vegetable oil spray and set aside.

2. In a small bowl, combine the ricotta, basil, ¼ cup of the mozzarella, Parmesan, and egg. Stir until blended. Set aside.

3. Spread a thin layer of the tomato sauce in the reserved dish. On top of the sauce, layer half of the gnocchi and spinach. Using half of the ricotta mixture, place small dollops on top of the spinach. Cover with another thin layer of sauce. Repeat the process, ending with sauce. Sprinkle on the remaining ¼ cup mozzarella.

4. Bake for 40 minutes, or until the top is bubbly and the cheese is lightly browned. Let stand for 15 minutes before serving.

MAKES 6 SERVINGS

Per serving: 250 calories, 25 g carbohydrate, 11 g protein, 12 g fat, 6 g saturated fat, 65 mg cholesterol, 400 mg sodium, 4 g fiber

Carbohydrate Choices: 2

Dietary Exchanges: 1 starch, 1½ vegetable, 1 meat, 2 fat

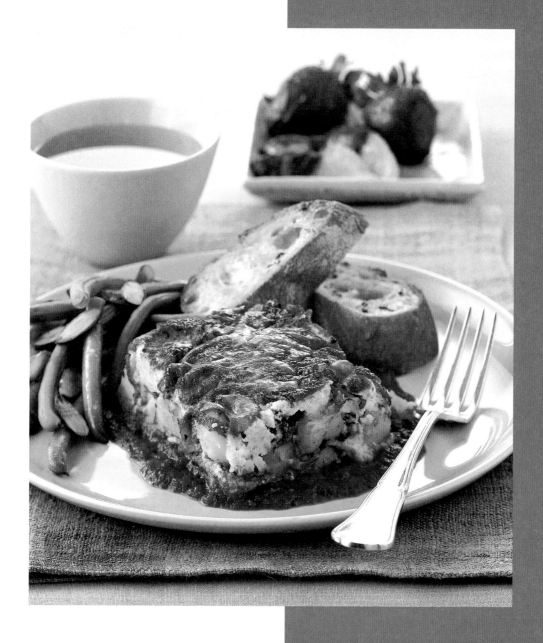

Basic Tomato Sauce

You'll rely on this recipe often as a healthier alternative to bottled sauces that often contain too much added sweetener and sodium.

Preparation time: 10 minutes ● **Cooking time: 20 minutes**

---

  2 **teaspoons olive oil, preferably extra virgin**
  ½ **cup chopped onion**
  ½ **cup chopped carrot**
  ½ **cup chopped celery**
  3 **cloves garlic, minced**
  1 **can (28 ounces) diced tomatoes**
  ¼ **teaspoon salt**
     Ground black pepper

Heat the oil in a medium saucepan over medium heat. Add the onion, carrot, celery, and garlic and cook for about 10 minutes. Add the tomatoes (with juice) and salt and cook for another 10 minutes. Season with pepper to taste. Remove from the heat. Puree the sauce in a blender in batches until smooth.

MAKES 6 SERVINGS (½ CUP PER SERVING)

Per serving: 54 calories, 10 g carbohydrate, 2 g protein, 2 g fat, 0 g saturated fat, 0 mg cholesterol, 184 mg sodium, 3 g fiber

Carbohydrate Choices: 1

Dietary Exchanges: 1½ vegetable, ½ fat

NOTE: The sauce can be refrigerated in an airtight container for up to 1 week.

NO-NEED-TO-HURRY VEGETABLE CURRY

You'll find curry paste in the ethnic section of some supermarkets or in Indian specialty food stores. You can replace it with dry curry powder if you like. Serve over basmati rice.

Preparation time: 20 minutes ● **Cooking time: 6–8 hours**

1 can (14 ounces) light coconut milk

¼ cup all-purpose flour

2½ tablespoons mild Indian curry paste or 2½ teaspoons curry powder

½ teaspoon salt

2 medium Yukon Gold potatoes (1 pound), cut into 1½" chunks

2 medium onions, halved and thinly sliced

1 bag (8 ounces) cauliflower florets

1 large red bell pepper, quartered and cut into ¾"-wide strips

8 ounces green beans, halved

1 cup frozen peas, thawed

½ cup chopped cilantro

Torn cilantro leaves (optional, for garnish)

Red bell pepper, finely chopped (optional, for garnish)

Sliced almonds, toasted (optional, for garnish)

1. In a 4-quart or larger slow cooker, whisk the coconut milk, flour, curry paste or powder, and salt until smooth. Add the potatoes, onions, cauliflower, and pepper strips. Toss to mix. Place the beans on top.

2. Cover and cook on the low setting for 6 to 8 hours, or until the vegetables are tender. Stir in the peas and chopped cilantro. Garnish with cilantro leaves, chopped pepper, and almonds, if desired.

MAKES 6 SERVINGS

Per serving: 200 calories, 34 g carbohydrate, 7 g protein, 5 g fat, 3.5 g saturated fat, 0 mg cholesterol, 385 mg sodium, 6 g fiber

Carbohydrate Choices: 2

Dietary Exchanges: 1 starch, 2½ vegetable

PASTA SHELLS WITH BROCCOLI, CHICKPEAS, AND TOMATOES

Recipes that rely on pantry staples are the kind you'll rely on in a pinch.

Preparation time: 10 minutes ● **Cooking time: 15 minutes**

1   **tablespoon olive oil, preferably extra virgin**

1   **can (15½ ounces) chickpeas, rinsed and drained**

1   **teaspoon minced garlic**

1   **teaspoon dried oregano**

⅛   **teaspoon red-pepper flakes**

1   **can (14½ ounces) no-salt-added diced tomatoes**

2   **cups pasta shells**

1   **bag (14 ounces) frozen cut broccoli**

¼   **cup (1 ounce) grated Pecorino Romano or Parmesan cheese**

1. Heat the oil in a large skillet over medium-high heat. Add the chickpeas, garlic, oregano, and red-pepper flakes. Cook for about 3 minutes, stirring gently, or until the chickpeas turn golden in spots. Stir in the tomatoes (with juice), cover, and cook 5 minutes over low heat.

2. Meanwhile, cook the pasta according to the package directions, omitting the salt. Two minutes before the pasta is cooked, add the broccoli to the pot. Before draining, ladle out and reserve ⅔ cup cooking liquid.

3. Drain the pasta and broccoli and return to the pot. Add the chickpea mixture and the reserved cooking water. Toss to blend. Spoon into bowls and top with cheese.

MAKES 4 SERVINGS

Per serving: 377 calories, 55 g carbohydrate, 14 g protein, 7 g fat, 1.5 g saturated fat, 5 mg cholesterol, 387 mg sodium, 10 g fiber

Carbohydrate Choices: 3½

Dietary Exchanges: 3 starch, 2 vegetable, 1 fat

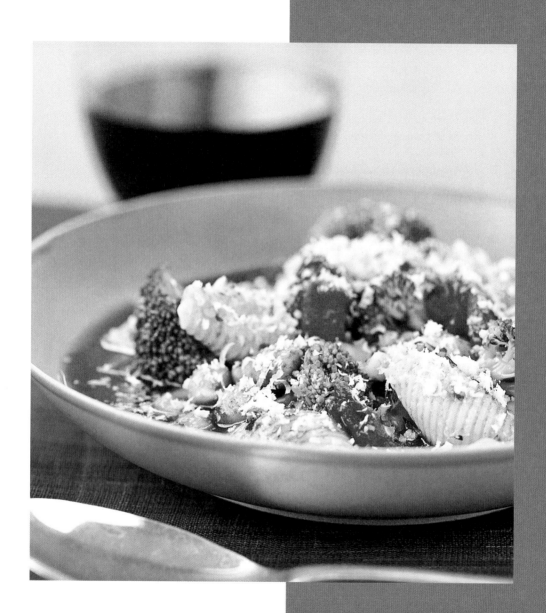

FUSILLI WITH MUSHROOMS AND CHARD

Chard, a cruciferous vegetable that's related to beets, grows large crinkly green leaves on celery-crisp ribs that vary in color from pale green to bright yellow to deep red. Chard is a good source of vitamins A and C, as well as iron.

Preparation time: 10 minutes ● **Cooking time: 15 minutes**

8 ounces tri-color or whole wheat fusilli pasta

3 tablespoons olive oil

4 large shallots, peeled and quartered lengthwise

1 large bunch green chard, trimmed; stems cut into ½"-thick slices; leaves (inner stems removed) sliced into long strips

10 ounces shiitake or brown mushrooms, stems removed and caps sliced

¼ teaspoon salt

¼ teaspoon ground black pepper

2 tablespoons chopped fresh parsley

⅓ cup (about 2¾ ounces) grated or shaved Parmesan cheese

1. Omitting the salt, cook the pasta according to the package directions.

2. Meanwhile, in a large skillet, heat the oil over medium heat. Add the shallots. Cook, tossing or stirring, for about 5 minutes, or until tender and golden brown. Add the chard stems. Cook for about 4 minutes, stirring often, until softened. Add the mushrooms, salt, and pepper. Cook for 2 to 3 minutes. Stir in the parsley and chard leaves and cook 1 minute longer, or until most of the liquid has evaporated and the leaves are wilted.

3. Drain the pasta, reserving ⅓ cup of the cooking water. Return the pasta and the reserved water to the pot. Add the chard mixture and the cheese. Toss well and serve immediately.

MAKES 6 SERVINGS

Per serving: 260 calories, 34 g carbohydrate, 9 g protein, 9 g fat, 2 g saturated fat, 5 mg cholesterol, 290 mg sodium, 5 g fiber

Carbohydrate Choices: 2

Dietary Exchanges: 2 starch, 1 vegetable, 1½ fat

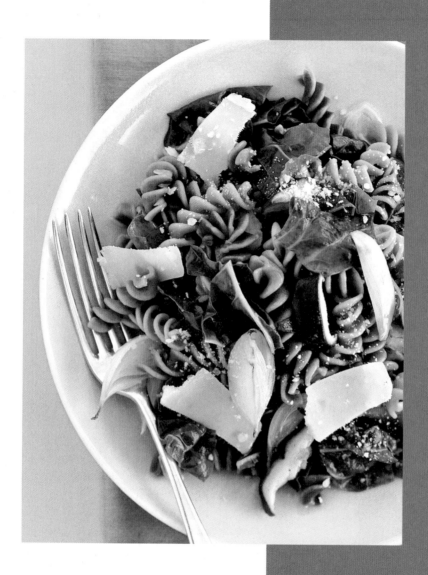

COOKING DRIED BEANS

Cooked dried beans are a nutritionist's dream date—a low-fat, cholesterol-free source of protein, carbohydrates, and soluble fiber. They appeal to creative cooks as well. Black beans, great Northern beans, cannellini beans, kidney beans, lima beans, pinto beans, and many other varieties offer different tastes and textures and adapt to a wide variety of seasonings and ethnic recipes.

Canned cooked dried beans are ultraconvenient but generally contain high levels of sodium (unless you seek out reduced-sodium brands sold in some supermarkets and natural food stores). To reduce the sodium in regular canned beans, dump the beans into a colander and rinse well under cold running water to drain off the thick canning liquid. A 15-ounce can yields about 1¾ cups beans.

If you prefer to cook your own dried beans from scratch (it's much cheaper), it pays to cook 1 or 2 pounds at a time. It's no more work, and you can freeze the cooked beans in convenient recipe-size portions. Beans can be cooked in a heavy pot on the stovetop, in the oven, in a slow cooker, or in a pressure cooker. (Follow the manufacturer's directions if using a slow cooker or pressure cooker.)

To prepare dried beans, first sort through them to remove any tiny pebbles and any cracked or shriveled beans. Place the beans in a colander and rinse them well under cold water. The next step prior to cooking is to rehydrate the dried beans by soaking them in water. Two methods can be used.

OVERNIGHT METHOD

Place the washed beans in a large bowl or pot. Cover with cold water, about three times as much water as beans. Let stand overnight. Drain the beans. Place in a pot and cover with three times as much fresh water as beans. Cook according to the package directions.

RAPID SOAK METHOD

Place the washed beans in a pot. Cover with three times as much water as beans. Bring to a boil. Cook for 2 minutes. Remove from the heat and let stand for 1 hour. Drain the beans, return to the pot, cover with three times as much fresh water as beans, and cook according to the package directions.

PROVENÇAL LENTIL RAGOUT

Turn to legume main dishes, like this lentil stew, more often to drastically reduce your intake of saturated fat and cholesterol. Broccoli, asparagus, kale, or another green vegetable is all you need to serve on the side.

Preparation time: 12 minutes ● **Cooking time: 32 minutes**

½ cup chopped carrot

½ cup chopped celery

½ cup chopped onion

2 tablespoons olive oil, preferably extra virgin

1½ teaspoons herbes de Provence

1 bay leaf

2 cups (8 ounces) dried lentils

1 tablespoon minced garlic

1 can (14½ ounces) chicken or vegetable broth

1 cup water

½ teaspoon salt

½ teaspoon ground black pepper

Balsamic vinegar

¼ cup finely chopped flat-leaf parsley

8 teaspoons grated Romano cheese

1. In a large pot over medium-high heat, combine the carrot, celery, onion, oil, herbes de Provence, and bay leaf. Stir. Cover and cook, stirring occasionally, for about 5 minutes, or until the vegetables start to soften.

2. Add the lentils and garlic. Cook, stirring, for 1 minute, or until the garlic is fragrant. Add the broth and water. Bring to a boil. Reduce the heat to low. Partially cover and simmer for about 25 minutes, or until the lentils are very soft but not mushy. Remove and discard the bay leaf.

3. Stir in the salt and pepper. Serve in pasta bowls. Drizzle about 1 teaspoon balsamic vinegar on each serving. Sprinkle on the parsley and cheese.

MAKES 8 SERVINGS (½ CUP PER SERVING)

Per serving: 180 calories, 24 g carbohydrate, 10 g protein, 5 g fat, 1 g saturated fat, 0 mg cholesterol, 270 mg sodium, 10 g fiber

Carbohydrate Choices: 1½

Dietary Exchanges: ½ vegetable, ½ meat, 1 fat

NOTES: Herbes de Provence is a blend of dried herbs that are characteristic of southern French cooking. The mixture typically contains basil, fennel, lavender, marjoram, rosemary, sage, savory, and thyme. If unavailable, replace with dried thyme, rosemary, and sage.

Refrigerate or freeze leftover lentils in ½ cup portions (without the garnishes). To serve as a lunch salad on radicchio or arugula leaves, thaw if frozen. Drizzle on ½ teaspoon each of olive oil and vinegar.

To serve as a soup, reheat with broth just to cover in a microwaveable bowl or a saucepan on the stove top.

CUBAN BLACK BEANS

Minced onion or scallion, with a splash of sherry vinegar, makes a sprightly garnish for this rich main dish.

Preparation time: 10 minutes ● **Cooking time: 20 minutes**

2 tablespoons olive oil, preferably extra virgin

1 cup chopped onion

1 cup chopped green bell pepper

1 tablespoon minced garlic

2 bay leaves

1½ teaspoons ground cumin

1 teaspoon dried oregano

¼ teaspoon salt

3 cups cooked black beans (page 312) or 3 cups canned black beans, rinsed and drained

1 cup chicken or vegetable broth

½ teaspoon hot-pepper sauce

2 cups hot cooked instant brown rice

1. In a large pot, combine the oil, onion, pepper, garlic, bay leaves, cumin, oregano, and salt. Cook over medium heat, stirring occasionally, for 4 minutes, or until softened. Stir in the beans. Cook for 1 minute to coat with the seasonings. Add the broth. Reduce the heat to medium-low. Cover and cook for about 15 minutes for the flavors to blend.

2. Remove and discard the bay leaves. Stir in the hot-pepper sauce. If desired, smash some of the beans with the side of a large spoon. Serve over the rice.

MAKES 4 SERVINGS

Per serving: 412 calories, 64 g carbohydrate, 17 g protein, 10 g fat, 1.5 g saturated fat, 0 mg cholesterol, 180 mg sodium, 14 g fiber

Carbohydrate Choices: 4

Dietary Exchanges: 4 starch, 1 vegetable, 1½ fat

MOROCCAN CHICKPEAS AND VEGETABLES WITH COUSCOUS

This skillet meal is one of the dishes that is adaptable to what you have on hand. Carrots can take the place of sweet potato, turnips can replace the bell pepper, and chopped broccoli stems can stand in for the peas.

Preparation time: 10 minutes ● **Cooking time: 13 minutes** ● **Standing time: 10 minutes**

1 tablespoon olive oil, preferably extra virgin

1 cup ½" cubed sweet potato

½ cup chopped onion

½ cup chopped bell pepper (any color)

1½ teaspoons ground cumin

¼ teaspoon salt

1 cup cooked chickpeas (page 312) or canned chickpeas, rinsed and drained

1 cup chicken broth or water

½ cup frozen baby peas

½ cup whole wheat couscous

2 tablespoons chopped fresh cilantro (optional)

Garlic chili sauce (optional)

1. Set a large skillet over medium-high heat for 1 minute. Add the oil and swirl to coat the pan bottom. Heat for 30 seconds. Add the sweet potato, onion, pepper, cumin, and salt. Cook, stirring occasionally, for 2 minutes, or until the onion is sizzling.

2. Add the chickpeas. Stir to coat with the seasonings. Add the broth or water and bring almost to a boil. Reduce the heat to a simmer. Cover and cook for 10 minutes, or until the sweet potatoes are tender.

3. Add the peas. Bring the mixture to a boil. Add the couscous and stir. Turn off the heat, cover, and let stand for 10 minutes.

4. Fluff the couscous with a fork. Serve, garnished with cilantro, if desired. Pass the garlic chili sauce at the table, if desired.

MAKES 4 SERVINGS

Per serving: 215 calories, 35 g carbohydrate, 9 g protein, 5 g fat, 1 g saturated fat, 0 mg cholesterol, 213 mg sodium, 8 g fiber

Carbohydrate Choices: 2

Dietary Exchanges: 2 starch, 1 vegetable, ½ meat, 1 fat

EGGPLANT ALLA PIZZAIOLA

If you're new to tofu, this is the dish for you. Seasoned with familiar Italian flavorings, it may become a permanent part of your repertoire.

Preparation time: 10 minutes ● **Cooking time: 45 minutes**

¼ cup (1 ounce) grated Parmesan and Romano cheese blend

1 tablespoon dried whole grain bread crumbs

2 teaspoons minced garlic

¾ teaspoon dried oregano

¼ teaspoon salt

¼ teaspoon ground black pepper

1¼ pounds Japanese or Italian eggplant, cut into ¼"-thick slices

4 ounces (one-quarter block) firm tofu, cut into ¼" pieces, patted dry

1 cup canned diced tomatoes

2 tablespoons olive oil, preferably extra virgin

1. Preheat the oven to 375°F. Coat a 12" × 8" baking dish with vegetable oil spray.

2. On a sheet of waxed paper, combine the cheese, bread crumbs, garlic, oregano, salt, and pepper. Dip both sides of the eggplant slices into the mixture. Shake off any excess. Arrange in slightly overlapping rows in the pan. Scatter on the tofu, tomatoes (with juice), and the remaining crumb mixture. Drizzle with the oil.

3. Bake for about 45 minutes, or until the eggplant is tender when pierced with a knife. If desired, broil 6" from the heat source for 2 to 3 minutes, or until browned on top.

MAKES 4 SERVINGS

Per serving: 187 calories, 12 g carbohydrate, 8 g protein, 11 g fat, 3 g saturated fat, 7 mg cholesterol, 420 mg sodium, 6 g fiber

Carbohydrate Choices: 1

Dietary Exchanges: 2 vegetable, 1 meat, 2 fat

NOTE: This dish can be assembled, covered with plastic wrap, and refrigerated for up to 24 hours before baking. Remove the plastic wrap before baking.

BLACK BEAN PATTIES

Replace meat cutlets every so often with these healthier vegetable patties. The patties in this recipe contain far less sodium than most frozen veggie burgers. Top with Salsa Fresca (page 119) and a dab of sour cream or stir-fried onion and bell peppers.

Preparation time: 15 minutes ● **Standing time: 1 hour 30 minutes** ● **Cooking time: 4 minutes**

1¾ cups cooked black beans (page 312) or 1 can (15½ ounces) canned black beans, rinsed and drained

¼ cup + 2 tablespoons whole wheat couscous

2 tablespoons finely chopped onion

2 tablespoons finely chopped parsley

1 egg

2 tablespoons olive oil, preferably extra virgin, divided

1½ teaspoons salt-free seasoning blend

½ teaspoon minced garlic

¼ teaspoon salt

1. In the bowl of a food processor fitted with a metal blade, combine the beans, couscous, onion, parsley, egg, 1 tablespoon oil, seasoning blend, garlic, and salt. Process for about 1 minute. Scrape down the sides of the bowl. Process for about 30 seconds, or until the mixture comes together but is still coarse. Transfer to a bowl. Cover with plastic wrap and refrigerate for about 1½ hours, or until firm enough to shape into patties.

2. Shape the mixture into 8 patties. Heat a skillet or griddle over medium-high heat. Add the remaining 1 tablespoon oil. Heat for 30 seconds. Place the patties in the pan. Cook for about 2 minutes, or until browned on the bottom. Flip and cook, reducing the heat slightly if the pan is too hot, for about 2 minutes, or until cooked through.

MAKES 8 SERVINGS

Per serving: 112 calories, 14 g carbohydrate, 5 g protein, 5 g fat, 1 g saturated fat, 26 mg cholesterol, 82 mg sodium, 4 g fiber

Carbohydrate Choices: 1

Dietary Exchanges: 1 starch, 1 fat

NOTE: The cooked, cooled patties can be frozen. Place them on a freezer-proof tray in a single layer. When frozen, pack the patties, separated by small pieces of waxed paper, into a resealable plastic freezer bag. To cook, microwave the frozen patties on high power for 1 to 1½ minutes, or until heated through.

LOUISIANA RED BEANS AND RICE

If you prefer a completely vegetarian main dish, simply leave out the sausage, and replace the chicken broth with vegetable broth.

Preparation time: 10 minutes ● **Cooking time: 25 minutes**

1	tablespoon olive oil
½	cup chopped onion
½	cup chopped green bell pepper
½	cup chopped celery
2	teaspoons minced garlic
1	teaspoon dried thyme
¼	teaspoon salt
2	bay leaves
4	ounces turkey sausage links, cut into chunks
3	cups cooked red beans (page 312) or canned red beans, rinsed and drained
½	cup chicken broth
	Hot-pepper sauce
2	cups hot cooked instant brown rice

1. Set a large pot over medium-high heat. Add the oil. Heat for 30 seconds. Add the onion, pepper, celery, garlic, thyme, salt, and bay leaves. Cook, stirring occasionally, for 3 minutes, or until starting to soften. Scrape the vegetables to one side of the pan. Add the sausage to the empty side. Cook, stirring occasionally, for about 5 minutes, or until the sausage is lightly browned.

2. Add the beans and broth. Cover and simmer over medium-low heat for about 15 minutes, or until the flavors blend. Remove and discard the bay leaves. Add up to 1 teaspoon of hot-pepper sauce. Serve over the rice. Pass the hot-pepper sauce at the table.

MAKES 4 SERVINGS

Per serving: 403 calories, 60 g carbohydrate, 21 g protein, 9 g fat, 1.5 g saturated fat, 21 mg cholesterol, 413 mg sodium, 12 g fiber

Carbohydrate Choices: 4

Dietary Exchanges: 4 starch, 1 vegetable, 1 meat, 1 fat

VEGETABLE AND BARLEY RAGOUT

Browning the vegetables to caramelize their natural sugars gives this meatless stew really good flavor.

Preparation time: 15 minutes ● **Cooking time: 25 minutes** ● **Standing time: 5 minutes**

---

1 tablespoon olive oil, preferably extra virgin

½ cup chopped onion

8 ounces small brown mushrooms, halved

1 medium sweet potato, cut into 1" chunks

1½ teaspoons minced fresh rosemary

½ teaspoon dried thyme

½ teaspoon salt

¼ cup dry red wine (optional)

1 cup vegetable or chicken broth

½ cup quick-cooking barley

8 ounces broccoli florets, cut into marble-size pieces

¼ teaspoon ground black pepper

1. Warm the oil in a large pot over medium-high heat. Add the onion, mushrooms, sweet potato, rosemary, thyme, and salt. Stir to mix. Cover and cook for about 5 minutes, stirring occasionally, until the mushrooms shrink and are glazed. Add the wine, if using. Cook for about 4 minutes, or until the liquid evaporates.

2. Add the broth and barley. Cover and reduce the heat to medium-low. Simmer for about 10 minutes, or until the barley is tender.

3. Meanwhile, place the broccoli in a medium skillet with enough water to come ½" up the pan sides. Cover and cook over high heat for 2 to 3 minutes, or until the broccoli is crisp-tender. Drain and stir into the stew. Add the pepper. Cover and let stand for 5 minutes for the flavors to blend.

MAKES 4 SERVINGS

Per serving: 194 calories, 34 g carbohydrate, 7 g protein, 5 g fat, 0.5 g saturated fat, 0 mg cholesterol, 440 mg sodium, 8 g fiber

Carbohydrate Choices: 2

Dietary Exchanges: 1½ starch, 2 vegetable, 1 fat

NOTES: The rosemary may be replaced with 1 teaspoon of crumbled dried rosemary.

If not using wine, drizzle a little bit of balsamic vinegar on the ragout just before serving. The acid will heighten the flavor.

The vegetable or chicken broth may be replaced with water.

CHAPTER 10

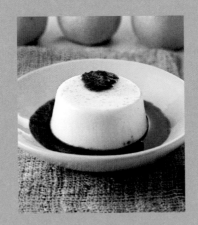

DESSERTS

MIXED BERRY COBBLER WITH CORNMEAL CRUST

No one will guess that you used frozen fruit in this easy, quick-to-make, and delicious dessert! (So don't tell.)

Preparation time: 10 minutes ● **Baking time: 40 minutes** ● **Standing time: 10 minutes**

BERRIES

- ¼ cup brown sugar
- 1½ tablespoons cornstarch
- 4 cups (about 1¼ pounds) frozen mixed berries, thawed

CRUST

- ¾ cup stone-ground cornmeal
- 2 tablespoons whole wheat pastry flour
- 1½ tablespoons brown sugar
- 1½ teaspoons baking powder
  Pinch of salt
- 2½ tablespoons cold Better Butter (page 323) or trans-fat free spread, cut into chunks
- ⅓ cup fat-free milk

1. Preheat the oven to 350°F. Coat an 8" × 8" baking dish with vegetable oil spray. Set aside.

2. To prepare the berries: In a mixing bowl, combine the sugar and the cornstarch. Stir to mix. Add the berries. Toss to combine. Transfer to the baking dish. Wipe the bowl clean with a paper towel.

3. To prepare the crust: In the bowl, combine the cornmeal, flour, sugar, baking powder, and salt. Stir with a fork or pastry blender. Add the Better Butter or spread. Cut into the dry ingredients until the pieces are the size of peas. Add the milk and stir quickly just to moisten. Dollop over the berries, leaving some bare patches.

4. Bake for about 40 minutes, or until the topping is golden and the fruit is bubbling. Let stand for 10 minutes before serving.

MAKES 6 SERVINGS

Per serving: 190 calories, 35 g carbohydrate, 3 g protein, 4.5 g fat, 1 g saturated fat, 0 mg cholesterol, 176 mg sodium, 4 g fiber

Carbohydrate Choices: 2

Dietary Exchanges: 1½ starch, 1 fruit, 1 fat

NOTE: In summer, fresh berries can replace the frozen.

RUM-GLAZED PINEAPPLE

This tropical fruit is perfect when you want a little dessert after a substantial dinner!

Preparation time: 4 minutes ● **Cooking time: 4 minutes**

2 tablespoons pineapple juice or water

1 tablespoon brown sugar

2 teaspoons Better Butter (below) or trans-fat free spread

¼ teaspoon rum extract

8 pineapple rings, fresh or canned packed in juice, drained

4 teaspoons sour cream

1 tablespoon finely chopped macadamia nuts

1. In a nonstick skillet set over medium heat, combine the juice or water, sugar, Better Butter or spread, and extract. Whisk to combine. Place the pineapple in the skillet. Cook for about 2 minutes on each side, or until sizzling.

2. Place 2 pineapple rings on each of 4 dessert plates. Drizzle the pan sauce over the pineapple. Top each serving with 1 teaspoon sour cream. Sprinkle on the nuts.

MAKES 4 SERVINGS

Per serving: 113 calories, 20 g carbohydrate, 1 g protein, 4 g fat, 1 g saturated fat, 3 mg cholesterol, 28 mg sodium, 1 g fiber

Carbohydrate Choices: 1

Dietary Exchanges: 1 fruit, 1 fat

A BETTER BUTTER

For those who love the taste of real butter and want to avoid the whole trans-fat issue (see page 34), there is a way to enjoy it in moderation while reducing the saturated fat content by 60 percent. Mix your own blend of monounsaturated canola oil and unsalted butter.

½ cup (1 stick) unsalted butter, at room temperature

¾ cup canola oil

Place the butter in a bowl. Beat with a spoon until fluffy. Continue beating, while gradually adding the oil, until smooth. Place in an airtight container. Refrigerate for up to 1 month or freeze for up to 3 months.

Makes 1¼ cups; 20 tablespoons

PEACHES IN WARM CUSTARD SAUCE

An easy vanilla custard sauce makes a creamy companion to just about any good ripe fruit. Try strawberries, raspberries, or pears when peaches go out of season.

Preparation time: 15 minutes ● **Cooking time: 4 minutes**

---

3 ripe peaches, peeled (if desired) and sliced

1 teaspoon brown sugar

½ teaspoon ground cinnamon

3 tablespoons confectioners' sugar

1½ tablespoons all-purpose flour

1 egg

1 cup whole milk

2 teaspoons vanilla extract

1. In a bowl, combine the peaches with the brown sugar and the cinnamon. Toss and set aside.

2. In a saucepan, combine the confectioners' sugar and flour. Whisk to mix. Break the egg into a small bowl. Beat with a fork until smooth. Add the milk and mix to combine. Whisking constantly, gradually add the milk mixture to the dry ingredients in the pan. Cook, whisking constantly, over medium-low heat for about 4 minutes, or until the mixture bubbles and thickens. Remove from the heat. Whisk in the vanilla.

3. Spoon the peaches and juice in the bowl into 4 large goblets or glass dessert dishes. Spoon the cream sauce over the peaches. Serve right away.

MAKES 4 SERVINGS

Per serving: 126 calories, 19 g carbohydrate, 5 g protein, 3.5 g fat, 1.5 g saturated fat, 59 mg cholesterol, 43 mg sodium, 1 g fiber

Carbohydrate Choices: 1

Dietary Exchanges: ½ starch, ½ fruit, ½ fat

NOTE: A flat spoon-shaped whisk, sold in kitchen supply stores, makes it foolproof to whisk the custard in the corners of the saucepan so it doesn't curdle.

GINGERED AUTUMN FRUIT CRISP

This homestyle classic is easy to prepare ahead of serving. The crystallized ginger adds that special flavor touch but doesn't overpower.

Preparation time: 25 minutes ● **Baking time: 55 minutes** ● **Standing time: 10 minutes**

FRUIT

- 3 tablespoons confectioners' sugar
- 2 teaspoons cornstarch
- 2 cups (about 1 pound) sliced Anjou or Bartlett pears
- 2 cups (about 1 pound) sliced McIntosh apples
- 2 cups (about 1 pound) sliced red or purple plums
- 2 tablespoons finely chopped crystallized ginger
- 2 teaspoons vanilla extract

TOPPING

- ¾ cup old-fashioned oats
- 2 tablespoons brown sugar
- ½ teaspoon apple pie spice
- 2 tablespoons cold Better Butter (page 323) or trans-fat free spread

1. Preheat the oven to 350°F. Coat an 8" × 8" baking dish with vegetable oil spray. Set aside.

2. To prepare the fruit: In a bowl, combine the confectioners' sugar and cornstarch. Stir until well blended. Add the pears, apples, plums, ginger, and vanilla. Toss to coat evenly. Transfer to the reserved dish. Set aside.

3. To prepare the topping: Wipe the bowl dry with a paper towel. Add the oats, brown sugar, and apple pie spice. Toss with a fork to mix. With the fork, break the Better Butter or spread into small chunks. Add to the mixture. Use the fork to cut into smaller pieces that blend with the oats mixture. Scatter over the reserved fruit.

4. Bake for about 55 minutes, or until golden and bubbly. Let stand for 10 minutes before serving. Serve warm or at room temperature.

MAKES 9 SERVINGS

Per serving: 152 calories, 32 g carbohydrate, 2 g protein, 2.5 g fat, 0.5 g saturated fat, 0 mg cholesterol, 22 mg sodium, 4 g fiber

Carbohydrate Choices: 2

Dietary Exchanges: 1 starch, 1½ fruit, ½ fat

NOTE: Apple pie spice is a ready-made blend of spices typically used to flavor apple pie: ground cinnamon, nutmeg, and allspice. If you don't have it, cinnamon may replace it.

RASPBERRY-ORANGE GELATIN MOLD

Serve this concoction in a martini glass with a dab of whipped cream sprinkled with a bit of finely grated orange peel for a light, refreshing dessert.

Preparation time: 15 minutes ● **Initial chilling time: 1 hour 30 minutes** ● **Final chilling: 2 hours**

2 cups cold water, divided
1 tablespoon plain gelatin
1 tablespoon sugar
1 cup orange juice with pulp
½ teaspoon orange extract
1 navel orange, peeled, sectioned, and cut into small chunks
1 cup raspberries, fresh or frozen loose-pack
Whipped cream (aerosol)

1. Place ½ cup water in a saucepan. Sprinkle on the gelatin. Allow to stand for 10 minutes.

2. Gradually add the remaining 1½ cups water while whisking constantly to partially dissolve the gelatin. Add the sugar. Cook over medium heat, whisking constantly, for 2 minutes, or until the gelatin is dissolved. Remove the saucepan from the heat. Stir in the orange juice and extract. Pour the mixture into an 8" × 8" baking dish. Refrigerate for 1½ hours, or until partially gelled.

3. Fold in the orange and raspberries. Cover and refrigerate for at least 2 hours, or until set. Serve with a spritz of whipped cream (2 tablespoons per serving).

MAKES 9 SERVINGS

Per serving: 66 calories, 10 g carbohydrate, 1 g protein, 2 g fat, 1.5 g saturated fat, 10 mg cholesterol, 3 mg sodium, 1 g fiber

Carbohydrate Choices: 1

Dietary Exchanges: ½ fruit, ½ fat

NOTE: One envelope of unflavored gelatin does not contain 1 tablespoon, so be sure to measure 1 level tablespoon of gelatin from several envelopes if necessary.

CANNOLI CREAM NAPOLEON

A cross between Italian cannoli (the filling) and French puff pastry, this dessert will leave you with a feeling of sweet sophistication.

Preparation time: 45 minutes ● **Baking time: 7 minutes**

---

4 tablespoons confectioners' sugar, divided + 1 teaspoon for garnish

3 sheets frozen whole wheat or regular phyllo dough, thawed

Vegetable oil in a spray bottle

1½ cups part-skim ricotta cheese

2 teaspoons grated orange peel

⅛ teaspoon orange extract

¼ cup natural pistachios, coarsely chopped

1 teaspoon unsweetened cocoa powder (optional)

1. Preheat the oven to 375°F. Transfer 2 tablespoons of the sugar to a small fine sieve, sifter, or dredger. On a work surface, lay out 1 sheet of dough so the shorter sides of the rectangle are left and right. Cut from top to bottom into 4 equal rectangles. Coat the top of 1 rectangle very lightly with vegetable oil. Dust very lightly with confectioners' sugar. Stack a second small rectangle on top of the first. Coat the top of the second rectangle very lightly with vegetable oil. Dust very lightly with confectioners' sugar. Repeat the procedure with the remaining 2 small rectangles. Spray and dust the top layer. Carefully transfer the pastry to a large nonstick baking sheet. Repeat cutting and layering with the remaining 2 whole sheets of phyllo dough to make 2 other layered pastries. Bake for about

7 minutes, or until crisp and browned. Let stand to cool.

2. In a bowl, combine the ricotta, 2 tablespoons sugar, orange peel, and extract. Stir with a wooden spoon until smooth. Place one of the reserved pastry on a rectangular serving plate or tray. Spread with half of the ricotta mixture. Sprinkle on half of the pistachios. Cover with the second pastry, the remainder of the ricotta mixture, and the remaining nuts. Top with the remaining pastry. In a small fine sieve, sifter, or dredger, combine the remaining 1 teaspoon sugar with the cocoa powder, if using. Sift over the top of the Napoleon. Cut with a serrated knife.

MAKES 8 SERVINGS

Per serving: 124 calories, 11 g carbohydrate, 7 g protein, 6 g fat, 2.5 g saturated fat, 14 mg cholesterol, 84 mg sodium, 1 g fiber

Carbohydrate Choices: 1

Dietary Exchanges: ½ starch, 1 meat, 1 fat

NOTE: This dessert is at its finest when served immediately after assembly, but it can be refrigerated, uncovered, for about 1½ hours without becoming soggy. Alternatively, you can bake the pastry and store it in a cool, dry spot for up to 24 hours. Prepare the ricotta mixture; cover and refrigerate for up to 24 hours. Assemble just before serving.

MANGO TREAT

Simple and luscious are two words that sum up this cool dessert. If you can't find mango sorbet in the supermarket, peach is equally good.

Preparation time: 3 minutes

⅓ cup low-fat vanilla yogurt

¼ cup mango sorbet

4 raspberries (garnish)

Place the yogurt in a bowl. Top with the sorbet. Garnish with raspberries.

MAKES 1 SERVING

Per serving: 133 calories, 31 g carbohydrate, 4 g protein, 1 g fat, 0.5 g saturated fat, 4 mg cholesterol, 59 mg sodium, 1 g fiber

Carbohydrate Choices: 2

Dietary Exchanges: 2 starch, ½ fat

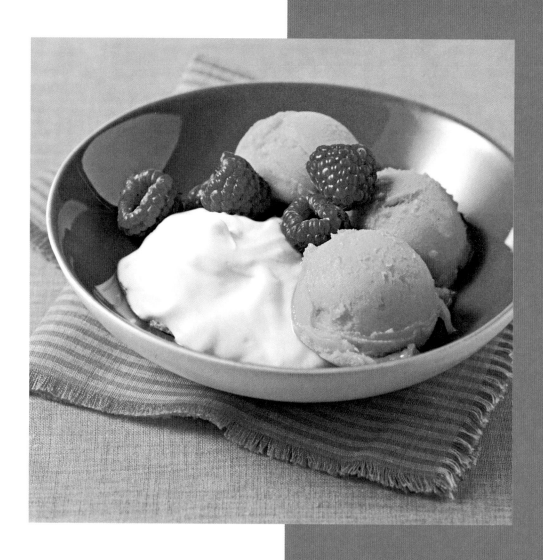

CHOCOLATE STRAWBERRIES

Choose firm but ripe strawberries for this decadent treat.

Preparation time: 3 minutes ● **Cooking time: 2 minutes** ● **Chilling time: 30 minutes**

3½ ounces high-quality dark chocolate
1 tablespoon fat-free milk
20 medium ripe strawberries with stems

1. Line a baking sheet with parchment paper.

2. Place the chocolate and milk in a microwaveable bowl. Microwave on high power for about 90 seconds, or until partially melted. Stir. If any chunks remain, microwave for an additional 20 seconds. Stir until smooth.

3. Holding the stem, dip each berry three-quarters into the chocolate mixture. Place on the prepared baking sheet, leaving 1" of space around each berry.

4. Refrigerate for 30 minutes, or until the chocolate sets.

MAKES 4 SERVINGS (5 STRAWBERRIES PER SERVING)

Per serving: 164 calories, 22 g carbohydrate, 2 g protein, 8 g fat, 5 g saturated fat, 2 mg cholesterol, 3 mg sodium, 4 g fiber

Carbohydrate Choices: 1½

Dietary Exchanges: 1 starch, ½ fruit, 1½ fat

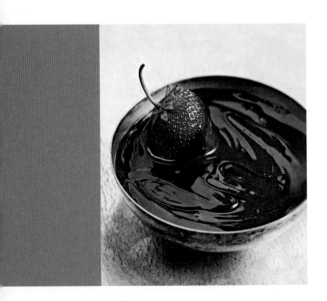

SPICY PUMPKIN MOUSSE
WITH MINI CHOCOLATE CHIPS

Although it may not be the first thing that comes to mind when you're indulging in this dessert, pumpkin is an outstanding source of vitamin A, a powerful compound that (among many other health benefits) boosts the immune system.

Preparation time: 15 minutes ● **Chilling time: 1 hour**

1 can (15 ounces) pumpkin puree
¼ cup pure maple syrup
1 teaspoon ground cinnamon
½ teaspoon ground ginger
¼ teaspoon ground cloves
2 cups frozen fat-free whipped topping, thawed
¼ cup semisweet mini chocolate chips

1. In a large bowl, combine the pumpkin, maple syrup, cinnamon, ginger, and cloves. Gently fold in the whipped topping until blended. Transfer to 4 individual serving bowls and top with the chocolate chips.

2. Chill for 1 hour or longer before serving.

MAKES 4 SERVINGS

Per serving: 202 calories, 41 g carbohydrate, 2 g protein, 3.5 g fat, 2 g saturated fat, 0 mg cholesterol, 29 mg sodium, 4 g fiber

Carbohydrate Choices: 3

Dietary Exchanges: 2 starch, ½ fat

LET YOURSELF GO/STRESS LESS

Sweet Dreams

Getting just the right amount of sleep each night could protect against type 2 diabetes. A Yale University study of 1,709 men found that those who regularly got less than 6 hours of shut-eye doubled their diabetes risk. Those who slept more than 8 hours tripled their odds. Previous studies have turned up similar findings in women. "When you sleep too little—or too long because of sleep apnea—your nervous system stays on alert," says lead researcher Klar Yaggi, MD, assistant professor of pulmonary medicine at Yale. This interferes with hormones that regulate blood sugar. A recent Columbia University study found that sleeping less than 5 hours also doubled the risk of high blood pressure. For a good night's rest, practice relaxation techniques or read nonstressful material before turning in. Avoid any novel by Stephen King and skip late-night TV and computer time.

CLEMENTINE LATTE COTTA
WITH BLUEBERRY SAUCE

The intense citrus in the cool, creamy gelatin accents the mellow blueberries. This dish is special enough for company.

Preparation time: 10 minutes • **Cooking time: 10 minutes** • **Chilling time: 3 hours**

CUSTARD

- 1¾ cups whole milk, divided
- 2 teaspoons plain gelatin
- 3 tablespoons sugar
- 2 tablespoons finely grated clementine or tangerine peel
- Pinch of salt
- 3 tablespoons fresh clementine or tangerine juice

SAUCE

- 1 cup frozen blueberries, thawed
- 1 tablespoon sugar
- 1 tablespoon water

1. Coat four 6-ounce custard cups or 5-ounce ramekins with vegetable oil spray.

2. To prepare the custard: Pour ¼ cup of the milk into a small, heatproof bowl, sprinkle with gelatin, and let stand for 5 minutes. Place the bowl in a larger bowl of hot water and stir until the gelatin dissolves.

3. Meanwhile, in a medium saucepan, combine the sugar, clementine or tangerine peel, salt, and the remaining 1½ cups milk. Bring just to a boil over medium heat. Reduce the heat to low and cook for 5 minutes, stirring frequently, at a bare simmer. Remove the saucepan from the heat. Stir in the gelatin mixture and the juice. Pour through a fine strainer into a 4-cup glass measuring cup.

4. Evenly divide the milk mixture among the custard cups. Chill, loosely covered, for at least 3 hours, or until set.

5. To prepare the sauce: In a medium saucepan, combine the blueberries, sugar, and water. Cook over medium heat, stirring, for about 5 minutes, or until softened and a sauce forms.

6. Dip the bottom of each custard cup into a bowl of hot water for about 10 seconds and run a table knife around the inner edge. Invert onto serving plates and serve with sauce.

MAKES 4 SERVINGS

Per serving: 149 calories, 26 g carbohydrate, 4 g protein, 4 g fat, 2 g saturated fat, 15 mg cholesterol, 65 mg sodium, 1 g fiber

Carbohydrate Choices: 2

Dietary Exchanges: 1 starch, ½ fruit

NOTE: If desired, the sauce can be refrigerated, tightly covered, up to 1 week.

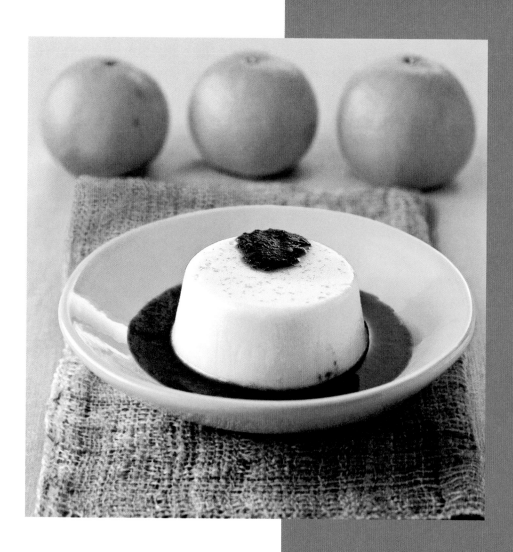

RED, WHITE, AND BLUE CHEESECAKE

For an Independence Day picnic or any special summer festivity, this dessert will make the event. Choose ripe berries that are bursting with sweet juices.

Preparation time: 20 minutes ● **Cooking time: 45 minutes** ● **Cooling time: 30 minutes** **Chilling time: 4 hours**

¼ cup dry bran cereal crumbs

3 packages (8 ounces each) fat-free cream cheese, at room temperature

1 cup confectioners' sugar

3 egg whites + 1 egg, separated

¾ cup fat-free plain yogurt

1 tablespoon + 1 teaspoon vanilla extract

1 teaspoon grated lemon peel

1 tablespoon cornstarch

¼ cup blueberries

1 pint medium strawberries, trimmed to uniform size (about 3 cups)

1. Arrange a rack in the bottom third of the oven. Preheat the oven to 325°F. Coat the bottom and sides of a 9" springform pan with vegetable oil spray. Sprinkle the crumbs evenly over the pan bottom. Set aside.

2. In the bowl of an electric mixer, combine the cream cheese and sugar. On medium speed, beat until smooth. (If lumps remain, use a spatula to smooth them before proceeding.) Reduce the speed to low, adding the egg whites and egg, one at a time, as you continue to mix. Add the yogurt, vanilla, and lemon peel. Mix to incorporate, being careful not to overbeat. Add the cornstarch and mix until just combined. Pour the batter into the reserved pan.

3. Bake for 40 to 45 minutes, or until the top is well set, but the center is still slightly soft and the edge is light golden brown.

4. Remove the pan from the oven. Run a butter knife around the inner edge but do not remove the pan side. Let stand to cool for 30 minutes before refrigerating. Chill at least 4 hours before serving.

5. Remove the pan side. With the berries, decorate the cake to resemble a flag: Place the blueberries in the upper left and then arrange the strawberries in horizontal rows to cover the remainder of the cake. Cut and serve.

MAKES 12 SERVINGS

Per serving: 140 calories, 21 g carbohydrate, 11 g protein, 0.5 g fat, 0 g saturated fat, 25 mg cholesterol, 320 mg sodium, 1 g fiber

Carbohydrate Choices: 1½

Dietary Exchanges: 1 starch, 1½ meat

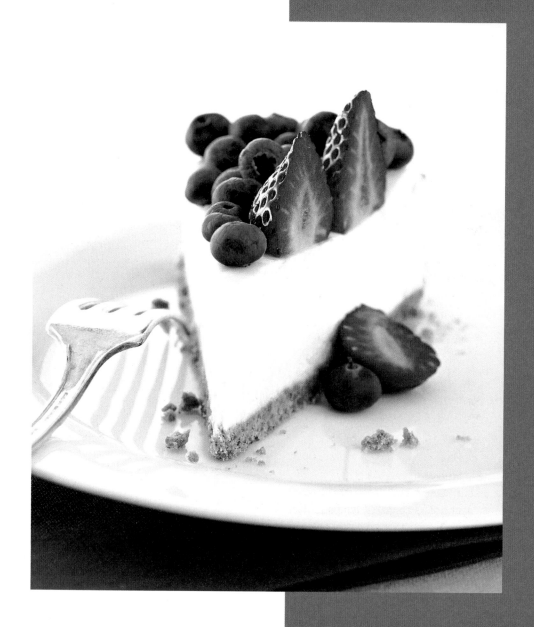

PARFAIT PRESTO

This treat is not only palate-pleasing, it's pretty to look at as well.

Preparation time: 7 minutes

½ cup raspberries

½ cup nonfat yogurt, divided

3 teaspoons granola

¼ cup banana slices

¼ cup kiwifruit slices

Fat-free whipped topping (optional)

Spoon a small handful of raspberries into the bottom of a parfait, pilsner, or tall wine glass. Top with about ¼ cup of yogurt, a teaspoon of granola, and banana and kiwifruit slices, followed by another dollop of yogurt. Continue layering, ending with granola. Top the parfait with fruit and fat-free whipped topping, if desired.

MAKES 1 SERVING

Per serving: 176 calories, 35 g carbohydrate, 8 g protein, 2.5 g fat, 0.5 g saturated fat, 3 mg cholesterol, 71 mg sodium, 7 g fiber

Carbohydrate Choices: 3

Dietary Exchanges: ½ starch, 2 fruit, ½ milk

UNLEASH NUTRIENTS

Dried Fruit Yogurt

In a classic case of mucking up a good thing, some food manufacturers now add so much sweetener to yogurt that it may as well be candy. For an everyday dessert that is naturally sweet but also loaded with calcium and fiber, mix cut-up dried fruits into plain fat-free yogurt. Select dried fruits that have no sugar added to them (they're sweet enough on their own because the natural sugars have been concentrated as the moisture content evaporates). Dates, raisins, apricots, and plums are all fine options. Chop them into small bits. Stir about 2 tablespoons of fruit into ½ cup of yogurt. Stir in ¼ teaspoon lemon, orange, or vanilla extract for additional flavor with no calories or carbohydrates.

COCONUT CUSTARD BRÛLÉE

For coconut lovers, this rich treat is the real deal for a once-in-awhile indulgence on the maintenance phase of your weight-loss program. The luscious coconut milk mimics the thick cream that would be used in a traditional crème brûlée.

Preparation time: 8 minutes   ●   Cooking time: 7 minutes   ●   Chilling time: 4 hours

---

⅓ cup confectioners' sugar

¼ cup cornstarch

2½ cups canned light coconut milk

3 eggs, beaten

Dash of salt

1½ teaspoons coconut extract

2 tablespoons brown sugar

1. Coat the insides of six ½-cup heatproof custard cups or ramekins with vegetable oil spray. Place them on a tray and set aside.

2. In a wide saucepan, combine the confectioners' sugar and cornstarch. While whisking constantly, gradually add the coconut milk until the mixture is smooth. Pass through a fine sieve set over a bowl or large measuring cup. With a spatula, press any lumps of cornstarch or sugar through the sieve. Return the milk mixture to the pan.

3. Add the eggs and salt. Whisk until smooth. Set over medium heat. Cook, whisking constantly, for 4 to 5 minutes, or until the mixture bubbles and thickens.

4. Remove the saucepan from the heat, continuing to whisk rapidly to cool down the mixture. Stir in the extract. Transfer the custard to the reserved dishes. With the back of a small spoon, smooth the tops to flatten. Cover with plastic and refrigerate for at least 4 hours, or until cold.

5. To serve the custards, preheat the broiler. Sprinkle the brown sugar evenly over the tops of the custards. Broil 6" from the heat source for 1 to 2 minutes, or until the sugar is caramelized. Watch carefully so the sugar doesn't burn.

MAKES 6 SERVINGS

Per serving: 159 calories, 20 g carbohydrate, 4 g protein, 2.5 g fat, 0.5 g saturated fat, 106 mg cholesterol, 86 mg sodium, 0 g fiber

Carbohydrate Choices: 1

Dietary Exchanges: 1 starch, ½ meat

NOTES: Be sure to purchase unsweetened coconut milk, not sweetened canned cream of coconut, for this recipe.

The custard must bubble vigorously to thicken. The cornstarch prevents the eggs from curdling.

BREAD PUDDING DRIZZLED WITH HONEY WHISKEY

This soufflé-like pudding gets a touch of pizzazz from the whiskey in the sauce. Vanilla extract can replace the whiskey if desired.

Preparation time: 15 minutes ● **Baking time: 35 minutes**

---

2 eggs, separated + 2 egg whites
Pinch of salt
1½ cups whole milk
¼ cup brown sugar
2 teaspoons vanilla extract
2 teaspoons Better Butter (page 323) or trans-fat free spread, melted
⅛ teaspoon ground nutmeg
3 cups cubed whole wheat bread
¼ cup honey
2 teaspoons whiskey
Pinch of ground cinnamon

1. Preheat the oven to 350°F. Coat an 8" × 8" baking dish with vegetable oil spray. Set aside.

2. Place the 4 egg whites and salt in the bowl of an electric mixer. Beat on low speed for about 1 minute, or until the whites are foamy. Increase the speed to high. Beat for about 1 minute, or until the whites hold soft peaks.

3. In another bowl, beat the egg yolks with a fork. Add the milk, sugar, vanilla, Better Butter or spread, and nutmeg. Beat to blend. Add the bread. Press with the back of a fork until the bread absorbs the liquid. Gently pour into the bowl with the beaten whites. Fold to incorporate. Transfer to the prepared pan.

4. Bake for about 35 minutes, or until risen and only slightly jiggly in the center. If the top is browning too fast, cover lightly with a sheet of aluminum foil.

5. Meanwhile, in a microwaveable bowl, combine the honey, whiskey, and cinnamon. Microwave on high power for about 1 minute, or until bubbling. Whisk until smooth. Spoon the warm pudding onto dessert plates. Drizzle with the honey whiskey.

MAKES 9 SERVINGS

Per serving: 130 calories, 20 g carbohydrate, 5 g protein, 3.5 g fat, 1.5 g saturated fat, 51 mg cholesterol, 132 mg sodium, 1 g fiber

Carbohydrate Choices: 1½

Dietary Exchanges: 1 starch, ½ meat, ½ fat

GERMAN APPLE PANCAKE

The right pan size is important to the success of this delightful homespun dessert. If you don't have an ovenproof 10" skillet that is at least 2" deep, cook the apples in a skillet and transfer to a deep 10" round baking dish.

Preparation time: 20 minutes ● **Cooking time: 15 minutes**

APPLES

- 2 tablespoons Better Butter (page 323) or trans-fat free spread
- 3 medium Golden Delicious apples, sliced (1 pound)
- 2 tablespoons brown sugar
- 1 teaspoon apple pie spice

PANCAKE

- 2 eggs, separated
- Pinch of salt
- 1 tablespoon confectioners' sugar + extra for dusting
- ¾ cup all-purpose flour
- ¼ cup soy flour
- 1 teaspoon baking powder
- ¾ cup whole milk
- 1½ teaspoons lemon extract

1. Preheat the oven to 375°F.

2. To prepare the apples: In an ovenproof 10" nonstick skillet, melt the Better Butter or spread over medium-high heat. Add the apples, brown sugar, and spice. Cover and cook, tossing frequently, for about 4 minutes, or until softened. Remove from the heat.

3. To prepare the pancake: While the apples are cooking, place the egg whites and salt in the bowl of an electric mixer. Beat on low speed for about 1 minute, or until foamy. Increase the mixer speed to high. Beat, adding 1 tablespoon confectioners' sugar, for 1 to 2 minutes, or until soft peaks form. Set aside.

4. In a mixing bowl, combine the flours and baking powder. Stir with a fork to mix. In a small bowl, use a fork to beat the milk with the egg yolks and extract. Add to the dry ingredients. Stir to blend. Transfer the whites to the bowl. Fold to mix. Dollop the batter over the apples.

5. Bake for about 15 minutes, or until puffed and golden. Dust lightly with confectioners' sugar. Cut into wedges.

MAKES 8 SERVINGS

Per serving: 151 calories, 22 g carbohydrate, 5 g protein, 5 g fat, 1.5 g saturated fat, 55 mg cholesterol, 131 mg sodium, 2 g fiber

Carbohydrate Choices: 1½

Dietary Exchanges: 1 starch, ½ fruit, 1 fat

CHOCOLATE CREAM BANANA PIE

Chocolate and bananas in a crunchy crumb crust is a mouthwatering creation. Although you need to allow time for cooling and chilling the pudding, the actual preparation is a snap. In fact, it's the kind of dessert you can prepare in stages.

Preparation time: 15 minutes • Chilling time: 5 hours 30 minutes • Cooking time: 5 minutes

½ cup all-fiber cereal crumbs
⅛ teaspoon ground cinnamon
1½ tablespoons cold Better Butter (page 323) or trans-fat free spread
¼ cup brown sugar
2½ tablespoons cornstarch
1 egg
2 cups fat-free milk
2 ounces bittersweet chocolate, chopped
1 teaspoon vanilla extract
1 ripe but firm banana
Whipped cream (optional)

1. Coat a pie pan with vegetable oil spray. In a bowl, combine the crumbs and cinnamon with a fork. Cut in the Better Butter or spread until well blended. Transfer to the prepared pan. Tilt the pan to coat the side with crumbs. Press the remaining crumbs with your knuckles to flatten evenly. Set in the freezer for 30 minutes.

2. Meanwhile, in a saucepan, combine the sugar and cornstarch. Whisk to mix. In a bowl, beat the egg with a fork. Add the milk and stir to blend. Add to the saucepan, whisking constantly, or until blended. Cook, stirring constantly, over medium heat for about 5 minutes, or until thickened. Remove from the heat. Add the chocolate and vanilla. Stir until the chocolate melts. Let stand, stirring occasionally, to cool completely.

3. Cut the banana into thin slices. Arrange on the bottom and sides of the reserved crust. Dollop the cooled pudding into the pan. Refrigerate for at least 5 hours, or until set.

4. Serve, garnished with 1 tablespoon of whipped cream (if using) per slice.

MAKES 8 SERVINGS

Per serving: 145 calories, 21 g carbohydrate, 4 g protein, 6.5 g fat, 3 g saturated fat, 33 mg cholesterol, 71 mg sodium, 3 g fiber

Carbohydrate Choices: 1½

Dietary Exchanges: 1 starch, 1 fat

NOW YOU KNOW

Sweets and desserts can be high in carbohydrates and raise glucose levels significantly. For better blood glucose control, include dessert with a low-carbohydrate meal. For instance, having cake with a meat and green vegetable dinner will not raise glucose levels as much as having cake with a pasta meal.

ICED LEMON CUPCAKES

Great with a cup of tea, these baked goods are sweet-tart, moist, and satisfying.

Preparation time: 15 minutes ● **Baking time: 15 minutes**

¾ cup all-purpose flour

⅓ cup fat-free soy flour

¾ teaspoon baking powder

½ teaspoon baking soda

   Pinch of salt

⅓ cup Better Butter (page 323) or trans-fat free spread + 2 teaspoons, divided, at room temperature

1 cup confectioners' sugar, divided

1½ teaspoons grated lemon peel

2 eggs

½ cup plain fat-free yogurt

½ teaspoon lemon extract

2–3 teaspoons lemon juice

1. Preheat the oven to 350°F. Line a 12-cup muffin pan with paper liners. Lightly coat the inside of the liners with vegetable oil spray.

2. In a mixing bowl, combine the flours, baking powder, baking soda, and salt. Stir to blend.

3. In the bowl of an electric mixer, beat ⅓ cup Better Butter or spread for 1 minute, or until smooth. Add ½ cup sugar and the lemon peel. Beat for 30 seconds, or until smooth. Add the eggs, one at a time, beating after each addition. Add the yogurt and lemon extract. Mix on low speed to blend. Gradually add the reserved dry ingredients, mixing on low speed to blend. Dollop the batter into the prepared cups.

4. Bake for about 15 minutes, or until the cupcakes are lightly browned and spring back when pressed. Remove to a rack to cool completely.

5. In a small bowl, combine the remaining ½ cup sugar, the remaining 2 teaspoons Better Butter or spread, and 2 teaspoons lemon juice. Whisk until smooth. Add up to 1 teaspoon more lemon juice if needed to make a spreadable consistency. Spread over the cupcakes.

MAKES 12 SERVINGS

Per serving: 134 calories, 18 g carbohydrate, 4 g protein, 5 g fat, 1.5 g saturated fat, 35 mg cholesterol, 147 mg sodium, 1 g fiber

Carbohydrate Choices: 1

Dietary Exchanges: 1 starch, 1 fat

NOTE: Store any leftover iced cupcakes in a tightly sealed plastic storage container in the freezer for up to 1 month. Let stand at room temperature for 1 hour to thaw.

DEVIL'S FOOD AND CHEESECAKE CUPCAKES

Two all-time favorite desserts in one cupcake make a doubly delicious treat. These little cakes freeze well if you don't have enough eaters for the whole batch.

Preparation time: 25 minutes ● **Baking time: 20 minutes**

1 cup all-purpose flour

⅓ cup unsweetened cocoa powder

¾ teaspoon baking soda

Dash of salt

3 tablespoons canola oil

2 tablespoons Better Butter (page 323) or trans-fat free spread, at room temperature

1 ounce unsweetened baking chocolate, chopped

⅔ cup + 3 tablespoons sugar

2 teaspoons vanilla extract, divided

1 egg, beaten

⅓ cup reduced-fat buttermilk

⅓ cup hot water

¼ cup (2 ounces) reduced-fat cream cheese, at room temperature

¼ cup (2 ounces) fat-free cream cheese, at room temperature

1. Preheat the oven to 350°F. Line a 12-cup muffin pan with paper liners. Lightly coat the inside of the liners with vegetable oil spray.

2. On a sheet of waxed paper, combine the flour, cocoa powder, baking soda, and salt. Stir to blend. Set aside.

3. In a microwaveable bowl, combine the oil, Better Butter or spread, and chocolate. Microwave on high power for 1 minute, or until hot. Stir until smooth. Transfer to a mixing bowl. Add ⅔ cup sugar and 1 teaspoon vanilla. Beat with a wooden spoon until smooth.

4. Measure 3 tablespoons of the egg and add to the batter. (Reserve the remainder.) Beat until smooth. Gradually add the reserved dry ingredients alternately with the buttermilk and water. Mix until blended. Dollop 1 heaping tablespoon of batter into each cup in the reserved pan.

5. In a bowl, beat the cream cheeses with a wooden spoon until very smooth. Add the remaining 3 tablespoons sugar, the remaining amount of the beaten egg, and the remaining 1 teaspoon vanilla. Blend slowly to incorporate and then beat until very smooth. Dollop the batter in equal amounts in the center of each cup. Cover evenly with the remaining chocolate batter. Swirl with the back of a spoon to even the tops.

6. Bake for about 20 minutes, or until a cupcake springs back when pressed lightly with a finger.

MAKES 12 SERVINGS (1 CUPCAKE PER SERVING)

Per serving: 185 calories, 25 g carbohydrate, 4 g protein, 8 g fat, 3 g saturated fat, 26 mg cholesterol, 159 mg sodium, 2 g fiber

Carbohydrate Choices: 1½

Dietary Exchanges: 1½ starch, 1½ fat

NOTE: Be sure to beat the egg well with a fork before measuring by tablespoonfuls. If the egg white clumps are too big, it may be hard to get an equal blend of yolk and white.

BLUEBERRIES AND LIME CREAM TART

Who knew a cheesecake could be this easy to make yet be so scrumptious? It offers just the right amount of creaminess and fruitiness.

Preparation time: 40 minutes ● **Chilling time: 3 hours 30 minutes**

---

2 tablespoons honey

2 teaspoons cornstarch

1½ cups blueberries, fresh or frozen

¼ cup all-fiber cereal crumbs

⅛ teaspoon ground cinnamon

1 tablespoon cold Better Butter (page 323) or trans-fat free spread

1 package (8 ounces) reduced-fat cream cheese, at room temperature

2 tablespoons confectioners' sugar
Grated peel and juice of 1 lime

1. Coat an 8" springform pan with vegetable oil spray. Set aside.

2. In a saucepan, combine the honey and cornstarch. Mix until blended. Add the blueberries. Cook over medium heat, stirring gently, for 4 to 5 minutes, or until the mixture bubbles. Remove and let stand until cooled to room temperature.

3. Meanwhile, in a bowl, combine the crumbs and cinnamon with a fork. Cut in the Better Butter or spread until well blended. Transfer to the prepared pan. Press with your knuckles to flatten evenly. Set in the freezer for 30 minutes.

4. Meanwhile, wipe the crumb bowl with a paper towel. Add the cream cheese, sugar, lime peel, and juice. Slowly mix to incorporate, then beat by hand until very smooth. Dollop into the pan. Spread evenly with a spatula. Dollop on the blueberry mixture. Spread evenly over the surface to the edge of the pan.

5. Cover and refrigerate for 3 hours, or until set.

MAKES 8 SERVINGS

Per serving: 114 calories, 15 g carbohydrate, 3 g protein, 6 g fat, 3 g saturated fat, 14 mg cholesterol, 130 mg sodium, 3 g fiber

Carbohydrate Choices: 1

Dietary Exchanges: ½ starch, ½ fruit, ½ meat, 1 fat

BANANA SNACK CAKE

The cake is destined to become a family favorite—moist, high, sweet enough, absolutely satisfying.

Preparation time: 25 minutes ● **Baking time: 30 minutes**

---

1 **cup whole wheat pastry flour**
½ **teaspoon baking soda**
½ **teaspoon baking powder**
  Pinch of salt
1 **egg, separated + 2 egg whites**
½ **cup granulated sugar, divided**
¼ **cup canola oil**
½ **cup mashed ripe banana**
¼ **cup low-fat buttermilk**
2 **teaspoons confectioners' sugar**
2 **teaspoons unsweetened cocoa powder**

1. Preheat the oven to 350°F. Coat an 8" × 8" baking pan with vegetable oil spray. Dust with flour; set aside.

2. On a sheet of waxed paper or in a bowl, combine the flour, baking soda, baking powder, and salt. Whisk to combine. Set aside.

3. Place the 3 egg whites in the bowl of an electric mixer. Beat on high speed for about 2 minutes, or until the whites are foamy. Continue beating, while adding 2 tablespoons granulated sugar, for about 1 minute, or until the whites hold their peaks. Set aside. Do not wash the beaters.

4. In a clean mixing bowl, combine the oil and remaining 6 tablespoons sugar. Beat until smooth. One at a time, beat in the egg yolk, banana, and buttermilk, mixing well. Gradually add the reserved dry ingredients, mixing on low speed until smooth. Stir a large spoonful of the reserved egg whites into the batter. Fold in the remaining whites. Pour the batter into the reserved pan; spread the top evenly.

5. Bake for 30 to 35 minutes, or until golden and the cake starts to come away from the sides of the pan. Allow to cool in the pan on a rack for 5 minutes. Turn onto the rack to cool completely.

6. To serve, in a small bowl, combine the confectioners' sugar and cocoa powder. Place in a small sieve and sift over the top of the cake.

MAKES 9 SERVINGS

Per serving: 176 calories, 25 g carbohydrate, 3 g protein, 7 g fat, 1 g saturated fat, 24 mg cholesterol, 136 mg sodium, 2 g fiber

Carbohydrate Choices: 2

Dietary Exchanges: 1 starch, 1 fat

NOTE: For a fancier dessert, garnish each piece with 1 tablespoon whipped cream dusted with a bit of unsweetened cocoa powder.

ORANGE SOUFFLÉ WITH SHAVED DARK CHOCOLATE

If you want a showstopper after a special occasion meal, here it is! It looks spectacular and tastes divine but is truly quick and easy to prepare.

Preparation time: 15 minutes ● **Baking time: 15 minutes**

---

1 teaspoon Better Butter (page 323) or trans-fat free spread

2 teaspoons sugar

½ cup chunky orange marmalade

1 tablespoon orange liqueur or 1 teaspoon orange extract

1 teaspoon grated lemon peel

6 egg whites, at room temperature Pinch of cream of tartar

1 ounce bittersweet chocolate, shaved

1. Preheat the oven to 400°F. Coat a 1½-quart (6 cups) soufflé dish or other baking dish with the Better Butter or spread. Sprinkle in the sugar. Tilt the dish to coat the bottom and sides. Set aside.

2. In a large bowl, combine the marmalade, liqueur or extract, and lemon peel. Whisk until blended. Set aside.

3. In the bowl of an electric mixer, combine the egg whites and cream of tartar. Beat on medium speed for about 2 minutes, or until foamy. Increase the speed to high and beat for about 1 minute, or until soft peaks form. Fold the beaten whites into the orange marmalade mixture. Some streaks of white can remain. Carefully transfer to the prepared baking dish. Level the top with a spatula. With a finger or thumb, create a shallow indentation around the inner side of the dish.

4. Bake for about 15 minutes, or until puffed and set near the sides (the center should be a bit jiggly). Spoon onto dessert plates. Sprinkle on the chocolate.

MAKES 6 SERVINGS

Per serving: 125 calories, 23 g carbohydrate, 4 g protein, 3 g fat, 1 g saturated fat, 0 mg cholesterol, 76 mg sodium, 1 g fiber

Carbohydrate Choices: 1½

Dietary Exchanges: 1½ starch, ½ meat, ½ fat

NOTES: The flavor of this dessert depends on choosing the best-quality orange marmalade, one that contains chunks of fruit.

If you own a good-quality electric mixer with a whisk attachment, you can easily prepare this glorious dessert.

Make sure your soufflé dish is big enough so the whites have room to rise. If you're unsure, pour 1½ quarts (6 cups) of water into the dish to test the volume before baking.

Before preheating the oven, make certain that one oven rack is positioned in the center of the oven with no other rack above it. You wouldn't want your masterpiece to run into a rack as it rises!

Over a plate or a sheet of waxed paper, shave the edge of the chocolate piece with a vegetable peeler. Reserve in a cool spot until serving time.

DARK CHOCOLATE SOUFFLÉ CAKES WITH RASPBERRIES

A great dessert for a special occasion. It is very easy to make, and the warm, soft chocolate just glides over your tongue.

Preparation time: 30 minutes ● **Baking time: 10 minutes**

½ cup unsweetened cocoa powder

⅓ cup whole wheat pastry flour

¼ cup brown sugar

1½ cups 1% milk

2 eggs, separated, at room temperature

¼ cup Better Butter (page 323) or trans-fat free spread

2 teaspoons raspberry or almond extract

2 egg whites, at room temperature
  Pinch of cream of tartar or salt

18 fresh raspberries (6 ounces)
  Confectioners' sugar (optional)

1. Preheat the oven to 375°F. Coat 8 individual brioche molds or other ½-cup baking dishes with vegetable oil spray. Set on a sturdy baking pan. Set aside.

2. In a saucepan, combine the cocoa powder, flour, and brown sugar. Whisk to blend. In a bowl, beat the milk and egg yolks with a fork until blended. Gradually whisk into the cocoa mixture until dissolved. Cook, whisking constantly, for 5 minutes, or until bubbling and thickened. Remove from the heat. Whisk in the Better Butter or spread and the raspberry or almond extract. Let stand to cool slightly.

3. In the bowl of an electric mixer, combine the 4 egg whites and the cream of tartar or salt. Beat on medium speed for about 2 minutes, or until foamy. Increase the mixer speed to high. Beat for 2 minutes, or until soft peaks form. Stir one-third of the whites into the reserved chocolate mixture. Pour the chocolate mixture into the bowl. Fold to incorporate. Dollop gently into the prepared pans.

4. Bake for 10 minutes, or until the cakes have risen and set on top but are still slightly soft in the center. Remove from the oven and let stand for 5 minutes. Turn each cake onto a dessert plate. Serve warm with raspberries and a dusting of confectioners' sugar if desired.

MAKES 8 SERVINGS

Per serving: 146 calories, 16 g carbohydrate, 6 g protein, 7 g fat, 2.5 g saturated fat, 55 mg cholesterol, 100 mg sodium, 4 g fiber

Carbohydrate Choices: 1

Dietary Exchanges: ½ starch, 1 fat

CLEMENTINE UPSIDE-DOWN CAKE

This scrumptious confection may look like it came from a professional bakery, but it's surprisingly easy to prepare.

Preparation time: 20 minutes • Baking time: 30 minutes

½ stick (¼ cup) butter, melted
¾ cup brown sugar
2 clementines, peeled
⅔ cup all-purpose flour
⅓ cup fat-free soy flour
1 teaspoon baking powder
½ teaspoon baking soda
½ teaspoon ground cinnamon
Dash of salt
2 eggs
½ cup fat-free plain yogurt
¼ cup canola oil
1 teaspoon orange extract

1. Preheat the oven to 350°F. Coat a 9" round cake pan with vegetable oil spray. Drizzle the butter evenly over the bottom. Scatter ¼ cup sugar into the pan bottom. Press with a fork to spread the sugar evenly. Separate the clementines into sections. With a small knife, cut each section in half lengthwise to create two skinny half-moons. Lay the section halves, cut side up, in a spiral starting at the outer edge of the pan. Continue laying the sections in spirals, not overlapping, until the pan bottom is completely covered. Set aside.

2. On a sheet of waxed paper, combine the flours, baking powder, baking soda, cinnamon, and salt. Blend with a fork. In a bowl, beat the eggs, yogurt, and oil with a fork until smooth. Add the remaining ½ cup sugar and the extract. Beat until smooth. Stir in the dry ingredients. Dollop the batter carefully into the prepared pan.

3. Bake for about 30 minutes, or until browned and a tester inserted in the center comes out clean. Remove from the oven. Let stand for 5 minutes. Place a heatproof platter over the pan. Holding the platter and the pan firmly with oven mitts, turn over the cake onto the tray. Using a serrated knife, cut the cake into wedges. Serve warm.

MAKES 12 SERVINGS

Per serving: 167 calories, 18 g carbohydrate, 4 g protein, 9 g fat, 3 g saturated fat, 45 mg cholesterol, 146 mg sodium, 1 g fiber

Carbohydrate Choices: 1

Dietary Exchanges: 1 starch, 2 fat

NOTE: Select fat-free (check the nutrition facts label) soy flour, which is now sold in many supermarkets and also natural food stores. It gives a protein boost to baked goods and adds moisture. Store the opened flour in the refrigerator or freezer.

CHEWY MOLASSES COOKIES

These are perfect little spice gems whether they're enjoyed with an afternoon glass of milk or an evening small glass of red wine.

Preparation time: 25 minutes ● **Baking time: 8 minutes**

---

2 cups whole wheat pastry flour

1½ teaspoons baking soda

1½ teaspoons ground cinnamon

1 teaspoon ground ginger

¼ teaspoon ground allspice

Pinch of salt

½ cup Better Butter (page 323) or trans-fat free spread

½ cup brown sugar

¼ cup dark molasses

1 egg white

1. Preheat the oven to 350°F. Lightly coat several cookie sheets with vegetable oil spray. On a sheet of waxed paper, combine the flour, baking soda, cinnamon, ginger, allspice, and salt. Stir with a fork to blend. Set aside.

2. In the bowl of an electric mixer, beat the Better Butter or spread until smooth. Add the sugar, molasses, and egg white. Mix slowly to incorporate, then beat until smooth. Gradually stir in the reserved flour mixture until well blended. The dough will be soft but not sticky.

3. Using your palms, roll the dough into ¾" balls (1 level teaspoon). Place, separated, on the prepared pans.

4. Bake for 8 minutes, or until the edges are set. Let stand on the sheet for 5 minutes, then remove to a rack to cool. Continue until all the dough is baked.

MAKES 70 COOKIES (3 COOKIES PER SERVING)

Per serving: 90 calories, 14 g carbohydrate, 1 g protein, 3.5 g fat, 1 g saturated fat, 0 mg cholesterol, 123 mg sodium, 1 g fiber

Carbohydrate Choices: 1

Dietary Exchanges: ½ starch, ½ fat

NOTE: The cookies can be stored in an airtight tin for up to a week or frozen for up to 3 months.

BABY BANANA SPLITS

When is the ultimate splurge not a splurge? When you have a Baby Banana Split.

Preparation time: 20 minutes

---

2 ounces bittersweet chocolate, chopped

1 tablespoon whole milk

1 ripe but firm banana

1⅓ cups Slow Churned Lite Ice Cream (4 small scoops)

8 strawberries or ½ cup sliced partially thawed loose-pack strawberries

½ cup chopped pineapple, fresh or canned in juice, drained

Whipped cream (aerosol)

2 tablespoons roasted unsalted peanuts, chopped

1. In a small microwaveable dish, combine the chocolate and milk. Microwave for 30 seconds, or until hot. Stir until smooth. Set aside.

2. Cut the banana in half through the middle. Slice each half lengthwise into 4 slices.

3. Set out 4 shallow dessert dishes. Place a scoop of ice cream in each dish. Put a banana slice on the sides of each scoop. Top with strawberries and pineapple. Drizzle on the reserved chocolate sauce. Top with a spritz (about 1 tablespoon) of whipped cream. Sprinkle on the peanuts. Serve right away.

MAKES 4 SERVINGS

Per serving: 250 calories, 35 g carbohydrate, 5 g protein, 12 g fat, 5.5 g saturated fat, 14 mg cholesterol, 33 mg sodium, 4 g fiber

Carbohydrate Choices: 2

Dietary Exchanges: 2 starch, 1 fruit, ½ meat, 2 fat

LOOSEN UP/GET MOVING

Movement Motivators

We all need an extra something to get going. Try these methods to energize your fitness program.

- Find an exercise buddy. Many people find that they are more likely to do something active if a friend or partner joins them.

- Keep track of your physical activity. Write down when you exercise and for how long in your blood glucose record book. You'll be able to track your progress and to see how physical activity affects your blood glucose.

- Reward yourself. Do something nice for yourself when you reach your activity goals. For example, treat yourself to a movie or buy a new plant for the garden.

CHOCOLATE ALMOND BISCOTTI

Light, crunchy, nutty, and layered with chocolate flavors, these Italian cookies are the perfect after-dinner treat.

Preparation time: 45 minutes ● **Baking time: 35 minutes**

1½ cups whole wheat pastry flour
½ cup Dutch cocoa powder
2 teaspoons baking soda
   Pinch of salt
½ cup sugar
⅓ cup packed brown sugar
3 eggs, at room temperature
1½ teaspoons vanilla extract
2 ounces unsweetened baking chocolate, chopped into small chunks
1½ cups sliced almonds

1. Place a rack in the center of the oven and preheat the oven to 350°F. Line a baking sheet with parchment paper.

2. Sift together the flour, cocoa powder, baking soda, and salt, and transfer to a large mixing bowl. Blend in the sugars with an electric mixer.

3. In a small bowl, whisk the eggs with the vanilla. Add to the dry ingredients. Blend on low speed until thoroughly combined. Scrape down the sides of the bowl with a rubber spatula as needed.

4. Add the chocolate and almonds and blend thoroughly. (The dough will be very stiff and sticky.)

5. Dust your hands with flour. Place the dough on a clean work surface liberally dusted with flour. Divide the dough into two equal pieces. Shape each into a 10" × 2" × ¾" log. Place on the prepared pan, 2" apart.

6. Bake for about 20 minutes, or until set. Remove from the oven and let rest for 10 minutes. Lower the oven temperature to 325°F.

7. Cut the logs diagonally into ½" slices. Place the slices on their sides on the baking sheet. Bake for 15 to 20 minutes, or until firm. Transfer the biscotti to racks to cool.

MAKES 18 SERVINGS (2 BISCOTTI PER SERVING)

Per serving: 159 calories, 21 g carbohydrate, 5 g protein, 9 g fat, 1.5 g saturated fat, 35 mg cholesterol, 162 mg sodium, 3 g fiber

Carbohydrate Choices: 1½

Dietary Exchanges: 1 starch, ½ meat, 1 fat

NOTE: Store in an airtight container at room temperature for up to 2 weeks.

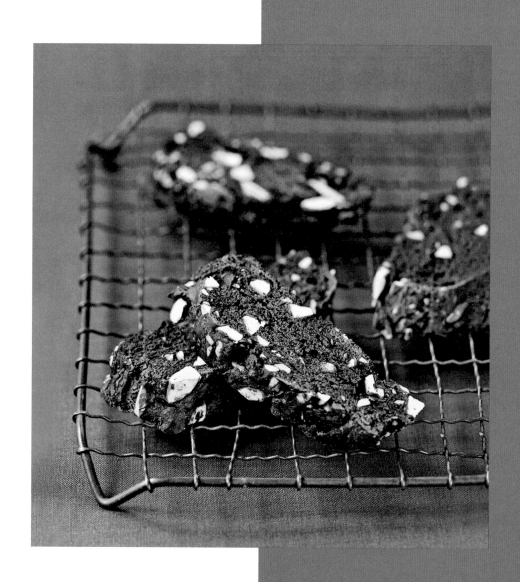

DARK CHOCOLATE MINT COOKIE BARS

These bars are a treat to savor with a steaming cup of tea or coffee.

Preparation time: 15 minutes ● **Baking time: 16 minutes** ● **Cooling time: 30 minutes**

---

4 ounces bittersweet chocolate, chopped

1 cup old-fashioned oats

⅓ cup packed brown sugar

2 tablespoons unsweetened cocoa powder

1 teaspoon baking powder

½ cup 1% cottage cheese

2 tablespoons Better Butter (page 323) or trans-fat free spread

1 egg

½ teaspoon mint extract

Confectioners' sugar

1. Preheat the oven to 350°F. Coat an 8" × 8" baking dish with vegetable oil spray. Place the chocolate in a small microwaveable bowl. Microwave on high power for about 1 minute, or until partially melted. Stir until smooth. Set aside.

2. Place the oats, sugar, cocoa powder, and baking powder in a food processor bowl fitted with a metal blade. Process for 3 minutes, or until the oats are finely ground. Transfer to a mixing bowl. Add the cottage cheese to the processor bowl. Process, scraping the bowl as needed, for about 2 minutes, or until smooth. Add the Better Butter or spread, egg, and extract. Process, scraping the bowl as needed, for about 1 minute, or until smooth.

Add to the oats mixture along with the reserved melted chocolate. Stir to mix. Dollop the batter into the prepared pan. Pat to spread evenly.

3. Bake for about 16 minutes, or just until the top is set. Do not overbake. Let stand to cool. Cut into 16 squares.

4. Dust lightly with confectioners' sugar just before serving.

MAKES 16 SERVINGS

Per serving: 100 calories, 13 g carbohydrate, 3 g protein, 5 g fat, 2 g saturated fat, 15 mg cholesterol, 75 mg sodium, 1 g fiber

Carbohydrate Choices: 1

Dietary Exchanges: 1 starch, 1 fat

NOTE: If not serving right away, store the bars in an airtight container in the freezer.

CRANBERRY SPICE AND WALNUT BISCOTTI

Biscotti were created for dunking! Whether your choice is a steaming cup of tea, coffee, or hot chocolate, these crispy cookies are sure to satisfy.

Preparation time: 25 minutes ● Chilling time: 3 hours ● Baking time: 1 hour
Cooling time: 10 minutes

¾ cup all-purpose flour

½ cup whole wheat pastry flour

¾ teaspoon baking powder

1 teaspoon apple pie spice

Pinch of salt

3 tablespoons Better Butter (page 323) or trans-fat free spread, softened

3 tablespoons honey

½ teaspoon orange extract

1 egg

3 tablespoons fat-free milk

3 tablespoons chopped walnuts

3 tablespoons chopped dried cranberries

1. On a sheet of waxed paper, combine the flours, baking powder, spice, and salt. Stir with a fork to mix. In a mixing bowl, combine the Better Butter or spread, honey, and orange extract. With a wooden spoon, beat until smooth and light. Add the egg, beating until smooth. Add the milk. Beat until smooth. Gradually add the dry ingredients, beating just until combined. Stir in the walnuts and cranberries. Cover with plastic wrap. Refrigerate for at least 3 hours, or longer if desired, until firm.

2. Preheat the oven to 325°F. Coat a baking sheet with vegetable oil spray. Turn the dough onto a lightly floured work surface. Divide the dough in half. Roll each piece of dough into a 1" diameter log. Place the logs, separated, on the sheet. Bake for 30 minutes, or until the logs are set. Remove to a rack to cool for 10 minutes.

3. Reduce the oven temperature to 300°F. On a cutting board with a serrated knife, cut each log into ½"-wide diagonal slices. Place the slices, cut sides down, on the baking sheets.

4. Bake for 18 minutes, or until toasted on top. Turn the cookies and bake for about 10 minutes, or until toasted on top. Remove to racks to cool.

MAKES 10 SERVINGS (2 BISCOTTI PER SERVING)

Per serving: 133 calories, 19 g carbohydrate, 3 g protein, 5 g fat, 1 g saturated fat, 21 mg cholesterol, 88 mg sodium, 1 g fiber

Carbohydrate Choices: 1

Dietary Exchanges: ½ starch, 1 fat

NOTE: Biscotti may be stored in an airtight container for several weeks or frozen in an airtight container for several months.

GOOEY DATE WALNUT CLUSTERS

These treats are wonderful to have on hand in your refrigerator when you need a little "sweet hit."

Preparation time: 15 minutes • **Cooking time: 4 minutes** • **Cooling time: 5 minutes**
Chilling time: 2 hours

---

1 bag (8 ounces) dried pitted dates
3 tablespoons water
1 egg white, lightly beaten
2 teaspoons Better Butter (page 323) or trans-fat free spread
1 teaspoon vanilla extract
⅓ cup walnuts, toasted and finely chopped

1. Coat a plate with vegetable oil spray. Set aside. Chop the dates into very small pieces.

2. In a small nonstick saucepan, combine the dates, water, egg white, and Better Butter or spread. Cook, stirring constantly, over low heat for about 4 minutes, or until the mixture is thickened. Continually squash the dates with a heatproof spatula or the back of a wooden spoon. Stir in the vanilla. Dollop onto the reserved plate; spread into a thin layer. Let stand for about 5 minutes, or until cool to the touch.

3. Place the walnuts on a sheet of waxed paper. Coat your hands lightly with vegetable oil spray. With a butter knife, score the date mixture into 18 sections. Scoop up and roll each section into a ball. Dip the ball into the walnuts to lightly coat. Place in a rectangular plastic storage container. Repeat until all the mixture is shaped and coated with nuts. Put waxed paper between the layers in the container. Cover. Refrigerate for several hours to allow the flavors to mellow.

MAKES 18 SERVINGS (1 CLUSTER PER SERVING)

Per serving: 55 calories, 10 g carbohydrate, 1 g protein, 2 g fat, 0 g saturated fat, 0 mg cholesterol, 8 mg sodium, 2 g fiber

Carbohydrate Choices: 1

Dietary Exchanges: ½ fruit, ½ fat

NOTES: Start with whole pitted dates and chop them yourself. It takes a few more minutes, but the end result will be moister than if you started with prechopped dates.

Toasting brings out the flavor and crisps the texture of nuts. To toast walnuts, spread them on a baking sheet in a single layer. Bake in a preheated 350°F oven, stirring occasionally, for about 10 minutes, or until sizzling. Let stand to cool.

Vary the flavorings by replacing the vanilla extract with 1 tablespoon finely chopped crystallized ginger or 1 teaspoon grated orange peel.

BUTTERSCOTCH CHIP MACADAMIA COOKIES

These goodies are sure to be a big hit at your next potluck or backyard get-together.

Preparation time: 25 minutes ● **Baking time: 10 minutes**

---

1 cup + 2 tablespoons all-purpose flour

½ teaspoon baking soda

Dash of salt

½ cup Better Butter (page 323) or trans-fat free spread, at room temperature

½ cup brown sugar

1 egg yolk

1 teaspoon vanilla extract

½ cup (3 ounces) butterscotch chips

¼ cup macadamia nuts, finely chopped

1. Preheat the oven to 350°F. On a sheet of waxed paper, combine the flour, baking soda, and salt. Stir with a fork to mix.

2. In a mixing bowl, beat the Better Butter or spread with a wooden spoon until smooth. Add the sugar and beat until smooth. Add the egg yolk and vanilla. Beat until smooth. Add the reserved dry ingredients. Stir to mix. Add the butterscotch chips and nuts. Stir to mix.

3. Roll the dough into 24 equal balls. Place the dough balls, 1" apart, on a nonstick baking sheet.

4. Bake for about 10 minutes, or until puffed and golden on the bottom. Remove and allow to cool on the sheet before removing to a rack.

MAKES 24 SERVINGS (1 COOKIE PER SERVING)

Per serving: 93 calories, 10 g carbohydrate, 1 g protein, 5 g fat, 2 g saturated fat, 9 mg cholesterol, 173 mg sodium, 0 g fiber

Carbohydrate Choices: 1

Dietary Exchanges: ½ starch, 1 fat

FILL UP ON WHOLE FOODS

Flours for Baked Goods

When preparing the baked goods recipes in this chapter, be sure to use the exact type of flour or flours that are listed. We've incorporated whole wheat pastry flour, 100 percent stone-ground cornmeal, ground oats, and soy flour whenever possible, but some all-purpose flour is required for best results in some recipes, especially with cakes. These items are, after all, once-in-a-while treats and not intended to be a major source of nutrients. These flours are now commonly available in most supermarkets thanks to the renewed emphasis on whole grains with the most recent government dietary guidelines.

BRAND NAMES OF RECOMMENDED WHOLE FOODS

Crunchies

These snacks have 3 to 6 grams of fiber per serving and five ingredients or less:

> Erin's Popcorn
>
> In the Shell Edamame (Sunrich Naturals)
>
> Que Pasa Whole Grain Tortilla Chips
>
> Terra Exotic Vegetable Chips
>
> Trader Joe's Popcorn
>
> Trader Joe's Stone Ground Tortilla Chips

These snacks have 2 grams of fiber per serving and five ingredients or less:

> Garden of Eatin' Blue Chips
>
> Guiltless Gourmet Blue Corn Tortilla Chips
>
> Kettle Tortilla Chips
>
> Mexi-Snax Tortilla Chips
>
> Yaya's Popcorn

Flour and Ground Grains

> Arrowhead Mills flaxseed meal and whole grain flours
>
> Bob's Red Mill low-fat soy flour and whole grain flours
>
> Hodgson Mill fat-free soy flour and whole grain flours
>
> King Arthur Flour 100 percent white whole wheat flour and other whole grain flours

Hot Cereal

> Bob's Red Mill Whole Oats Groats, Steel-Cut Oats, and other whole grain cereals
>
> Quaker Oat Bran
>
> Quaker Oatmeal (4 minutes)

Nut Butters

> Adam's/Smucker's 100 Percent Natural Peanut Butter
>
> Kettle nut butters
>
> Maranatha nut butters
>
> Trader Joe's Almond, Cashew, Cashew Macadamia, and Peanut Butters

Soups and Broths

> Amy's Organic canned soups
>
> Health Valley Low-Fat Chicken or Beef Broth, No Salt Added
>
> Pacific organic soups and broths
>
> Walnut Acres organic soup

Sweets

> Dreyer's/Edy's Slow Churned Lite Ice Cream

Whole Grain Bread

> Alvarado St. Bakery Sprouted Sour Dough Bread

Ezekiel 4:9 Sprouted 100 Percent Whole Grain Bread, English Muffins, or Tortillas

Silver Hill Sprouted Grain Bread and Bagels

Tam-X-ico 100 Percent Whole Wheat Tortillas

Whole Grain Crackers

Ak-Mak

Good Health's Low Sodium Quilts

Mary's Gone Crackers

100 Percent Whole Wheat Matzos

Trader Joe's Low Fat Rye Mini Toasts

Triscuits

Wasa

Whole Grain Crispbreads

Finn Crisp

Kavli

Ryvita

Whole Grain Pasta

Annie's Whole Wheat Spaghetti

DeBoles Whole Wheat Pasta

Gia Russa Whole Wheat Lasagna

Organic BioNaturae Pasta

Organic Spelt Pasta VitaSpelt

Pasta Joy Brown Rice Pasta

Trader Joe's Organic 100 Percent Whole Wheat Spaghetti, Penne, Rotelle

Westbrae Natural Organic Whole Wheat Pasta and Lasagna Noodles

Yogurt

Plain, low-fat yogurt is the healthiest choice. However, for sweetened yogurts, look for ones that contain 30 grams of carbohydrate or less per serving and have no artificial colors or flavorings.

For example:

All Natural Brown Cow

Cascade Fresh

Dannon

Horizon

Nancy's Yogurt

Redwood Hill Farm Goat Milk Yogurt

Stonyfield Farm Organic Yogurt

Wallaby Organic Yogurt

Whole Soy and Company Soy Yogurt

BODY MASS INDEX TABLE

Body mass index (BMI) is a tool that health professionals use to determine if someone's weight is unhealthfully high or low. Generally, the higher BMIs are associated with unhealthy amounts of body fat—not just total pounds. To determine your BMI, find your height in the column at the left and then move across until you find your weight. Your BMI is the number at the bottom of the column.

Height	Weight (lb)										
4'10"	86	91	96	100	105	110	115	119	124	129	134
4'11"	89	94	99	104	109	114	119	124	128	133	138
5'	92	97	102	107	112	118	123	128	133	138	143
5'1"	96	100	106	111	116	122	127	132	137	143	148
5'2"	99	104	109	115	120	126	131	136	142	147	153
5'3"	102	107	113	118	124	130	135	141	146	152	158
5'4"	105	110	116	122	128	134	140	145	151	157	163
5'5"	109	114	120	126	132	138	144	150	156	162	168
5'6"	112	118	124	130	136	142	148	155	161	167	173
5'7"	116	121	127	134	140	146	153	159	166	172	178
5'8"	120	125	131	138	144	151	158	164	171	177	184
5'9"	123	128	135	142	149	155	162	169	176	182	189
5'10"	126	132	139	146	153	160	167	174	181	188	195
5'11"	130	136	143	150	157	165	172	179	186	193	200
6'	134	140	147	154	162	169	177	184	191	199	206
6'1"	138	144	151	159	166	174	182	189	197	204	212
6'2"	141	148	155	163	171	179	186	194	202	210	218
6'3"	145	152	160	168	176	184	192	200	208	216	224
6'4"	149	156	164	172	180	189	197	205	213	221	230
BMI	18	19	20	21	22	23	24	25	26	27	28

Underweight: Less than 18
Normal:18–24
Overweight: 25–29

Obese: 30–34
Very obese: 35–39
Extremely obese: 40 and above

29	30	31	32	33	34	35	36	37	38	39	40
138	143	148	153	158	162	167	172	177	181	186	191
143	148	153	158	163	168	173	178	183	188	193	198
148	153	158	163	168	174	179	184	189	194	199	204
153	158	164	169	174	180	185	190	195	201	206	211
158	164	169	175	180	186	191	196	202	207	213	218
163	169	175	180	186	191	197	203	208	214	220	225
169	174	180	186	192	197	204	209	215	221	227	232
174	180	186	192	198	204	210	216	222	228	234	240
179	186	192	198	204	210	216	223	229	235	241	247
185	191	198	204	211	217	223	230	236	242	249	255
190	197	203	210	216	223	230	236	243	249	256	262
196	203	209	216	223	230	236	243	250	257	263	270
202	209	216	222	229	236	243	250	257	264	271	278
208	215	222	229	236	243	250	257	265	272	279	286
213	221	228	235	242	250	258	265	272	279	287	294
219	227	235	242	250	257	265	272	280	288	295	302
225	233	241	249	256	264	272	280	287	295	303	311
232	240	248	256	264	272	279	287	295	303	311	319
238	246	254	263	271	279	287	295	304	312	320	328
29	30	31	32	33	34	35	36	37	38	39	40

PHOTO CREDITS

INDEX

Underscored page references indicate boxed text and tables. **Boldface** references indicate photographs.